AF711390

Pediatric Echocardiography Review

A Q&A REVIEW FOR THE ARDMS PEDIATRIC ECHOCARDIOGRAPHY EXAM

Register Your Book!

It's quick and easy, and it will connect you to the free video component of this book (more than 60 video clips), study alerts, expert advice, exclusive promotions, and premium content. Register toll-free by phone at 1-877-792-0005 or at DaviesPublishing.com/book-registration. It will be helpful to have the last three digits of your book's ISBN at hand. Need help? Call us toll-free between 9 AM and 5 PM Pacific time. Thank you!

Pediatric Echocardiography Review

A Q&A REVIEW FOR THE ARDMS PEDIATRIC ECHOCARDIOGRAPHY EXAM

Hui Gao, MB, RDCS (AE, FEc, PE)
Children's Hospital Los Angeles
Los Angeles, California

Pierre C. Wong, MD
Children's Hospital Los Angeles
Los Angeles, California

Novel A. Castillo, RDCS (AE, FEc, PE)
Children's Hospital Los Angeles
Los Angeles, California

DAVIES PUBLISHING

Copyright © 2026, 2023, 2020 by Davies Publishing, Inc.

All rights reserved. No part of this work may be reproduced, stored in a retrieval system, or transmitted in any form or by any means, electronic or mechanical, including photocopying, scanning, and recording, without prior written permission from the publisher. If you receive a photocopy or web-based copy of this or any other Davies book, please call toll-free to report it—1-877-792-0005 during business hours, 9am–5pm Pacific time. Thank you!

Davies Publishing, Inc.
32 South Raymond Avenue
Pasadena, California 91105-1961
Phone 626-792-3046
Facsimile 626-792-5308
e-mail info@daviespublishing.com
www.daviespublishing.com

Michael P. Davies, Publisher

Christina J. Moose, Editorial Director
Charlene Locke, Production Manager
Janet Heard, Operations Manager
Satori Design Group, Inc., Design

Printed and bound in the United States of America.

ISBN 978-0-941022-18-7

Library of Congress Cataloging-in-Publication Data

Names: Gao, Hui, 1963- author. | Wong, Pierre C., author. | Castillo, Novel A. (Novel Amilcar), 1979- author.
Title: Pediatric echocardiography review : a Q&A review for the ARDMS pediatric echocardiography exam / Hui Gao, Pierre C. Wong, Novel A. Castillo.
Description: Pasadena, California : Davies Publishing, Inc., 2020. | Includes bibliographical references and index. | Summary: "Pediatric Echocardiography Review is a mock examination consisting of more than 600 multiple-choice questions, answers, explanatory text, and references designed to aid students and clinicians taking the ARDMS Pediatric Echo registry exam. It is designed to improve both knowledge and test-taking skills, covering the material on the ARDMS exam content outline for the Pediatric Echocardiography specialty exam in effect as of 2019. Covers pediatric cardiac anatomy and physiology, pathology and pathophysiology, congenital anomalies, postoperative anatomy, clinical standards and guidelines, and measurement techniques and quantification. This mock exam is also approved by the Society of Diagnostic Medical Sonography as a continuing medical education activity worth 12 credit hours"-- Provided by publisher.
Identifiers: LCCN 2019033416 | ISBN 9780941022187 (paperback)
Subjects: MESH: Echocardiography--methods | Child | Infant | Adolescent | Examination Question
Classification: LCC RC683.5.U5 | NLM WG 18.2 | DDC 616.1/207543076--dc23
LC record available at https://lccn.loc.gov/2019033416

Contributors and Reviewers

Contributors

Brandy Hattendorf, MD, FACC, FASE, FAAP
Associate Professor of Clinical Pediatrics
Keck School of Medicine of USC
Division of Cardiology
Children's Hospital Los Angeles
Los Angeles, California

Grace C. Kung, MD, FACC, FASE
Clinical Professor of Pediatrics
Keck School of Medicine of USC
Division of Cardiology
Fellowship Program Director
Children's Hospital Los Angeles
Los Angeles, California

Jay D. Pruetz, MD
Associate Professor of Clinical Pediatrics and Obstetrics & Gynecology
Keck School of Medicine of USC
Director, Fetal Cardiology Program
Division of Cardiology
Children's Hospital Los Angeles
Los Angeles, California

Andrew T. Souza, DO
Assistant Professor of Clinical Pediatrics
Keck School of Medicine of USC
Division of Cardiology
Children's Hospital Los Angeles
Los Angeles, California

Reviewers

Ruben J. Acherman, MD
Professor of Pediatrics
University of Nevada Las Vegas
Director of Fetal Cardiology Program
Children's Heart Center Nevada
Las Vegas, Nevada

Fariborz Behzadian, MD, RDCS (AE, PE, FEc), RVT
Pediatric Cardiac Sonographer
Children's Hospital Los Angeles
Los Angeles, California

Louis I. Bezold, MD
Professor of Pediatrics
Division Chief of Pediatric Cardiology
Kentucky Children's Hospital
University of Kentucky College of Medicine
Lexington, Kentucky

Aarti H. Bhat, MD, FASE, FACC
Associate Professor
Director, Heart Center Quality Improvement
Pediatric Cardiology
Seattle Children's Hospital
University of Washington
Seattle, Washington

Xiaoling Cao, MB, RDCS (AE, PE)
Senior Cardiac Sonographer
Heart and Vascular Institute
Hoag Memorial Hospital
Newport Beach, California
IAC Technical Director
Heart Services Echocardiography Laboratory
CHOC Children's Hospital
Orange, California

Andrew L. Cheng, MD, FAAP, FACC
Attending Physician, Division of Pediatric Cardiology
Children's Hospital Los Angeles
Assistant Professor of Clinical Pediatrics
Keck School of Medicine, University of Southern California
Los Angeles, California

Joseph Daniel, BS, RDCS (AE, PE)
Cardiac Sonographer II
Children's Hospital Los Angeles
Los Angeles, California

John Ho, MD
Pediatric Cardiologist
Pacific Pediatric Cardiology Medical Group
Pasadena, California

Kristin Kennedy, RDCS (AE, PE)
Staff Sonographer
Lucile Packard Children's Hospital Stanford
Stanford, California

Frederic J. Leong, MD, FACC
Pediatric Cardiologist
Pediatric Cardiology Medical Associates
Thousand Oaks, California

Katie Jo Stauffer, BS, RDCS (AE, PE, FEc), FASE
Lead Pediatric Cardiac Sonographer
Lucile Packard Children's Hospital Stanford
Stanford Children's Health
Palo Alto, California

Xiaohong Su, RDCS (AE, PE, FEc)
Echo Tech II
Boston Children's Hospital
Boston, Massachusetts

Adam Sutherland, RDCS (AE, PE), RVT
Pediatric Cardiac Sonographer
Children's Hospital Los Angeles
Los Angeles, California

Shuo (Sue) Wang, MD
Pediatric Cardiology Advanced Imaging Fellow
Children's Hospital Los Angeles
Los Angeles, California

Yin Tao Wang, MB, RDCS (AE, PE, FEc)
Technical Director, Pediatric Echocardiography Lab
Pediatric Cardiology
Sanger Heart & Vascular Institute
Charlotte, North Carolina

Preface

THIS MOCK EXAM is a question/answer/reference review of Pediatric Echocardiography for those candidates who plan to take the PE specialty examination for the Registered Diagnostic Cardiac Sonographer (RDCS) credential administered by the American Registry for Diagnostic Medical Sonography (ARDMS). Those sitting for the Registered Cardiac Sonographer (RCS) exam administered by Cardiac Credentialing International (CCI) will likewise find that these items will bolster and solidify their preparation. Designed as an adjunct to your regular study, this mock exam will help you precisely determine your strengths and weaknesses so that you can study more effectively. This mock exam is also an SDMS-approved CME activity worth 12 credits (see Part 8).

Facts about *Pediatric Echocardiography Review*

- This mock exam covers the material on the ARDMS exam content outline in effect as of the time of printing. Readers are advised to check the ARDMS website at www.ardms.org for the latest updates. The mock exam itself is continuously updated and revised as necessary, and readers can check Davies' website for the latest Study Alerts and other product updates by visiting http://www.daviespublishing.com/Product-Updates-C220.aspx. We send these alerts and updates to all customers who have registered their book or purchased it directly from us.
- The mock exam focuses exclusively on the Pediatric Echocardiography (PE) specialty exam to ensure thorough coverage of even the smallest subtopic and clinical task on the exam. (For those preparing for the Sonography Principles and Instrumentation exam, see Davies' *Ultrasound Physics Review: SPI Edition*, available in either print or interactive format at www.daviespublishing.com.)
- We use the most current ARDMS content outline as a guideline for coverage. It is, in fact, the foundation for our table of contents.

- This mock exam contains 603 questions*, many of which are accompanied by sonographic and other images, anatomic illustrations, and schematics—more than 150 image-based cases. More than 60 of these are real-time video clips accessible by registering your book at DaviesPublishing.com/book-registration, or by calling us toll-free in the U.S. at 1-877-792-0005.

Register your book.

- Items are presented in ARDMS exam format to give you an educational tool that will exercise those neural pathways in more than one direction. Registry candidates who master the key underlying facts, concepts, and principles will be exceptionally well prepared for the actual exam.
- The answer key located in Part 7 contains not only the answers but also concise explanations that are abundant, clear, and authoritatively referenced for further study. We recommend that you have a copy of a standard pediatric echocardiography review text at your side when using this mock exam to study for the PE exam—you will see several of these referenced in both the answer section and the "Suggested Readings" in Part 9.
- This mock examination has been approved by the Society of Diagnostic Medical Sonography (SDMS) as a CME activity. A CME application form, quiz, and full submission instructions are included in Part 8. Passing this quiz will qualify the applicant for 12 CME credits. A modest administrative processing fee applies at the time of submission, and more than one sonographer may use the forms in this book to submit this activity for CME credit. These credits are accepted by ARDMS, APCA, CCI, and other organizations toward meeting their CME requirements. Some credentials carry stipulations regarding specialty areas in which CME credits may be earned. Always check with the organization that governs your credential(s). All the credits in this activity may be applied to maintain the ARDMS RDCS credential.

*The exam itself contains 150 questions.

- The expanded ARDMS exam content outline, complete with all questions that apply to specific clinical tasks, appears in Part 10. Under each task we have indexed the question numbers in this mock exam that are related to that task, for your convenience in targeting your study on specific exam topics. (To ensure that your study is targeted at the most current examination outline, be sure to visit the ARDMS website at www.ardms.org.)

ARDMS Advanced Item Type (AIT) Questions

All the ARDMS exams now include Advanced Item Type (AIT) questions that assess practical instrumentation skills. For the PE specialty exam, these AIT questions include what ARDMS calls "Hotspot" questions. Hotspot items display an image with the question and ask you to indicate the correct answer by marking directly on the image using your cursor; this type of question is called "advanced" because it involves a higher level of thinking and processing than you perform when answering a conventional multiple-choice question. In Davies' mock exam, similar questions are identified as "AIT—Hotspot" questions. These items ask you to identify what an arrow in the image is pointing at or to indicate the label on an image that corresponds to the correct answer.

Another type of AIT question, the Semi-Interactive Console (SIC) item, requires the examinee to use a semi-interactive console to correct a problem with the image presented. Currently these items do not appear on the PE exam, but as a bonus feature we have identified such items as "AIT—SIC" questions.

Finally, PACSim items—case-based Picture Archive and Communication Simulation questions—are not included in this mock exam because currently this type of question is specifically designed for and limited to the Physician in Vascular Interpretation (PVI) and the Ob/Gyn exams—the former under the jurisdiction of the Alliance for Physician Certification and Advancement (APCA).

How to Use This Mock Exam

Pediatric Echocardiography Review effectively simulates the content of the Pediatric Echocardiography (PE) exam. Current ARDMS standards call for 150 multiple-choice questions to be answered during a three-hour period. That is, you will have an average time of approximately one minute to answer each question. Timing your practice sessions according to the number of questions you need to finish will help you prepare for the pressure experienced by PE candidates taking this exam. It also helps to ensure that your practice scores accurately reflect your strengths and weaknesses so that you can study more efficiently in the limited time you are able to devote to preparation.

> ***Important note:*** *Although many of our customers remark on similarities between our questions and those of the actual exam, do not be misled into thinking you should memorize these questions and answers. They are here to give you practice, to teach you things you may not know, and to reveal your strengths and weaknesses so that you know where to put your energy as you prepare for the exam. They also provide a means of assessing your progress as you study.*

ARDMS test results are reported as a "scaled" score that ranges from a minimum of 300 to a maximum of 700. A scaled score of 555 is the passing score—the "passpoint" or "cutoff score" for all ARDMS examinations. The scaled score is simply a conversion of the number of correct answers that also, in part, takes into account the difficulty of a particular question. You can search on the Internet for the "Angoff scoring method" if you want to learn more about scaled scoring. Suffice it to say that it helps to ensure the fairness of the exams.

We include below and strongly recommend that you read *Taking and Passing Your Exam*, by Don Ridgway, RVT, who offers useful tips and practical strategies for taking and passing the ARDMS examinations.

A work of this scope would not have been possible without the contributions of so many of our colleagues, who are listed in the "Contributors and Reviewers" section above. We wish to express our deepest appreciation to them, along with the many friends and family who extended their support during the writing, editing, and production of this book.

Finally, you have not only our best wishes for success but also our admiration for taking this big and important step in your career!

Hui Gao, MB, RDCS

Pierre C. Wong, MD

Novel A. Castillo, RDCS

Taking and Passing Your Exam

by Don Ridgway, RVT*

Preparing for Your Exam . . .

Study. And then study some more. Knowing your stuff is the most important factor in your success. Start early, set a regular study schedule, and stick to it. Make your schedule specific so you know exactly what to study on a particular day. Write it down. Establish realistic goals so that you don't build a mountain you can't climb.

As to what you study, don't just read aimlessly. Focus your efforts on what you need to know. Rely on a core group of dependable references, referring to others as necessary to firm up your understanding of specific topics. Let the ARDMS exam outline guide you. And use different but complementary study methods—texts, flashcards, and mock exams—to exercise those neural pathways.

Ease down on studying the week before. Wind down, reduce stress, build confidence, and rest up. Don't cram! And no studying the night before. You had your chance. Watch a movie, relax, go to bed early, and sleep well.

Organize your things the night before. Lay out comfortable clothes (including a sweater or sweatshirt in case the testing center is cold), your photo ID, car and house keys, glasses, prescriptions, directions to the test center, and any other personal items you might need. Remember that the only thing you can take into the testing room is you—there will be lockers for your personal items. And read about necessary documentation and examination admission compliance requirements for your exam at www.ardms.org. Be prepared!

---

*Don Ridgway is the author of *Introduction to Vascular Scanning: A Guide for the Complete Beginner* and editor of *Vascular Technology Review*. He is Professor Emeritus at Grossmont College in El Cajon, California.

The Day of Your Exam . . .

Eat lightly. You do not want to fall asleep during the exam. Go easy on the coffee or tea so your bladder doesn't distract you halfway through the exam.

Arrive early. Plan to arrive at the test center early, especially if you haven't been there before. Take directions, including the telephone number of the testing center in case you have to make contact en route. You don't need a wrong-offramp adventure.

Be confident. As you wait for the exam to begin, smile, lift both hands, wave them toward yourself, and say, "Bring it on."

During the Exam . . .

Read each question twice before answering. Guess how easy it is to get one word wrong and misunderstand the whole question!

Try to answer the question before looking at the choices. Formulating an answer before peeking at the possibilities minimizes the distraction of the incorrect answer choices, which in the test-making business are called—guess what?—distractors.

Knock off the easy ones first. First answer the questions you feel good about. Then go back for the more difficult items. Next, attack the really tough ones. Taking notes on long or tricky questions often can jog your memory or put the question in new light. For questions you just cannot answer with certainty, eliminate the obviously wrong answer choices and then guess.

Guessing. Passing the exam depends on the number of correct answers you make. Because unanswered questions are counted as incorrect, it makes sense to guess when all else fails. The ARDMS itself advises that it is to the candidate's advantage to answer all questions. Guessing alone improves your chances of scoring a point from zero (for an unanswered question) to 25% (for randomly picking one of four possible answers). Eliminating answer choices you know or suspect are wrong further improves your odds of success. For example, by using your knowledge and skill to eliminate two of the four answer choices before guessing, you increase your odds of scoring a point to 50%.

Pace yourself; watch the time. Work methodically and quickly to answer those you know, and make your best guesses at the gnarly ones. Leave no question unanswered.

Don't despair 50 minutes into the exam. At some point you may feel that things just aren't going well. Take 10 seconds to breathe deeply—in for a count of five, out for a count of five. Relax. Recall that you need to get only about three out of four answers correct to pass. If you've prepared reasonably well, a passing score is attainable even if you feel sweat running down your back.

Taking the Exam on Computer . . .

Some candidates express concern about taking the registry exam on a computer. Most folks find this to be pretty easy; some find it offputting, at least in prospect. But the computerized exams are quite convenient: You know whether or not you passed before you leave the testing center (compare that to waiting weeks and even months, as used to be the case), and if you don't pass the exam the first time, you can usually take it again after a couple months. Another good point: The illustrations are said to be clearer on computer than in the booklets at a Scantron-type exam.

Taking the test on computer is not complicated. The test center even has a tutorial to be sure you know what you need to do. You sit in a carrel with a computer and answer the multiple-choice questions by pointing and clicking with a mouse. There is a clock on the display letting you know how much time is left. Use it to pace yourself. A white board (today's equivalent of scratch paper) is available upon request, and it's a good idea to have one at your side for notes. You can mark questions for answering later. A display shows which questions have not been answered so you can return to them. When you have finished, you click on "DONE," and you find out immediately whether you passed.

It's nothing to be afraid of. The principles are the same as those for any exam. Be methodical and keep breathing.

Summary . . .

Preparing for the exam:

- Study.
- Use flashcards.
- Join a study group.
- Wind down a week before.
- Don't cram.
- Relax!

The day of your exam:

- Eat lightly; avoid too much caffeine.
- Arrive early.
- Take a sweater.
- Be confident!

During the exam:

- Read each question twice.
- Answer the question before looking at the answer choices.
- Answer the easy ones first.
- Guess when necessary.
- Pace yourself.
- Don't despair.

Taking the exam on computer:

- Just point and click.
- Take notes.
- Mark and return to the hard questions.
- Use the onscreen clock to pace yourself.
- Be methodical.
- Breathe!

Contents

Color Plates

We have included this section of color images to enhance the black-and-white versions used with some of the questions and answers in this mock exam. These images go with the questions and/or answers referenced below, and you will see that the questions and answers also include a cross-reference to the color versions of the images that appear here. For fuller information, we encourage you to refer to the image in the context of its question as well as its corresponding answer in Part 7, "Answers, Explanations, and References."

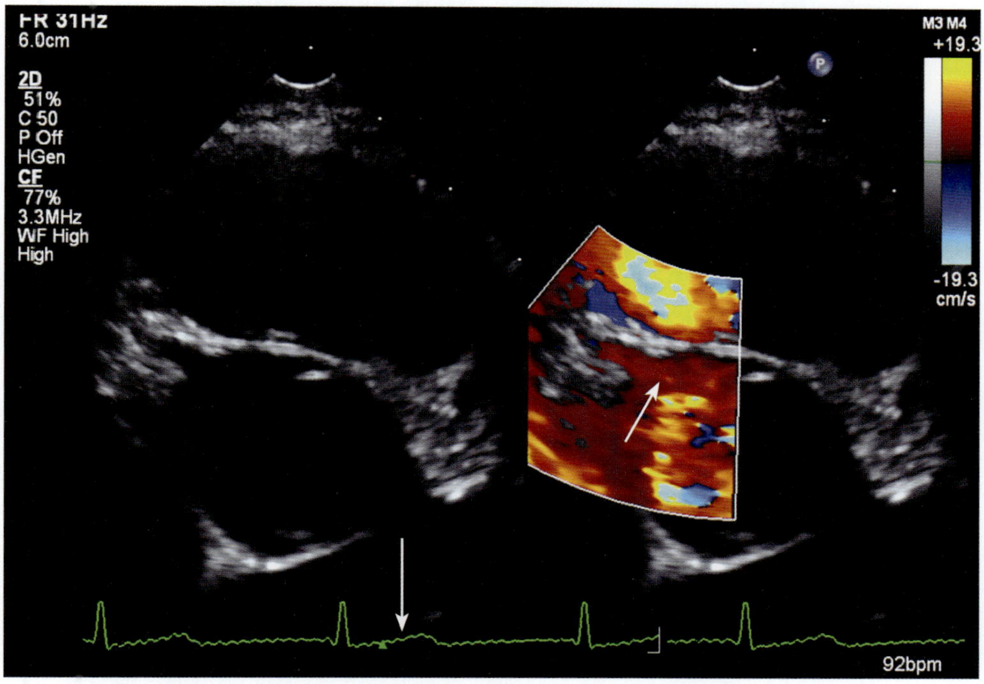

Color Plate 1 (page 7, question 25; page 10, question 32; page 185, answer 25; page 188, answer 32)

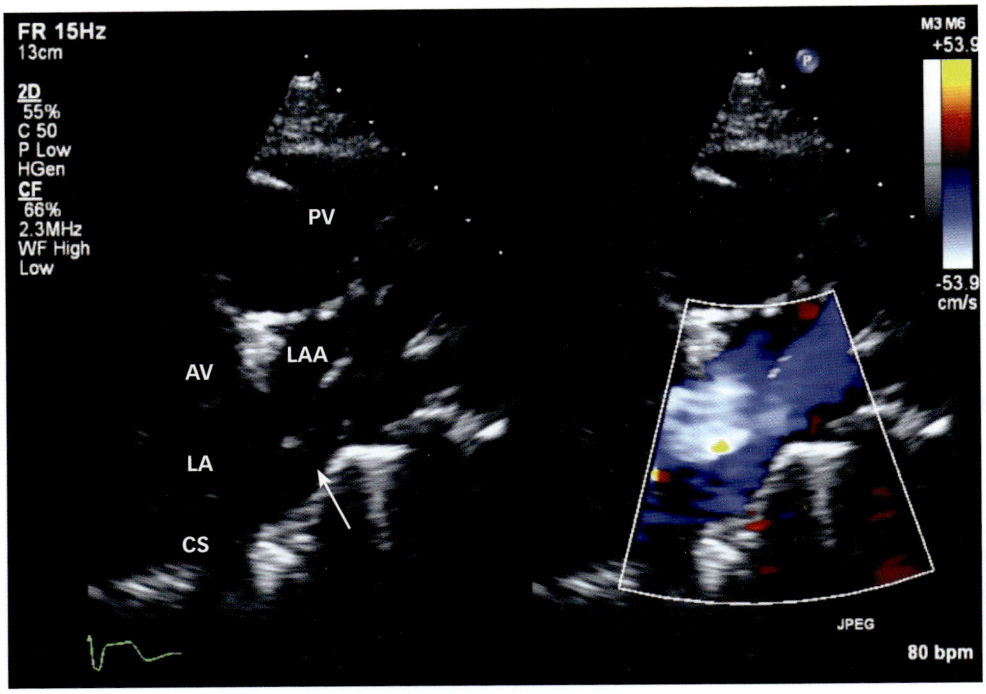

Color Plate 2 (page 11, question 34; page 189, answer 34)

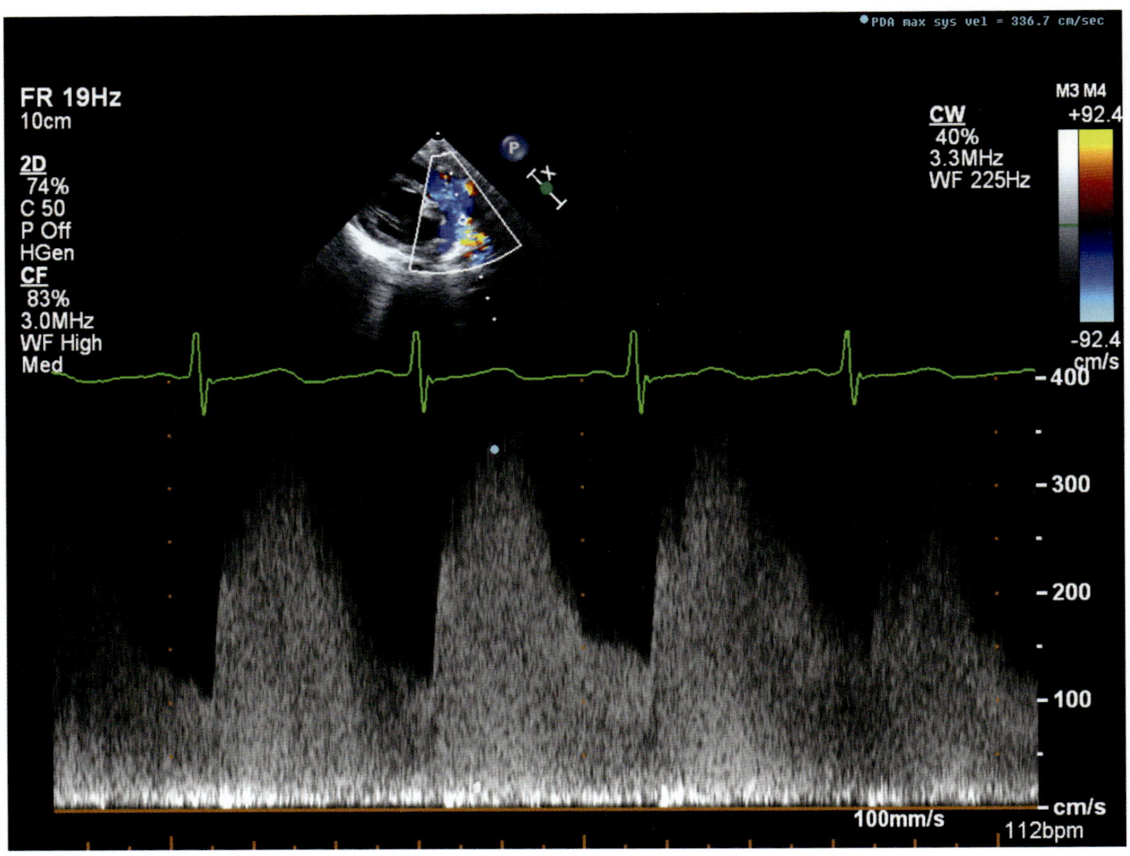

Color Plate 3 (page 17, question 58; page 198, answer 58)

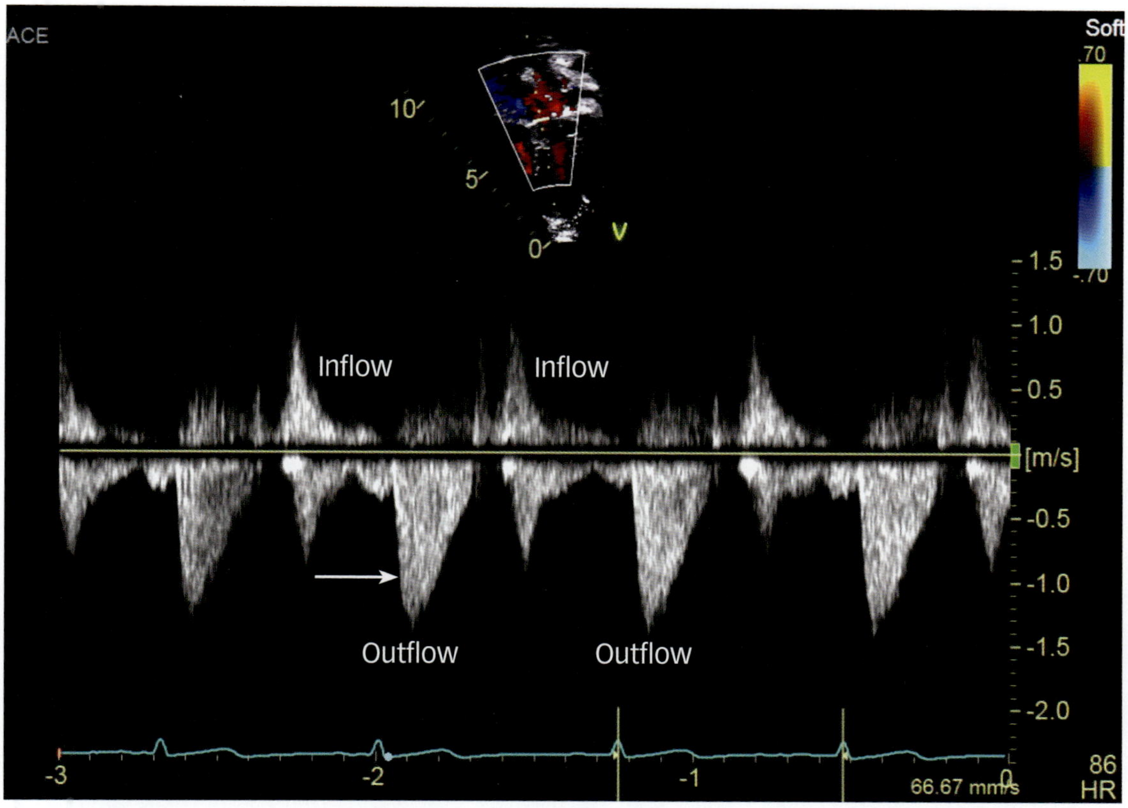

Color Plate 4 (page 17, question 59; page 199, answer 59)

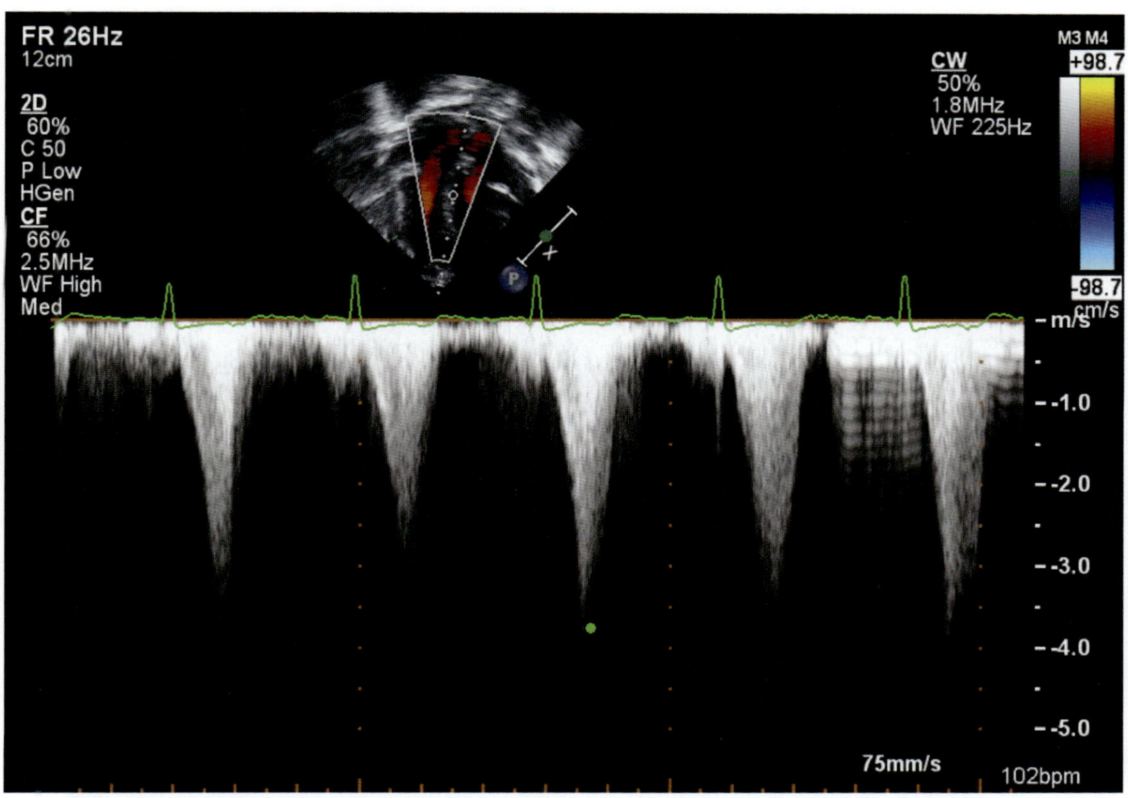

Color Plate 5 (page 21, question 64; page 202, answer 64)

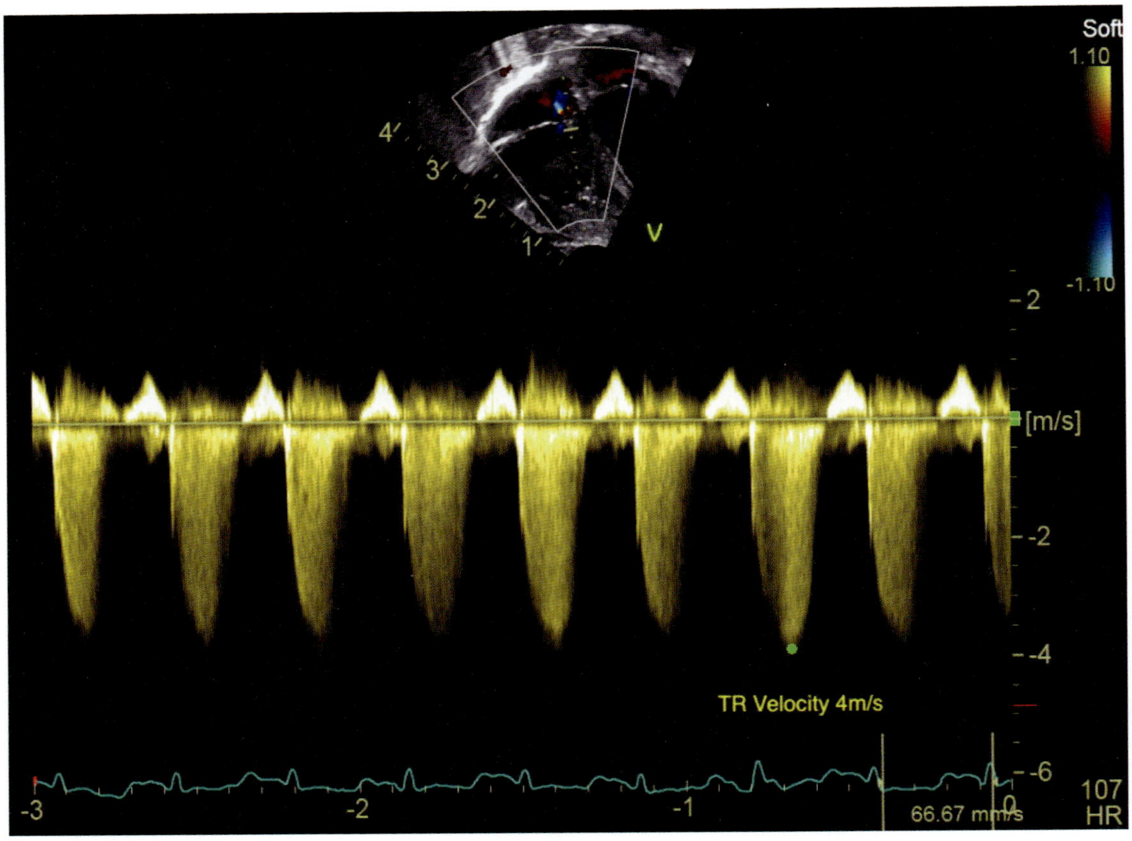

Color Plate 6 (page 24, question 73, image B; page 206, answer 73, image B)

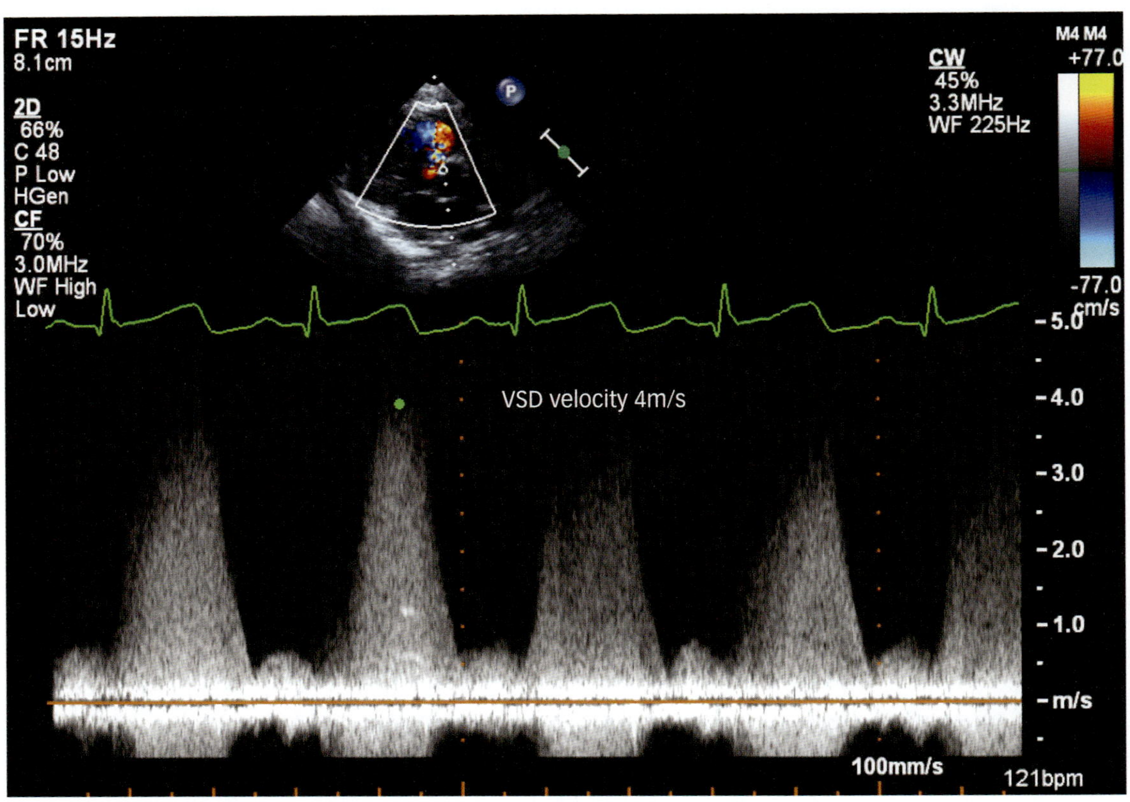

Color Plate 7 (page 25, question 75; page 207, answer 75)

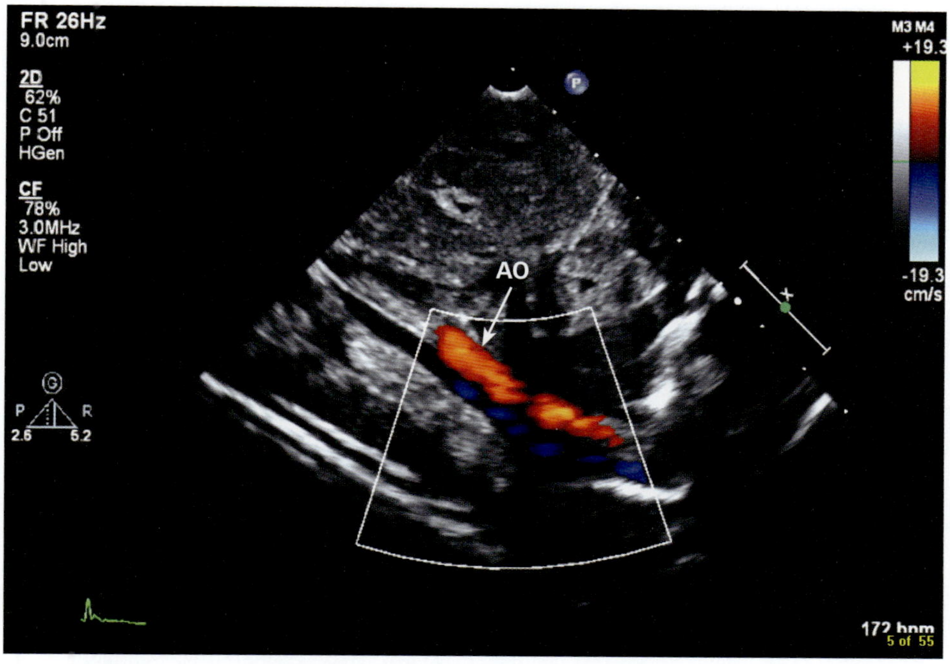

Color Plate 8 (page 38, question 126; page 227, answer 126)

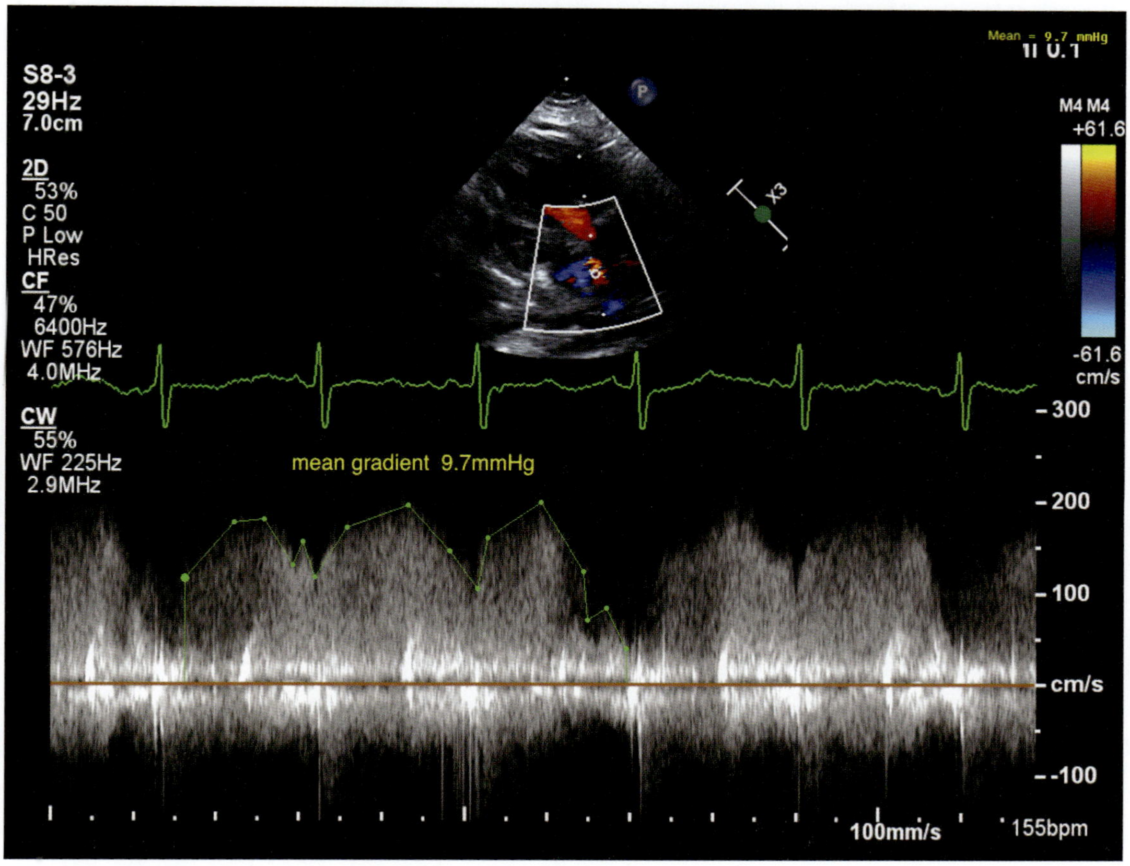

Color Plate 9 (page 64, question 223; page 266, answer 223)

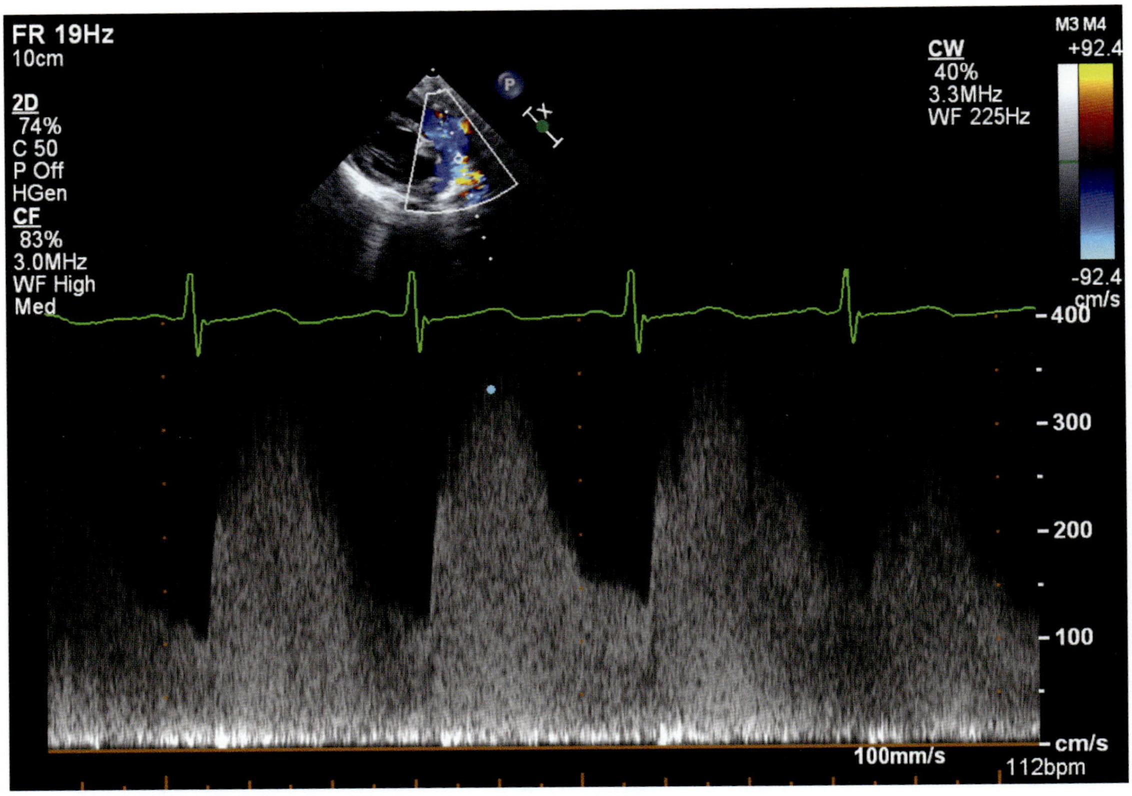

Color Plate 10 (page 74, question 265; page 282, answer 265)

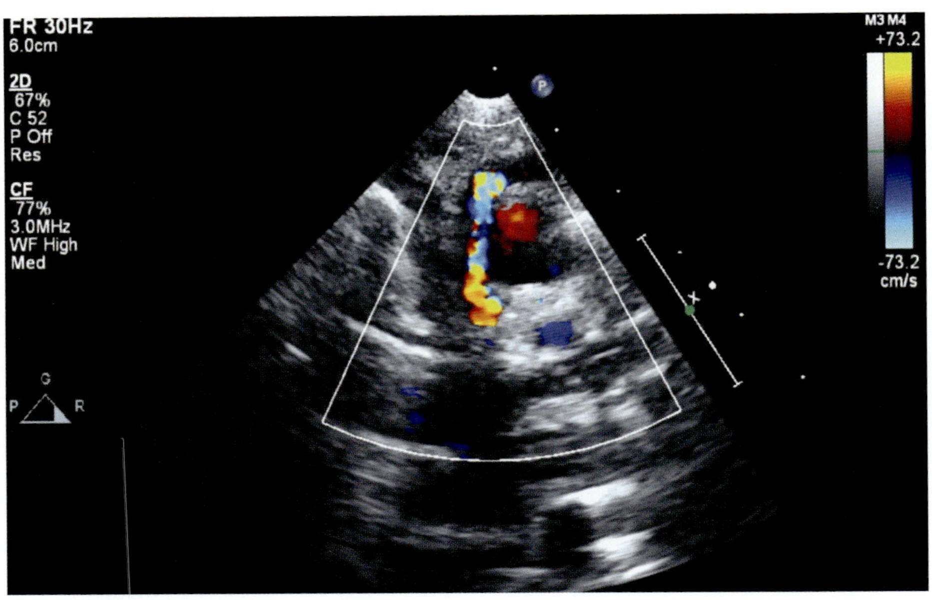

Color Plate 11 (page 95, question 346; page 311, answer 346)

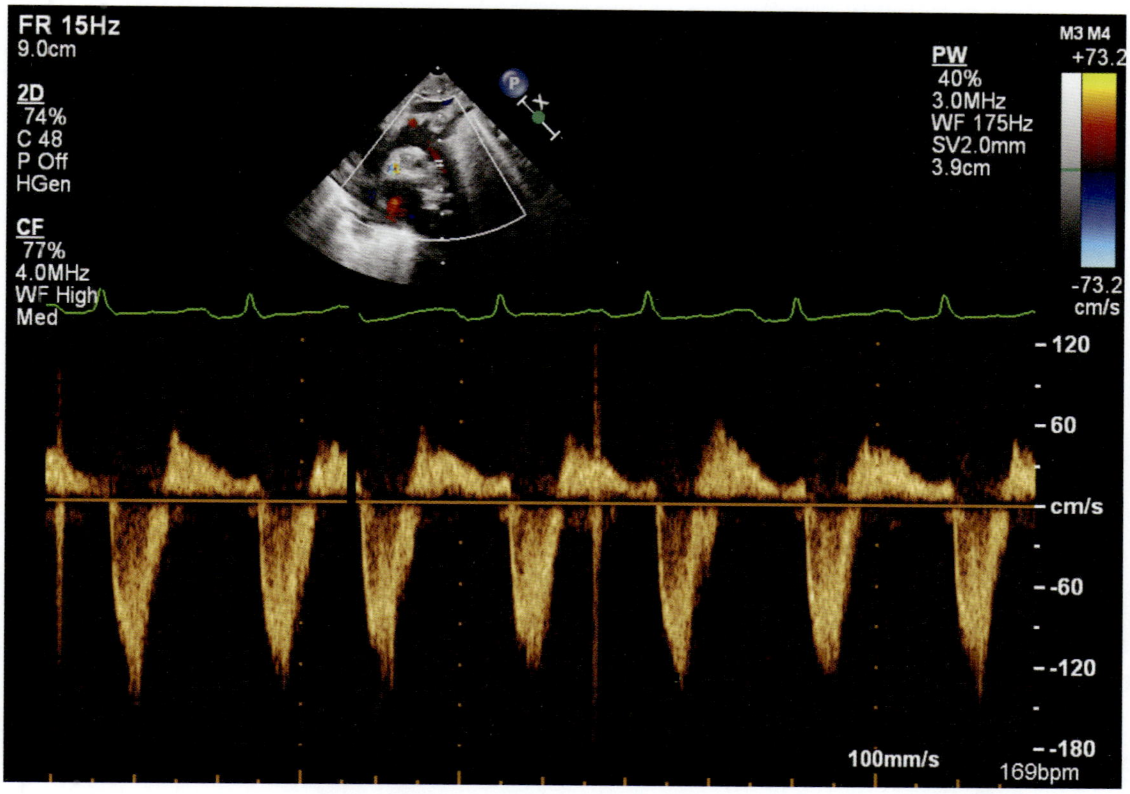

Color Plate 12 (page 95, question 347; page 311, answer 347)

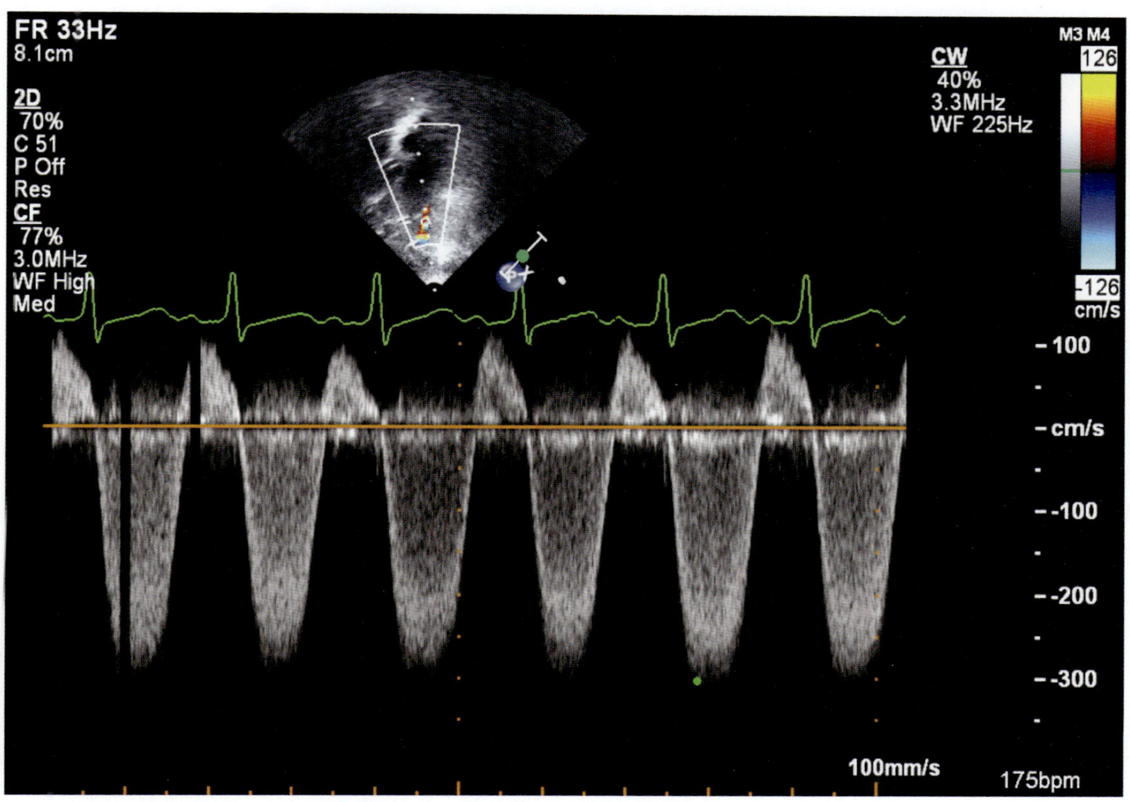

Color Plate 13 (page 97, question 352; page 313, answer 352)

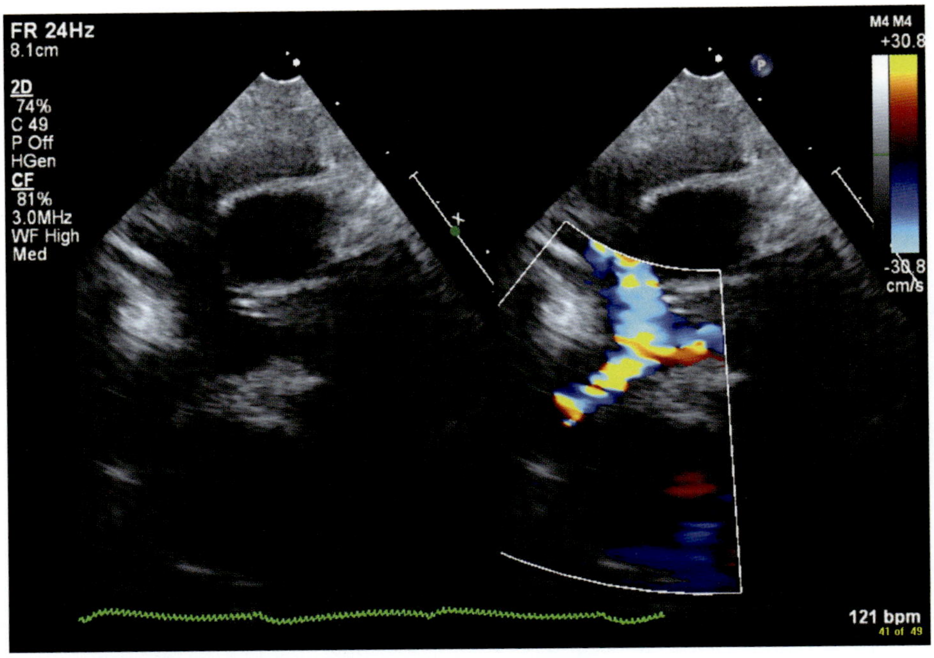

Color Plate 14 (page 98, question 356; page 314, answer 356)

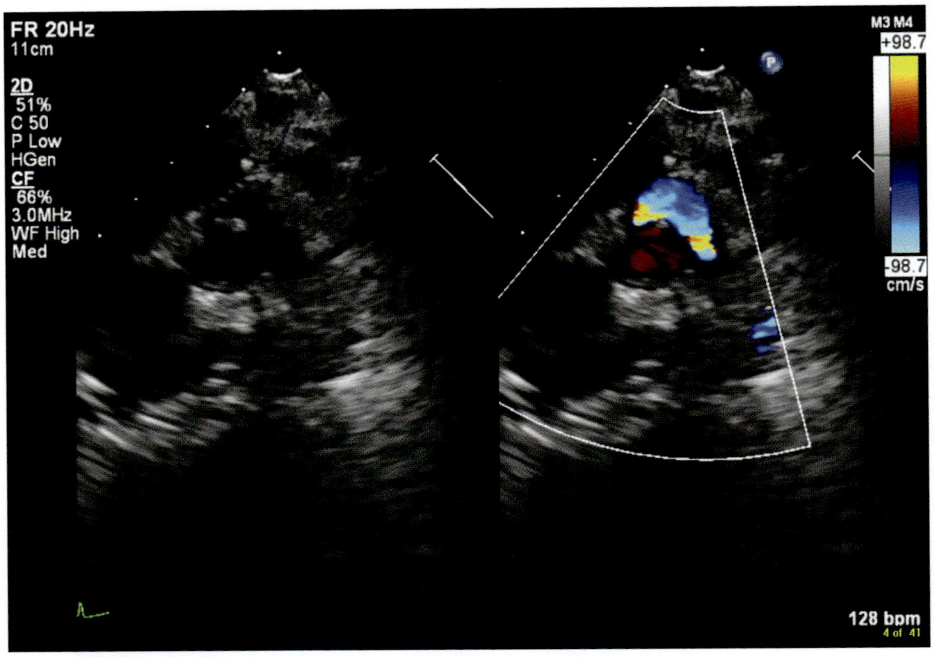

Color Plate 15 (page 99, question 361; page 316, answer 361)

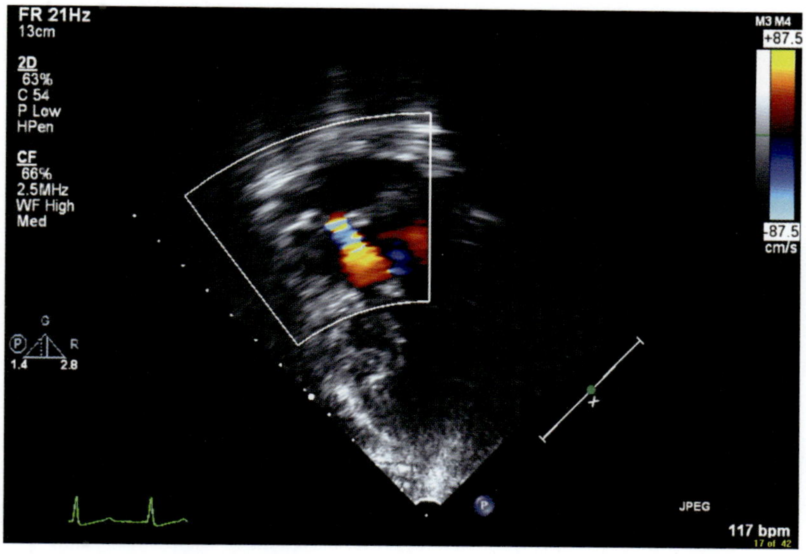

Color Plate 16
(page 102, question 369, image B; page 320, answer 369, image B)

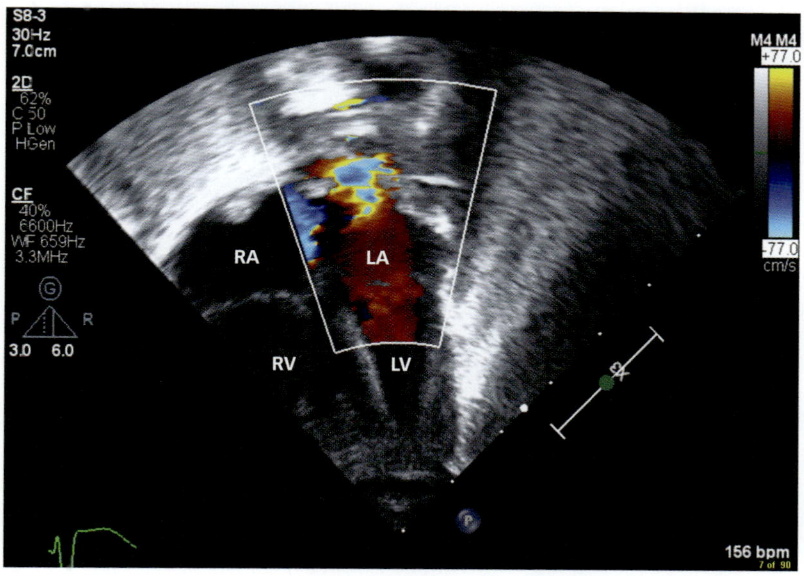

Color Plate 17
(page 328, answer 385)

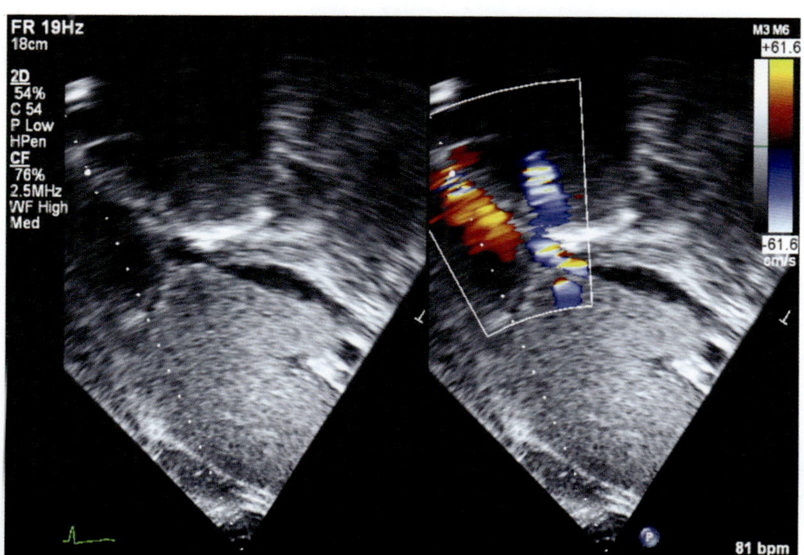

Color Plate 18
(page 108, question 387, image A; page 329, answer 387, image A)

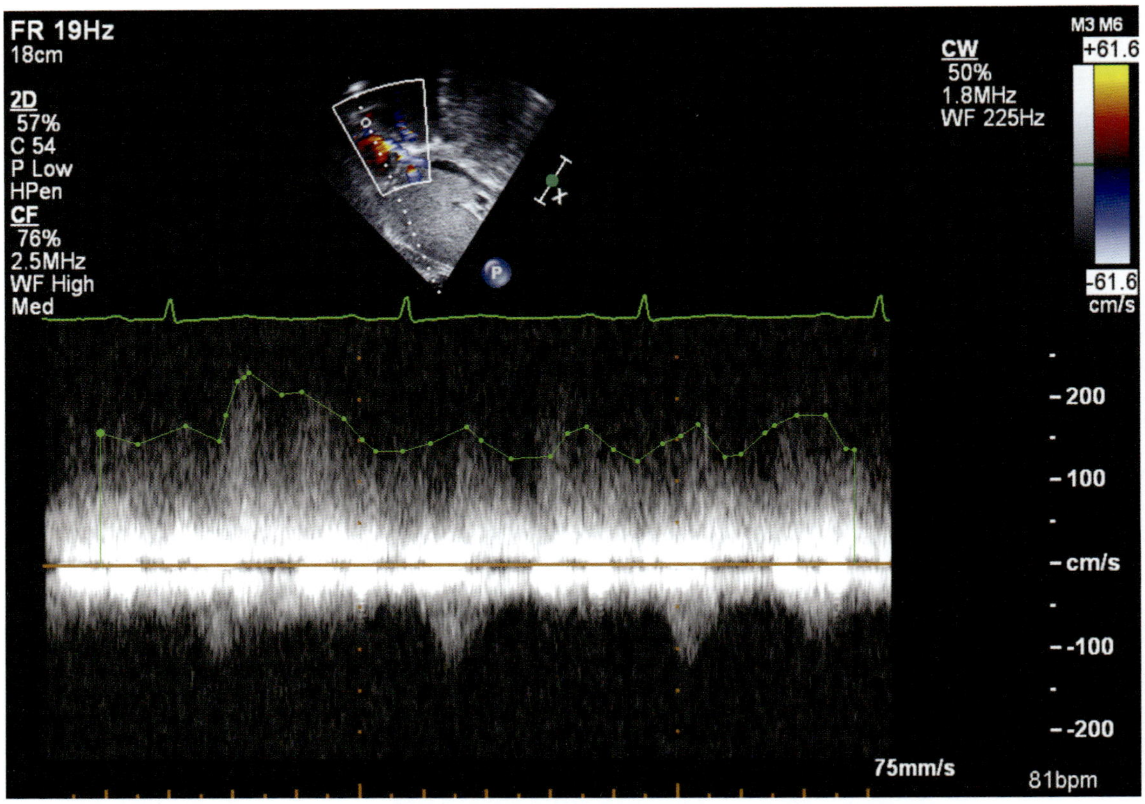

Color Plate 19 (page 108, question 387, image B; page 329, answer 387, image B)

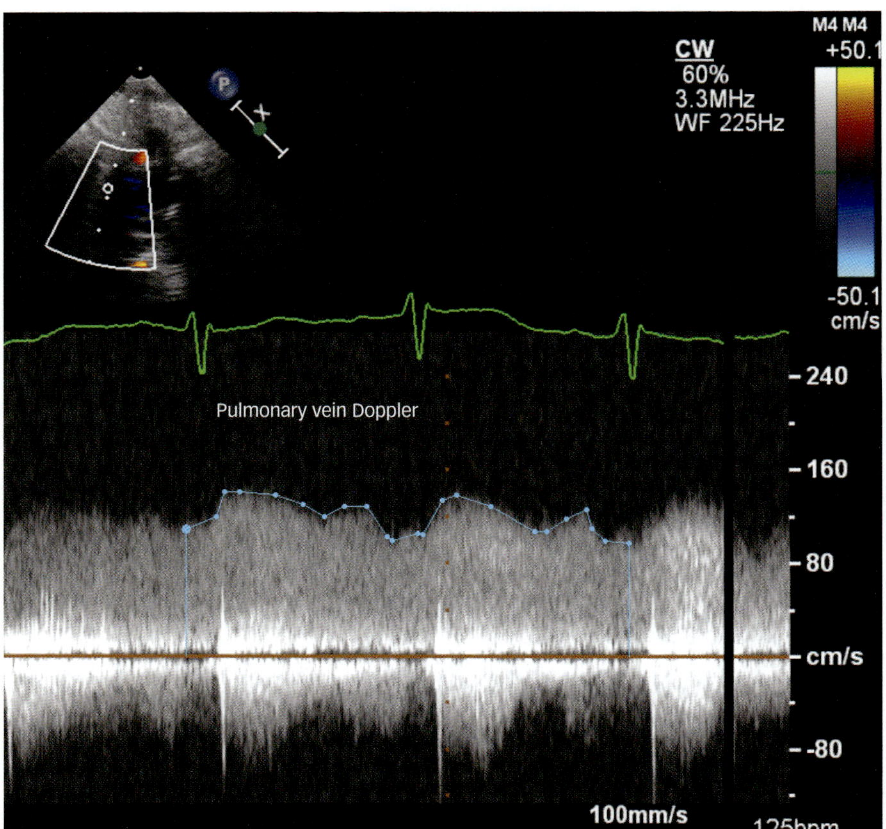

Color Plate 20 (page 109, question 388; page 330, answer 388)

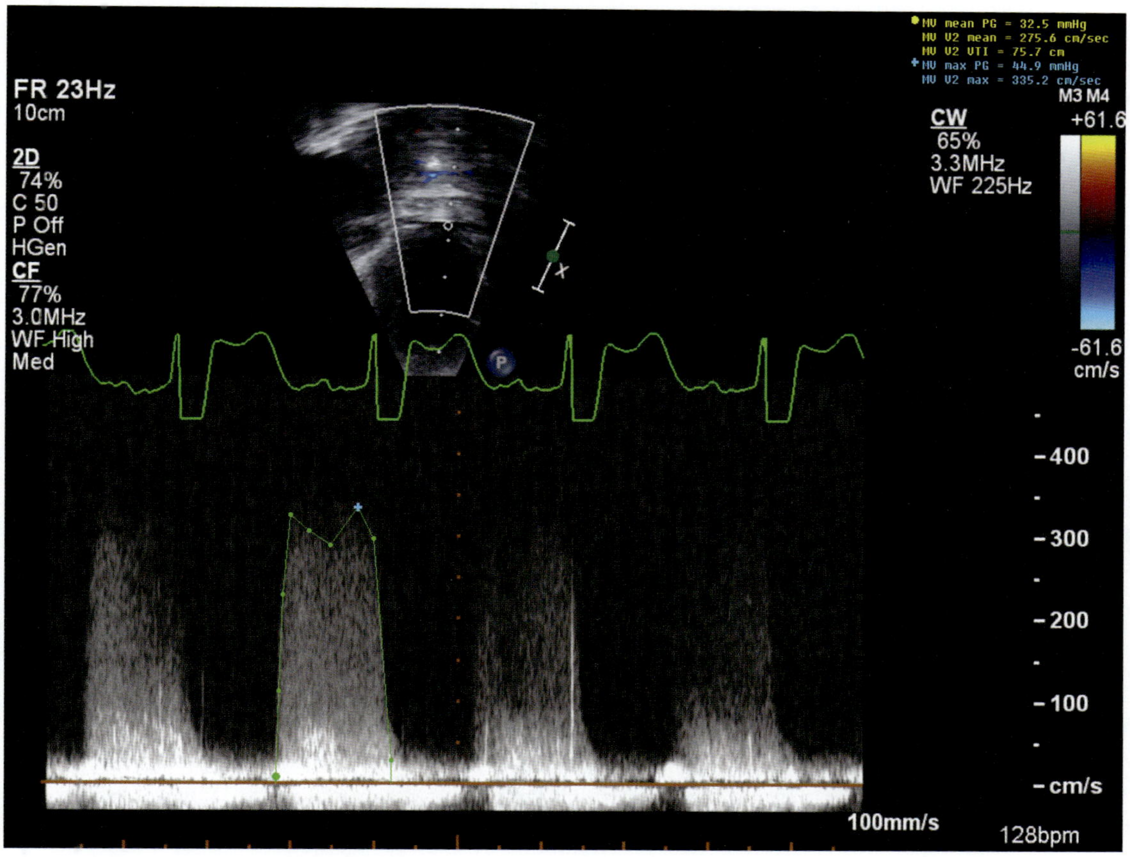

Color Plate 21 (page 121, question 434; page 350, answer 434)

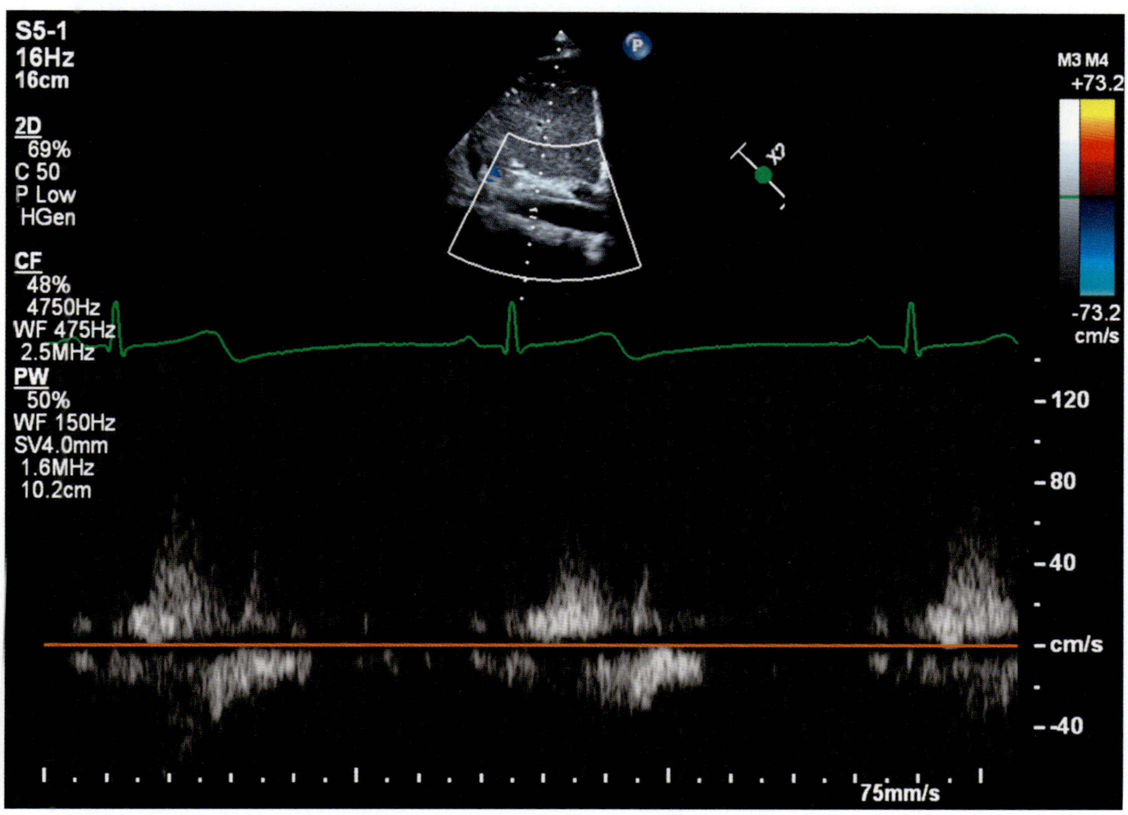

Color Plate 22 (page 128, question 452; page 358, answer 452)

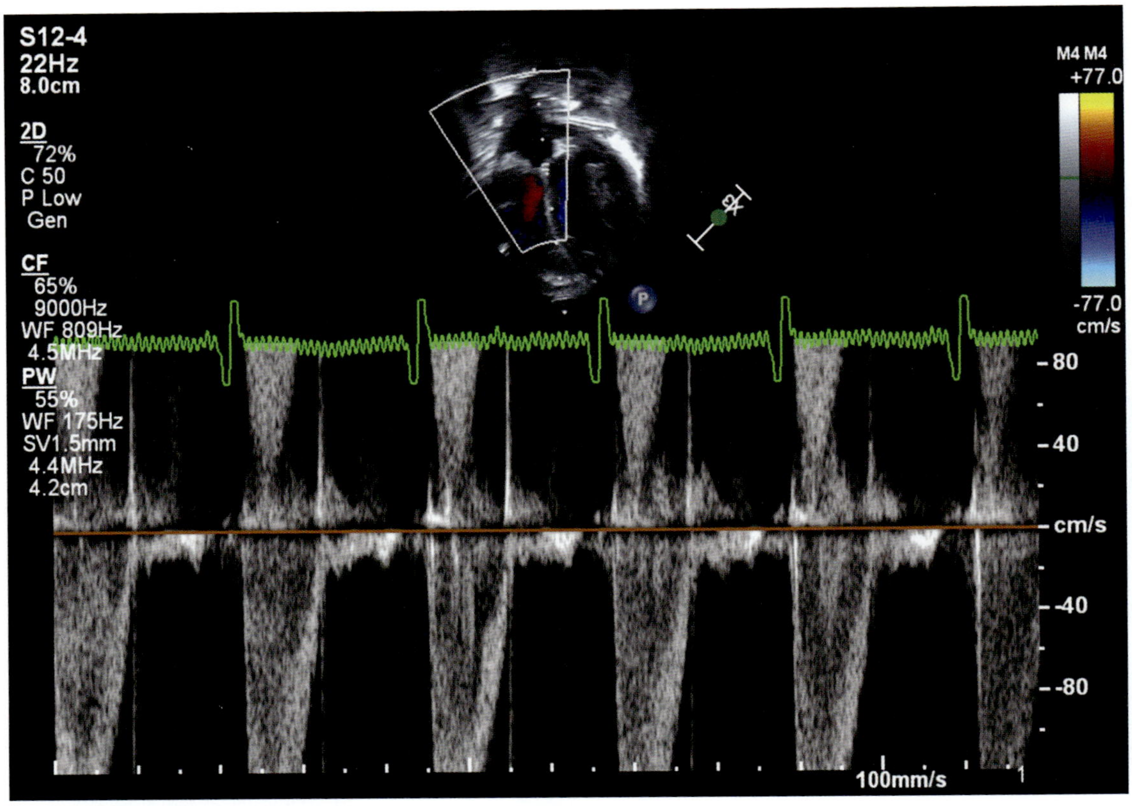

Color Plate 23 (page 129, question 455; page 360, answer 455)

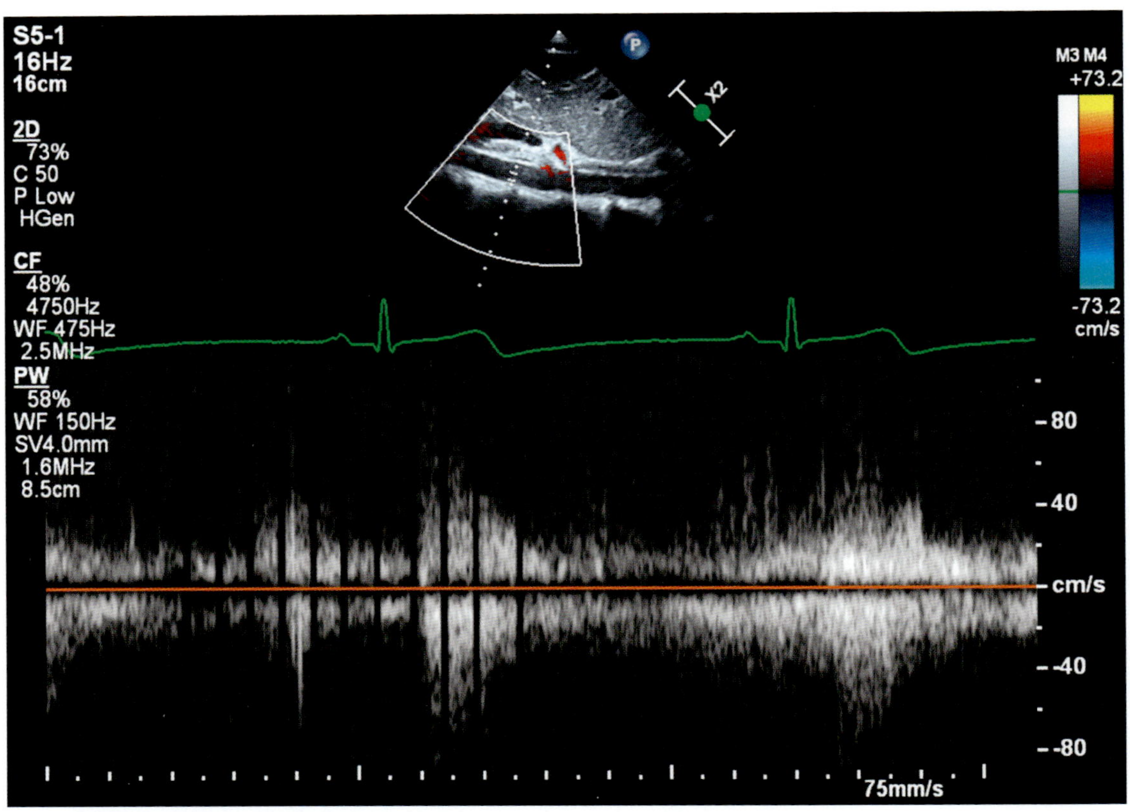

Color Plate 24 (page 130, question 458; page 362, answer 458)

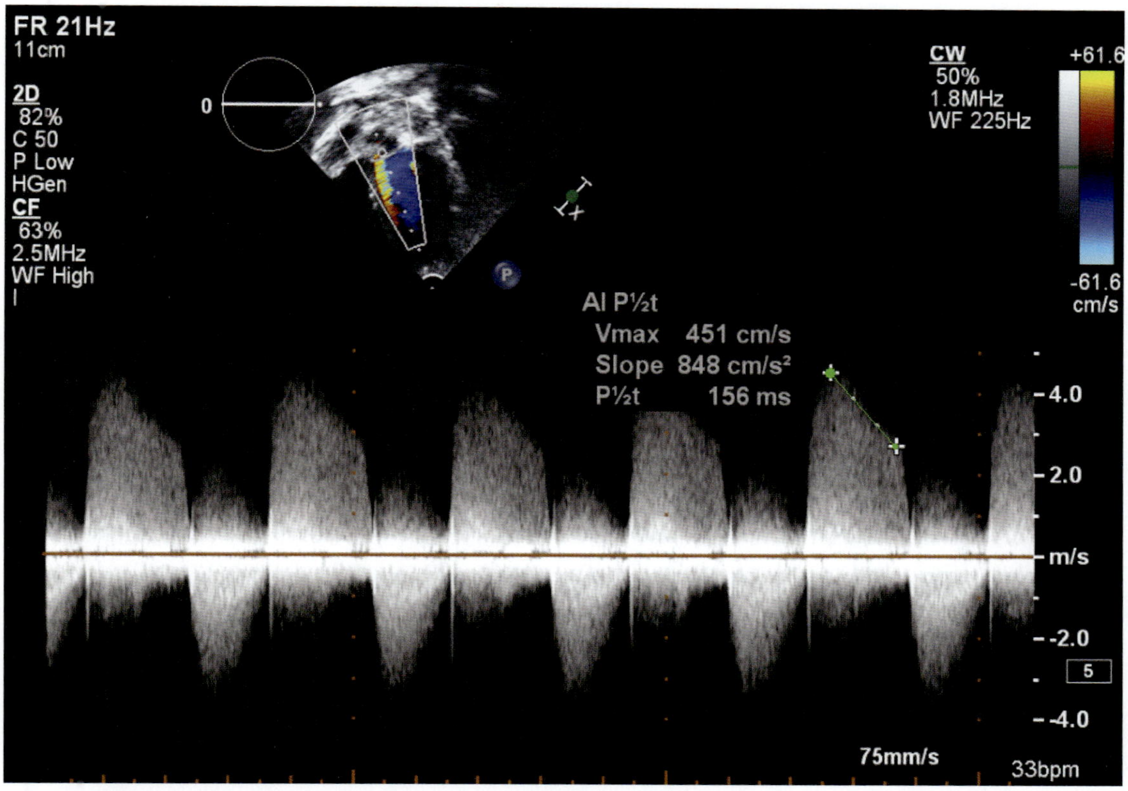

Color Plate 25 (page 145, question 507; page 385, answer 507)

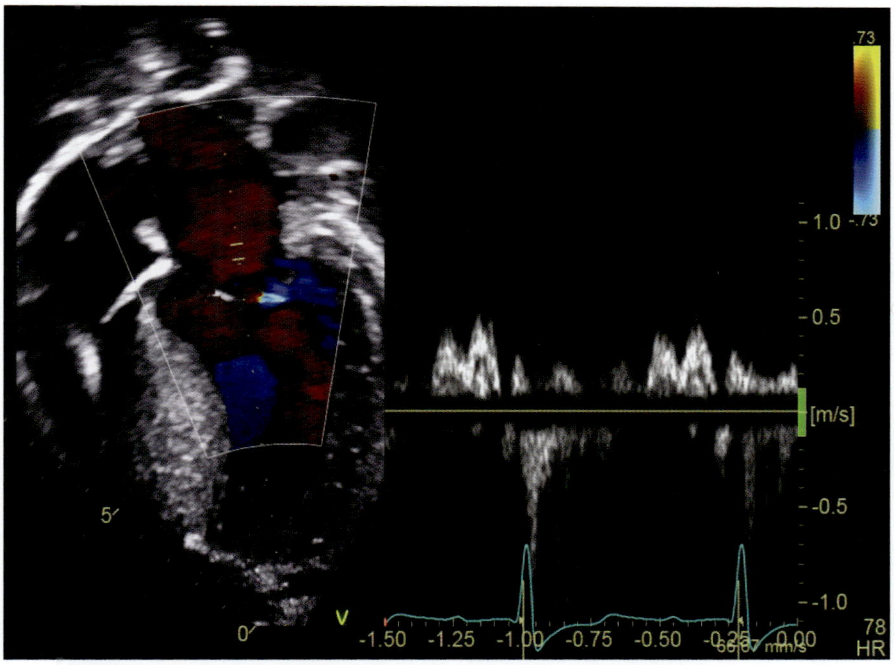

Color Plate 26 (page 154, question 543; page 399, answer 543)

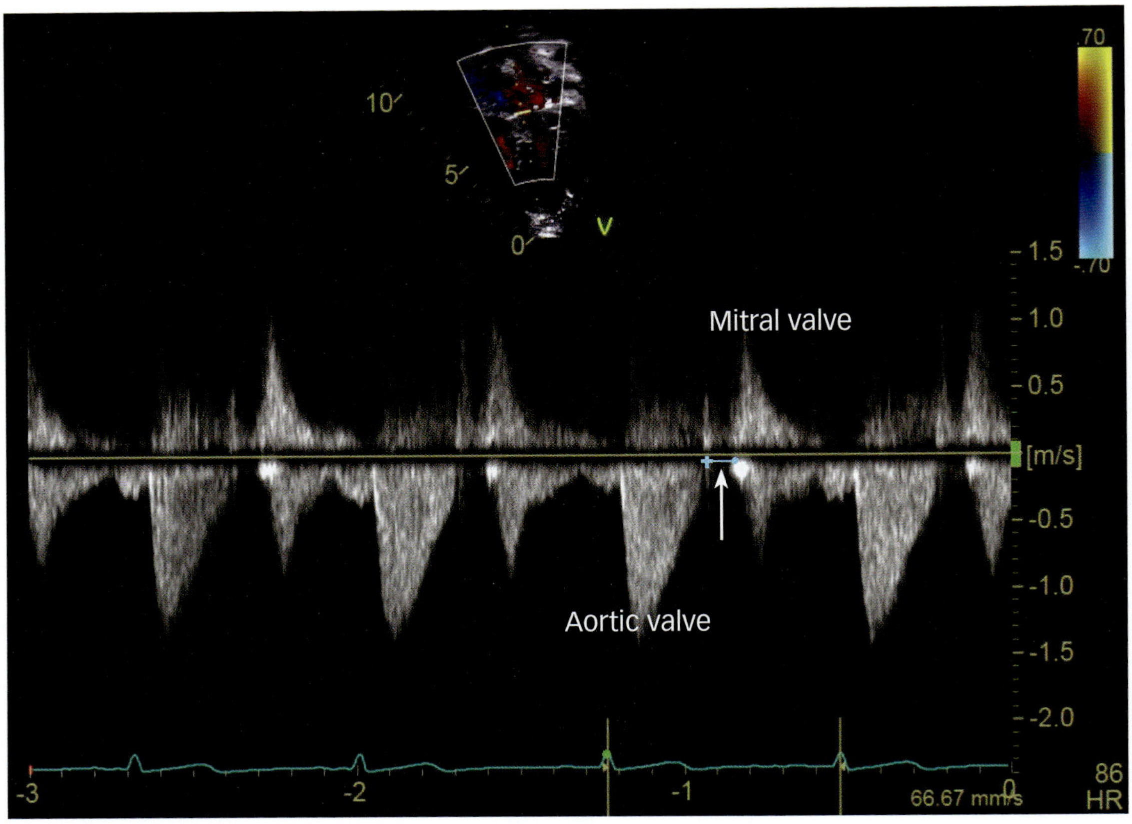

Color Plate 27 (page 154, question 544; page 400, answer 544)

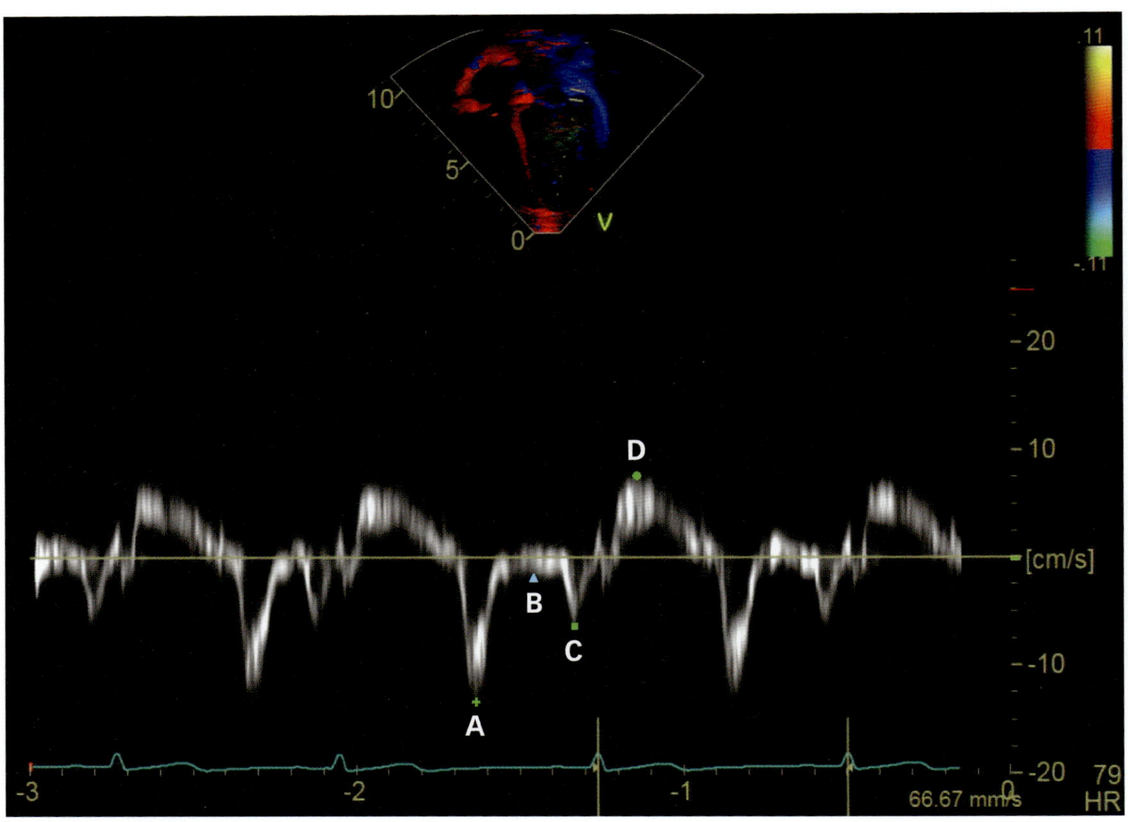

Color Plate 28 (page 156, question 549; page 402, answer 549)

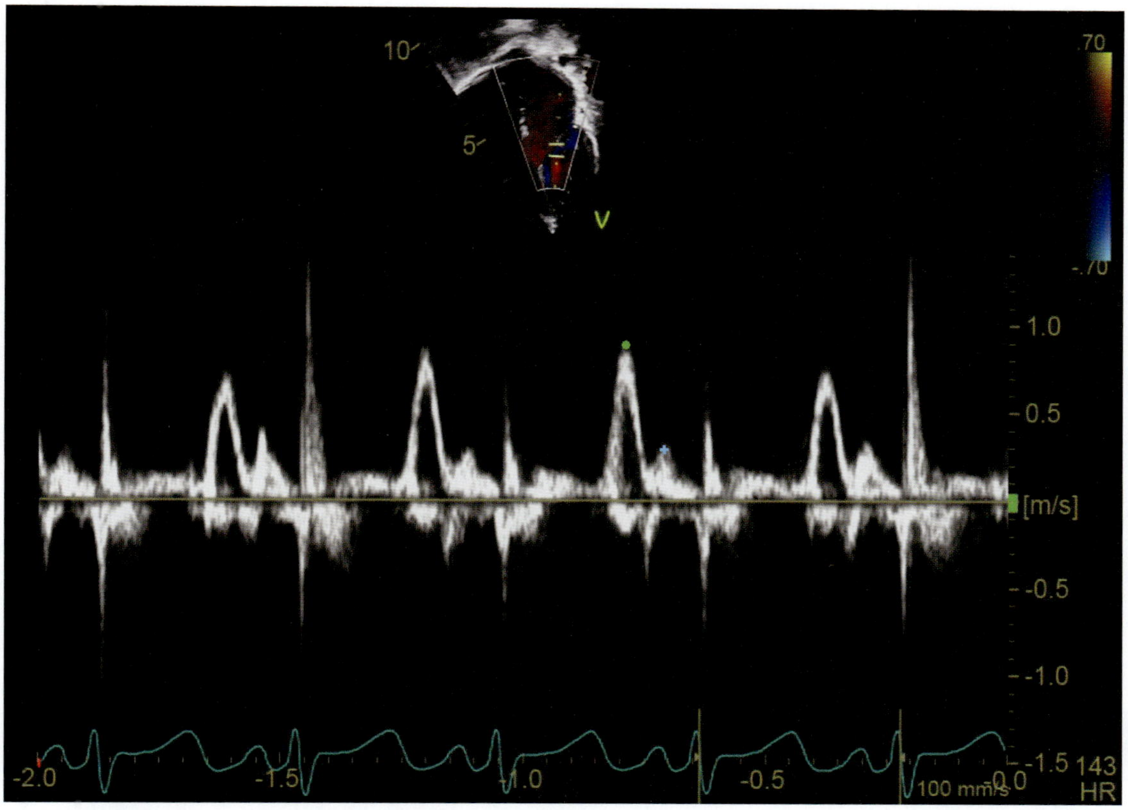

Color Plate 29 (page 158, question 557; page 405, answer 557)

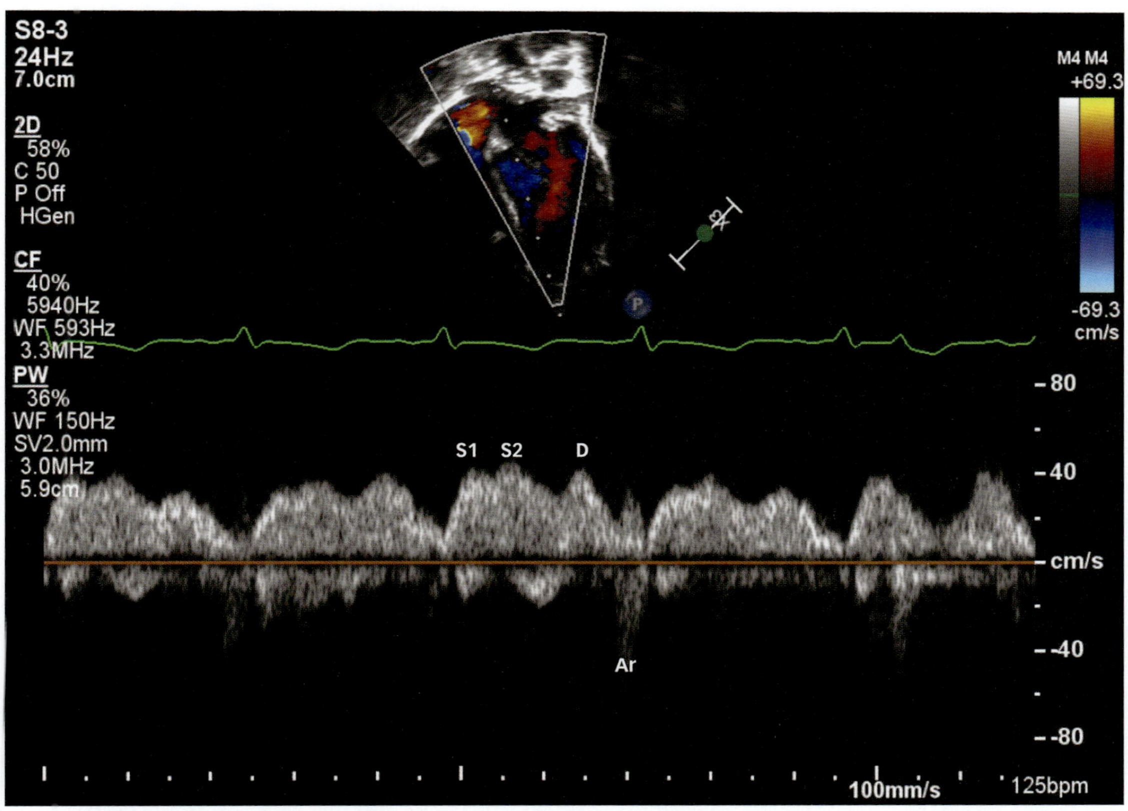

Color Plate 30 (page 159, question 560; page 406, answer 560)

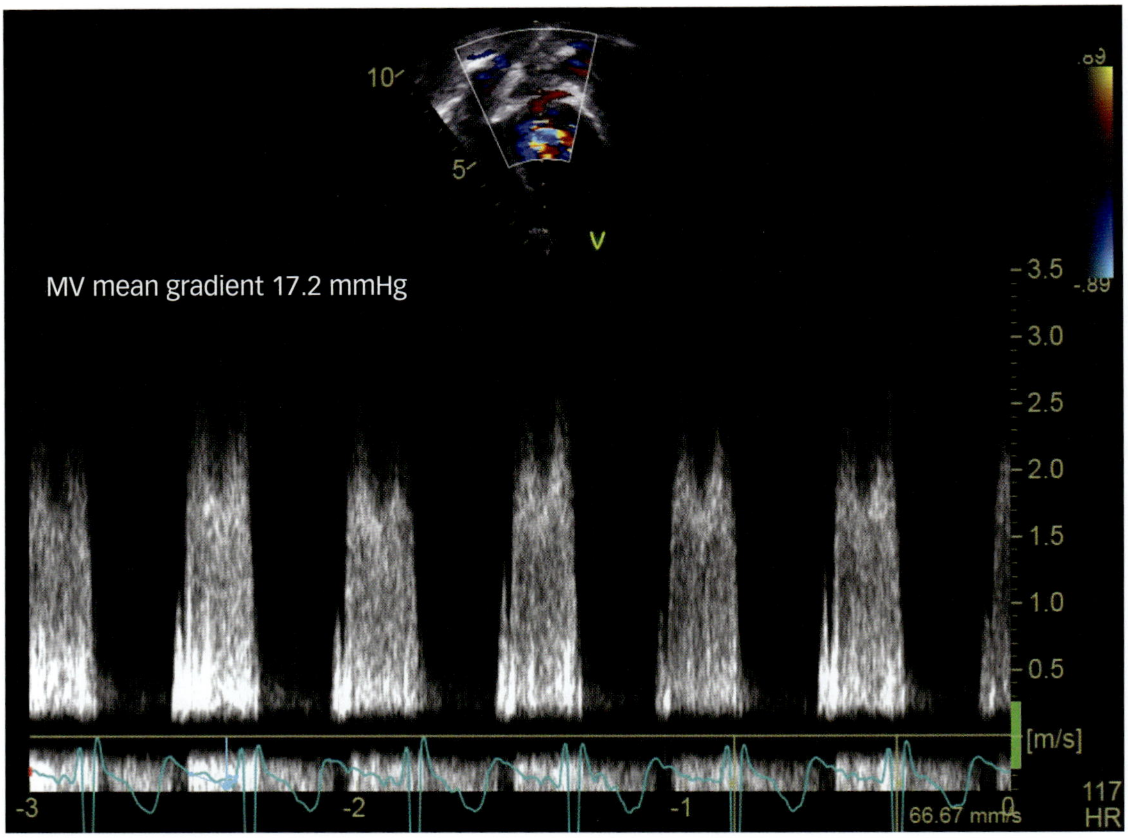

Color Plate 31 (page 163, question 571; page 411, answer 571)

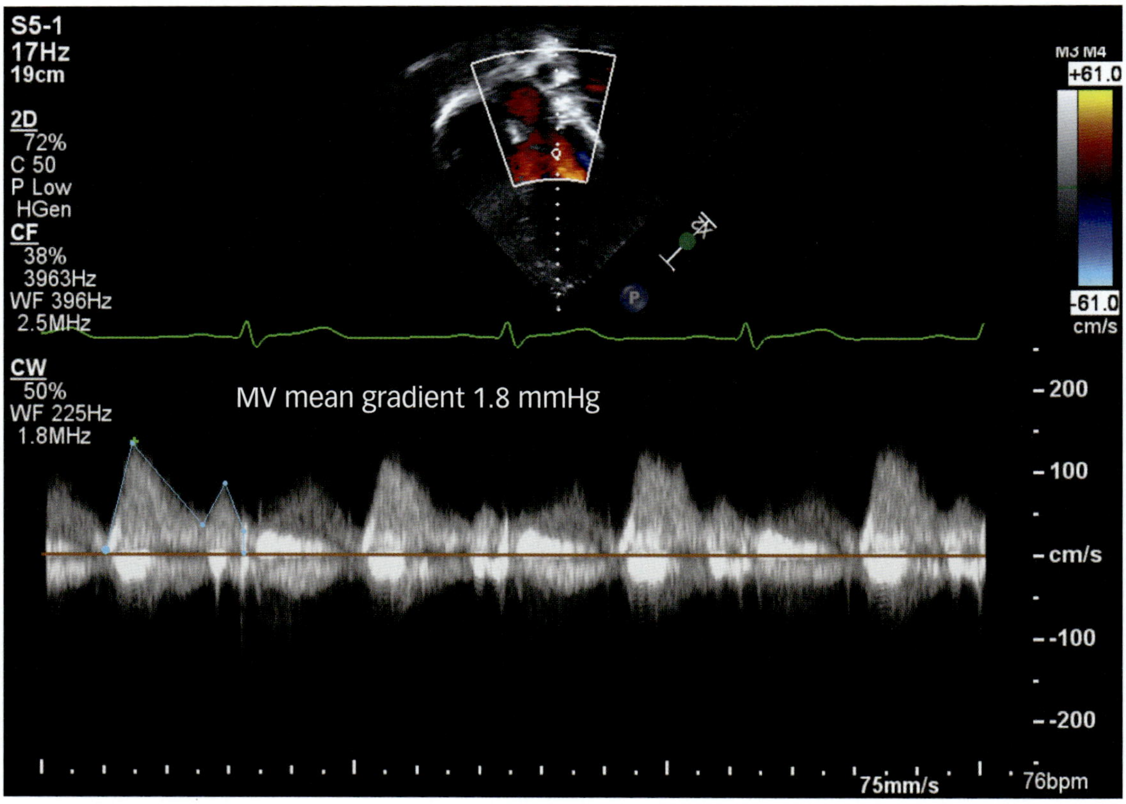

Color Plate 32 (page 164, question 574; page 412, answer 574)

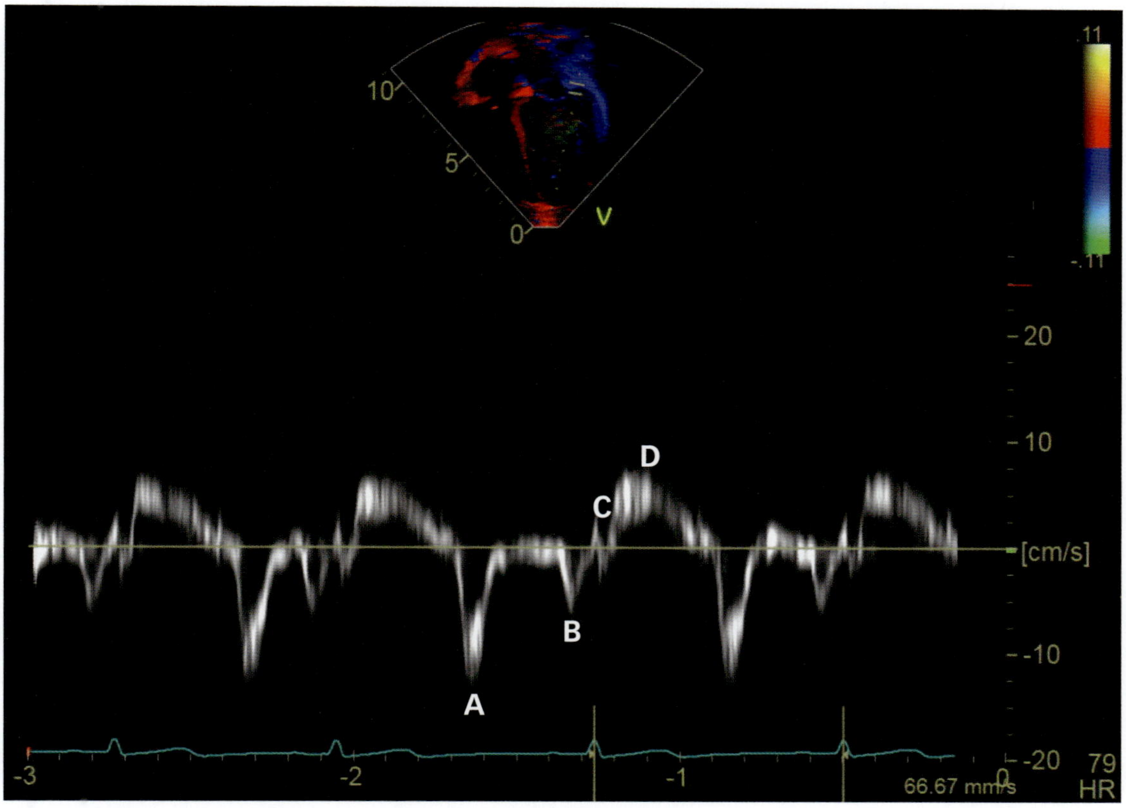

Color Plate 33 (page 173, question 602; page 425, answer 602)

PART 1

Anatomy and Physiology

1. By which week of embryonic development is the cardiovascular system completed?
   A. Fourth week
   B. Sixth week
   C. Eighth week
   D. Twelfth week

2. In the developing embryo the left aortic arch is formed by:
   A. The right fourth aortic arch and left dorsal aorta
   B. Persistence of the fifth aortic arch and seventh intersegmental artery
   C. The left fourth aortic arch and left dorsal aorta
   D. Involution of the left dorsal aorta

3. Aortic arch sidedness is defined by:
   A. The side where there is persistence of the third aortic arch
   B. The side where the ascending aorta ascends
   C. The side where the aortic arch passes over the mainstem bronchus
   D. The side where there is involution of the dorsal aorta

4. A patent ductus arteriosus results from the persistence of the:
   A. Fifth aortic arch
   B. Proximal left third aortic arch
   C. Left seventh intersegmental artery
   D. Right and/or left sixth aortic arch

5. In this image, what is the arrow pointing to?

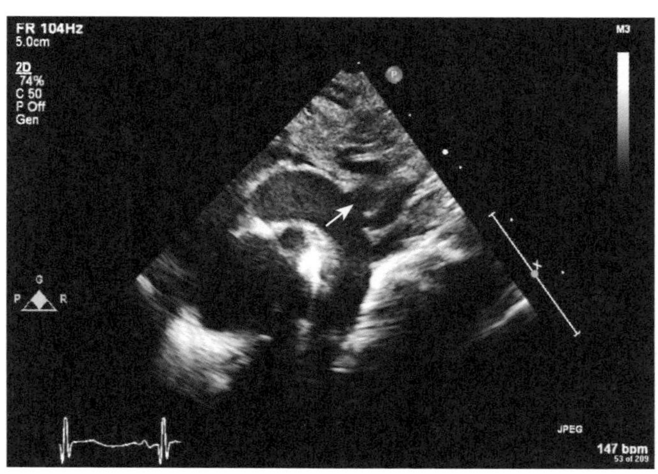

A. Innominate artery
B. Transverse aortic arch
C. Left subclavian artery
D. Innominate vein

AIT—Hotspot*

6. Which of these structures can be used to identify the aorta?
   A. Branch pulmonary arteries
   B. Coronary arteries and head and neck arteries
   C. Conal septum
   D. Concordant ventriculoarterial connections

7. Which of the following will help you identify the pulmonary artery in a neonate?
   A. Patent ductus arteriosus (PDA)
   B. Presence of a carina
   C. Trileaflet semilunar valve
   D. Bifurcation of the great artery

8. Fine ventricular trabeculations and a smooth septal surface are definitive characteristics of which of these structures?
   A. Right ventricular infundibular chamber
   B. Left ventricle
   C. Right ventricle
   D. Univentricular sinus

9. While performing a four-chamber view, you visualize a moderator band and coarse trabeculations on a left-sided ventricle. This morphology characterizes which of the following structures?
   A. Unknown
   B. Left ventricle
   C. D-looped ventricle
   D. Right ventricle

---

*Questions that are similar to the ARDMS Advanced Item Type (AIT) Hotspot items are marked throughout this mock exam. On the actual exam, Hotspot items require you to indicate the correct answer by marking directly on the image using your cursor; you can adjust the position of the mark (an X) as many times as you like before clicking on "Next" to submit the answer. In this Davies mock exam, similar questions are identified as ***AIT—Hotspot***. These ask you to identify what an arrow in the image is pointing at or to indicate the label on an image that corresponds to the correct answer.

Refer to video PER-Q10.

10. In this video clip the motion of the interventricular septum is consistent with:
    A. Normal right ventricular pressures
    B. Increased left ventricular preload
    C. Increased right ventricular volume and pressure
    D. Restrictive patent ductus arteriosus (PDA)

11. *Preload* is best described as:
    A. The pressure at the beginning of systole
    B. The time elapsed during ventricular contraction
    C. The load at the end of diastole and before contraction
    D. The load at the end of systole

12. Left ventricular afterload is most increased in which of the following disease processes?
    A. Aortic stenosis
    B. Mitral stenosis
    C. Mitral regurgitation
    D. Aortic regurgitation

13. During a bedside scan in the pediatric cardiothoracic intensive care unit, you visualize a right aortic arch with mirror-image branching. How did this arch form?
    A. Persistence of the left dorsal aorta and left third aortic arch
    B. Dissolution of the left dorsal aorta distal to the origin of the seventh intersegmental artery, persistence of the right fourth aortic arch, and persistence of the right dorsal aorta
    C. Persistence of the right fifth aortic arch
    D. Persistence of the right sixth aortic arch

14. During a parasternal long-axis sweep into the right ventricular inflow tract view, you visualize a broad-based structure that looks like it is incorporated into the right atrium. Which structure are you visualizing?
    A. Right atrial appendage
    B. Left atrial vestibule
    C. Right arterial pole
    D. Right vitelline vein

15. In a normal patient, the coronary sinus drains to the:
    A. Left atrium
    B. Right atrium
    C. Right atrial appendage
    D. Left atrial vestibule

16. What mechanism causes the patent ductus arteriosus (PDA) to close after birth?
    A. An increase in pulmonary venous return to the left atrium
    B. An increase in prostaglandin E1 (PGE1)
    C. An increase in arterial oxygen
    D. An increase in pulmonary vascular resistance

17. In the normal fetal circulation atrial-level shunting flows:
    A. Left to right
    B. Bidirectionally
    C. Right to left
    D. Nowhere; there is no atrial-level shunt.

18. Which choice best describes why the foramen ovale closes after birth?
    A. Decrease in systemic venous return
    B. Increase in systemic venous return
    C. Decrease in systemic venous oxygenation
    D. Increase in left atrial pressure

19. You are in the neonatal intensive care unit, scanning a patient with situs inversus totalis. You see the septum primum flopping into a right-sided atrium. Which statement best describes the morphology of this right-sided atrium?
    A. Morphologic right atrium
    B. Common atrium due to septum primum visualization
    C. Morphologic left atrium
    D. Left isomerism due to visualization of the septum primum

20. Identify the atrioventricular (AV) valve the arrow in this image is pointing to:

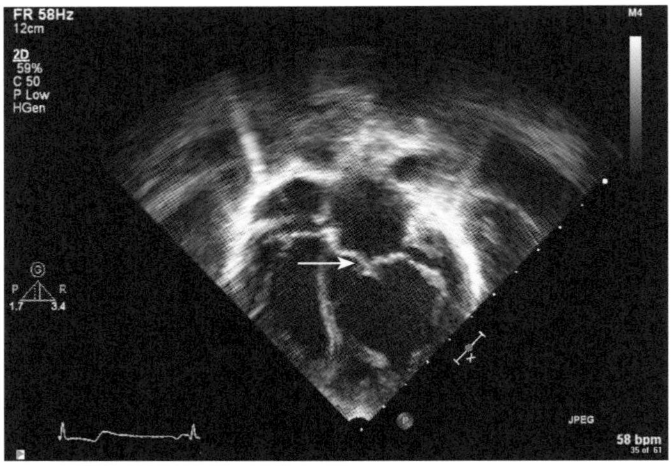

A. Aortic valve

B. Tricuspid valve

C. Mitral valve

D. Pulmonary valve

AIT—Hotspot

21. A 16-week-old patient is scheduled for an echocardiogram to evaluate a loud systolic heart murmur. You find a small restrictive muscular ventricular septal defect (VSD) with a peak pressure gradient (PPG) of 88 mmHg. In this patient when is it most likely that pulmonary vascular resistance (PVR) decreased the most?

A. 1–2 weeks

B. 6–8 weeks

C. 3–4 weeks

D. 14–16 weeks

22. Name the looping pattern of the ventricles in this image:

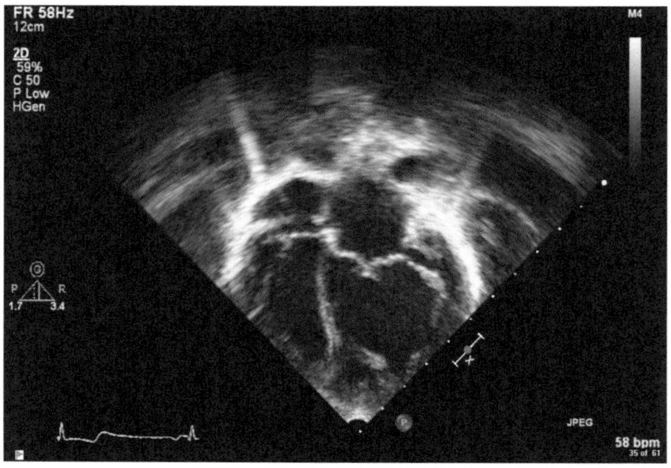

A. L-looped
B. D-looped
C. A-looped
D. X-looped

23. When does the ductus arteriosus usually close?
    A. 24 hours after birth
    B. 36–48 hours after birth
    C. 48–72 hours after birth
    D. 72–96 hours after birth

24. Ductal tissue is LEAST likely to close in the presence of:
    A. Oxygen
    B. Acetaminophen (Tylenol)
    C. Indomethacin
    D. Prostaglandin E1 (PGE1)

25. In this image, which anatomic structure is the arrow pointing to?

See Color Plate 1 on page xix.

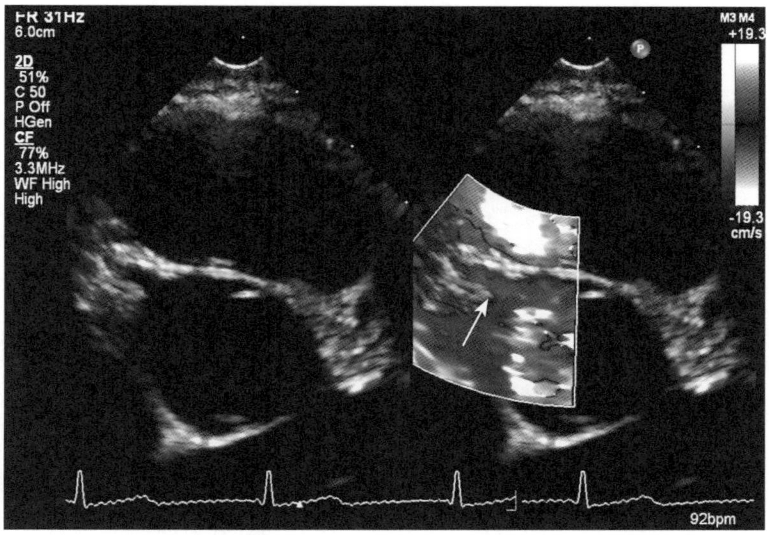

A. Left main coronary artery
B. Right coronary artery
C. Left anterior descending coronary artery
D. Posterior descending coronary artery

AIT—Hotspot

26. Which anatomic structure is the arrow in this image pointing to?

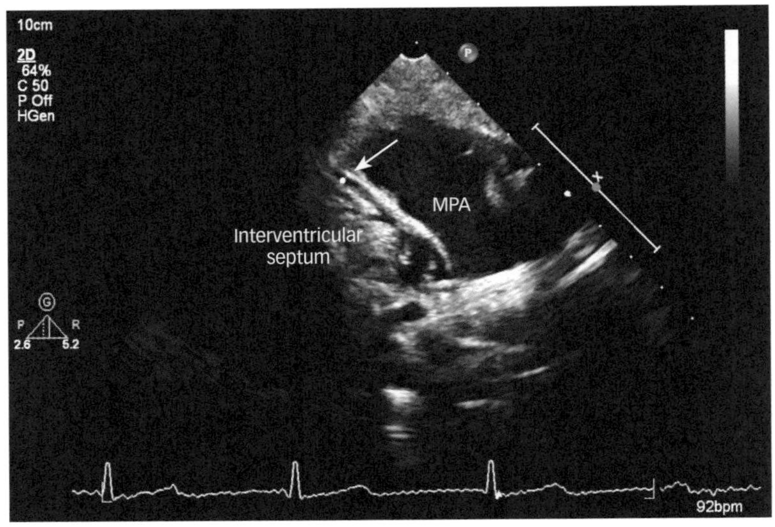

A. Left anterior descending coronary artery (LAD)
B. Left main coronary artery (LMCA)
C. Circumflex coronary artery (Cx)
D. Left main coronary artery fistula

AIT—Hotspot

27. Which anatomic structure is the arrow in this image pointing to?

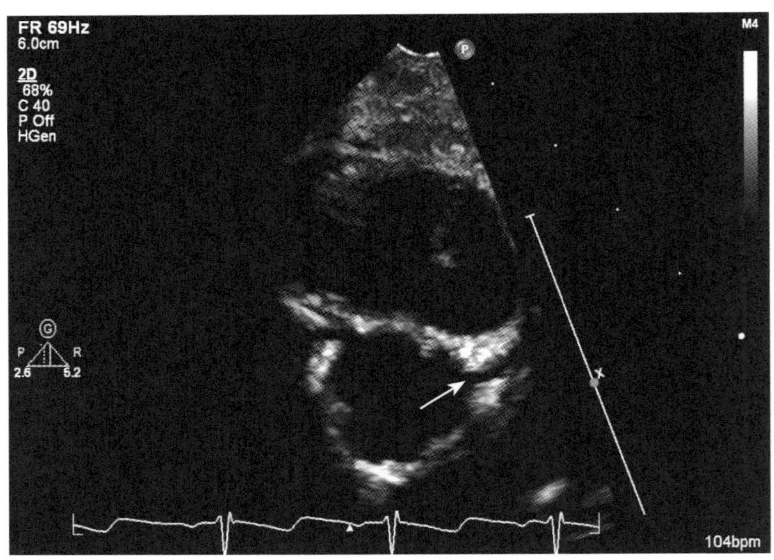

A. Left anterior descending coronary artery (LAD)
B. Circumflex coronary artery (Cx)
C. Left main coronary artery (LMCA)
D. Septal perforator coronary artery (SPCA)

AIT—Hotspot

Refer to video PER-Q28.

28. The patient in this video clip has transposition of the great arteries (d-TGA). Which anatomic structure is the arrow pointing to?
    A. Single left coronary artery
    B. Circumflex from the right coronary artery
    C. Conal branch off the right coronary artery
    D. Posterior descending coronary artery

AIT—Hotspot

29. In this image, which aortic anatomic structure is the arrow pointing to?

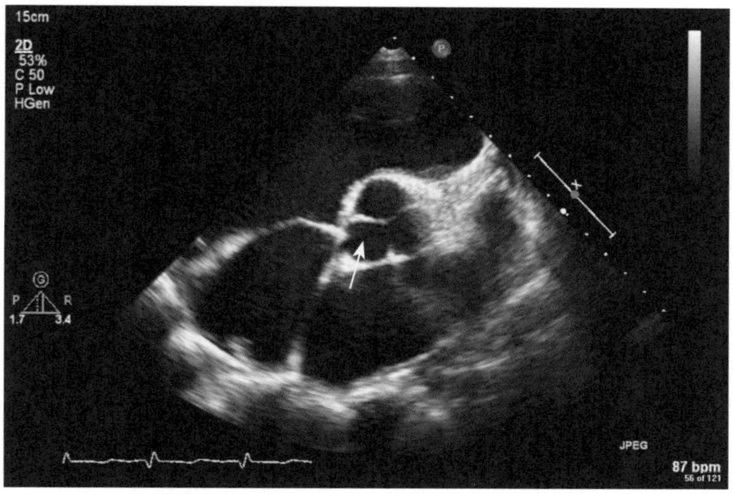

    A. Left coronary cusp (LCC)
    B. Right coronary cusp (RCC)
    C. Right and left commissural post
    D. Noncoronary cusp (NCC)

AIT—Hotspot

30. Which of these imaging methods, when paired with 2D imaging, helps locate the origins of the coronary artery?
    A. Spectral Doppler
    B. Power Doppler
    C. Color flow Doppler
    D. M-mode

31. Left main coronary artery filling is best seen during:
    A. Diastole
    B. Aortic valve opening
    C. Mitral valve closure
    D. Systole

32. This image demonstrates the right coronary artery (arrow) filling during which phase of the cardiac cycle?

See Color Plate 1 on page xix.

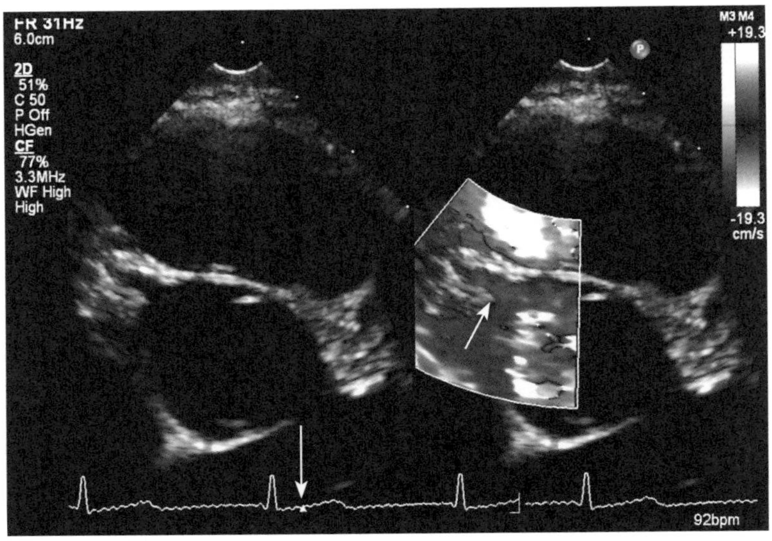

A. Isovolumic relaxation
B. Early diastolic filling
C. Late diastolic filling (atrial contraction)
D. Systole

AIT—Hotspot

33. The arrow in this image is pointing to the:

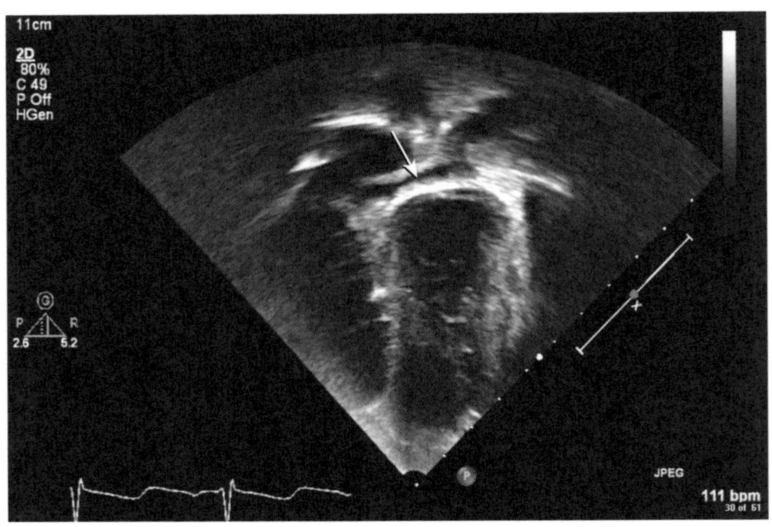

A. Left atrium
B. Coronary sinus
C. Thebesian valve
D. Circumflex coronary artery

AIT—Hotspot

34. In this image, what vascular structure is the arrow pointing to?

See Color Plate 2 on page xx.

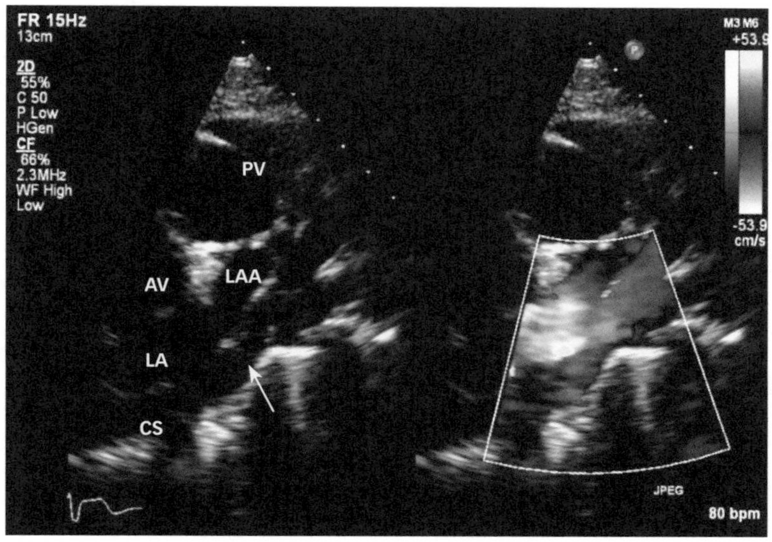

A. Left superior vena cava
B. Subclavian vein
C. Azygos vein
D. Hemiazygos vein

AIT—Hotspot

35. In this image, what vascular structure is the arrow pointing to?

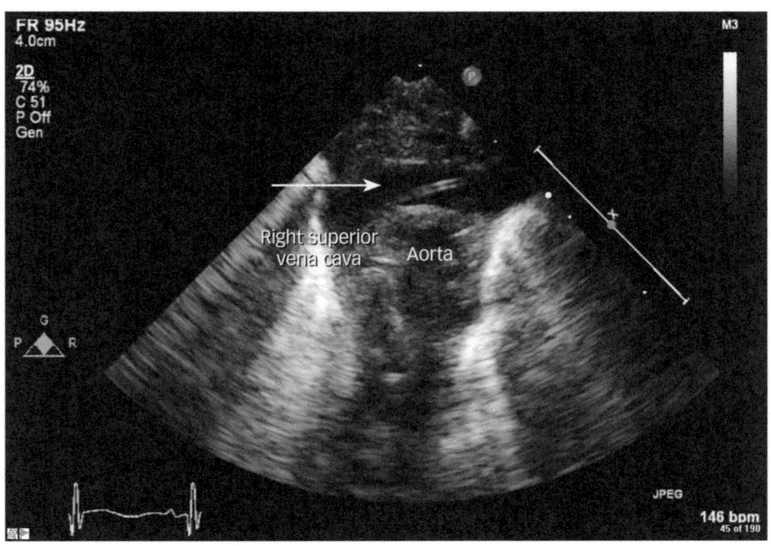

A. External jugular vein
B. Innominate vein
C. High intercostal vein
D. Innominate artery

AIT—Hotspot

36. Which anatomic structure is best visualized from the apical four-chamber view with posterior angulation of the transducer?
   A. Superior vena cava
   B. Circumflex coronary artery
   C. Left anterior descending coronary artery
   D. Coronary sinus

37. During embryologic development, the left horn of the sinus venosus eventually develops into which structure of the normal four-chambered heart?
   A. Eustachian valve
   B. Coronary sinus
   C. Levoatrial cardinal vein
   D. Superior vena cava

38. During embryologic development, the right horn of the sinus venosus eventually develops into which structure of the normal four-chambered heart?
   A. Left atrium
   B. Pulmonary veins
   C. Right atrium
   D. Left atrial appendage

39. Which structure is the arrow in this image pointing to?

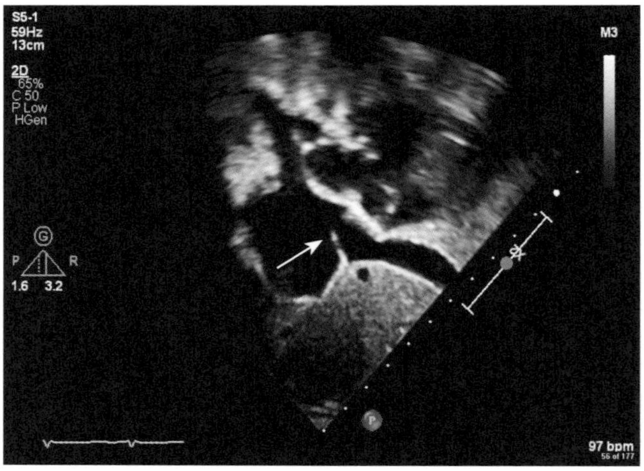

   A. Coumadin ridge
   B. Thebesian valve
   C. Eustachian valve
   D. Crista terminalis

AIT—Hotspot

40. Azygos continuation of the inferior vena cava (IVC) occurs when there is:
    A. Interruption of the hepatic portion of the IVC
    B. Interruption of the left vitelline vein
    C. Interruption of the levoatrial cardinal vein
    D. Interruption of the right anterior cardinal vein

41. You are scanning a newborn baby. You start with your subcostal views and pulsed-wave Doppler evaluation of the abdominal aorta and find prominent diastolic flow reversal. What do you suspect you will encounter during the remainder of the exam?
    A. Significant coarctation of the aorta (CoA)
    B. Unicuspid aortic valve with severe stenosis
    C. Bicuspid aortic valve (BAV) with mild stenosis
    D. Patent ductus arteriosus (PDA)

42. You are performing echocardiography on a patient in the neonatal intensive care unit and note a right-sided aortic arch with an aberrant left subclavian artery. Which of the following options would result in a vascular ring?
    A. A patent ductus arteriosus on the same side as the aortic arch
    B. A right-sided patent ductus arteriosus
    C. A left-sided patent ductus arteriosus
    D. A patent ductus arteriosus originating from the left innominate artery

43. Left atrial morphology is best established by which of the following characteristics?
    A. Site of pulmonary venous connection
    B. Crista terminalis
    C. Finger-like appendage
    D. Septum secundum

44. Which situs of the abdominal viscera is characterized by a right-sided liver, left-sided stomach, left-sided spleen, and right-sided cecum?
    A. Situs totalis
    B. Situs inversus
    C. Situs ambiguus
    D. Situs solitus

45. Which of the following terms describes a right-sided morphologic right atrium and left-sided morphologic left atrium?
    A. Asplenia
    B. Situs solitus
    C. Polysplenia
    D. Situs inversus

46. Which of the following terms best describes a right-sided morphologic left ventricle in the apical-four chamber view?
    A. X-looped ventricle
    B. D-looped ventricle
    C. L-looped ventricle
    D. A-looped ventricle

47. When you use your hand to determine ventricular looping, which cardiac structure does the thumb represent for the right ventricle?
    A. Tricuspid valve
    B. Pulmonary valve
    C. Right ventricular free wall
    D. Ventricular septum

48. Which of the following describes the arrangement of the great arteries in which the aorta is posterior, leftward, and normally connected/assigned to the left ventricle with its ascending segment crossing over the left-sided pulmonary artery?
    A. Normally related great arteries, situs solitus
    B. L-malposed great arteries
    C. A-malposed great arteries
    D. Normally related great arteries, situs inversus

49. Which of the following refers to a left-sided ventricle with an infundibulum connected to a pulmonary artery?
    A. Morphologic left ventricle in the setting of D-looped ventricles
    B. Morphologic right ventricle in the setting of L-looped ventricles
    C. Single-ventricle morphology with A-looped ventricles
    D. Morphologic left ventricle with pulmonary to tricuspid valve fibrous continuity

50. The two connecting segments described in the segmental approach to congenital heart disease are:
    A. Atrioventricular junction and great arteries
    B. Atrioventricular junction and ventricles
    C. Atrioventricular junction and atria
    D. Atrioventricular junction and ventriculoarterial junction

51. What are the three main segments described in the segmental approach to congenital heart disease?
    A. Ventricles, atrioventricular junction, and great arteries
    B. Ventricles, ventriculoarterial connection, and great arteries
    C. Atria, ventricles, and great arteries
    D. Atria, atrioventricular canal, and ventricles

Refer to video PER-Q52.

52. Describe the expected abdominal visceral situs seen in this video clip.
    A. Situs solitus
    B. Situs inversus
    C. Situs ambiguus
    D. Situs inversus totalis

53. What is the arrow in this image pointing to?

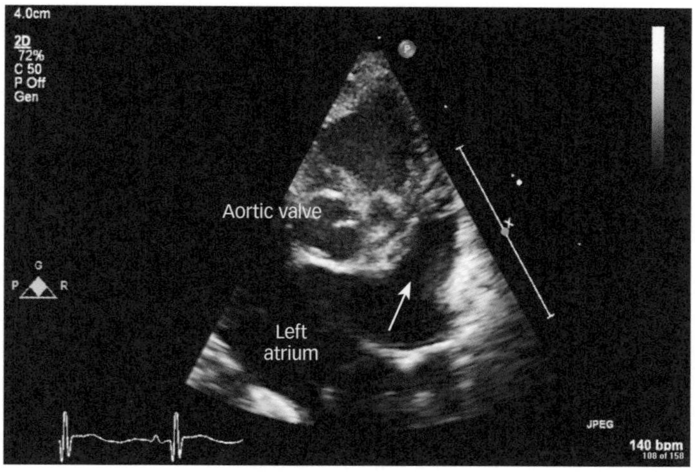

    A. Right upper pulmonary vein
    B. Right atrial appendage
    C. Left atrial appendage
    D. Right lower pulmonary vein

AIT—Hotspot

54. What is the arrow pointing to in this image?

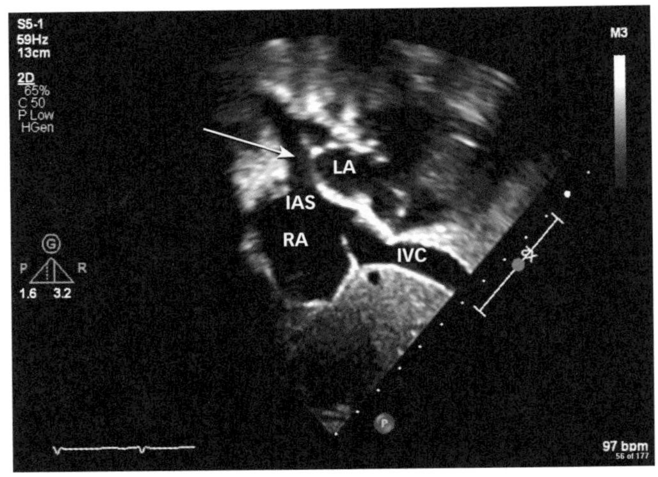

A. Left pulmonary vein

B. Septum secundum

C. Right juxtaposed left atrial appendage

D. Superior vena cava

AIT—Hotspot

Refer to video PER-Q55.

55. What does this video clip demonstrate?

A. Levocardia

B. Mesocardia

C. Dextrocardia

D. Dextroposition of the heart

56. What is the valve of the coronary sinus?

A. Eustachian valve

B. Thebesian valve

C. Crista terminalis

D. Chiari network

57. While scanning a patient in the neonatal intensive care unit, you see a floppy echogenic structure originating from the floor of the morphologic right atrium and stretching from the inferior vena cava valve to the atrial septum. This echogenic structure has multiple fenestrations. What does this structure most likely represent?

A. Eustachian valve

B. Chiari network

C. Umbilical vein catheter

D. Cor triatriatum dextrum

58. This spectral Doppler image is from a 2-week-old infant. What does this image most likely demonstrate?

See Color Plate 3 on page xx.

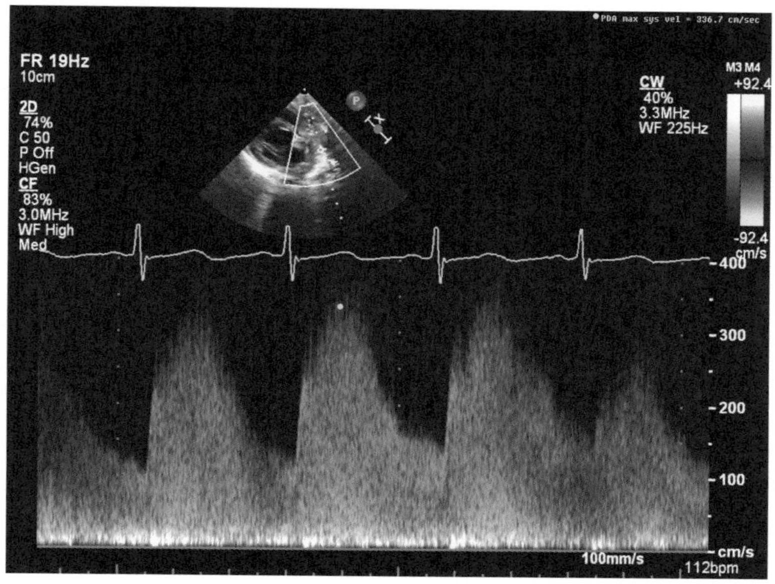

A. Small patent ductus arteriosus

B. Pulmonary vein

C. Superior vena cava

D. Left pulmonary artery

59. This is a spectral Doppler image of a structurally normal heart with no congenital heart disease. What structure is the flow going through, as indicated by the arrow?

See Color Plate 4 on page xxi.

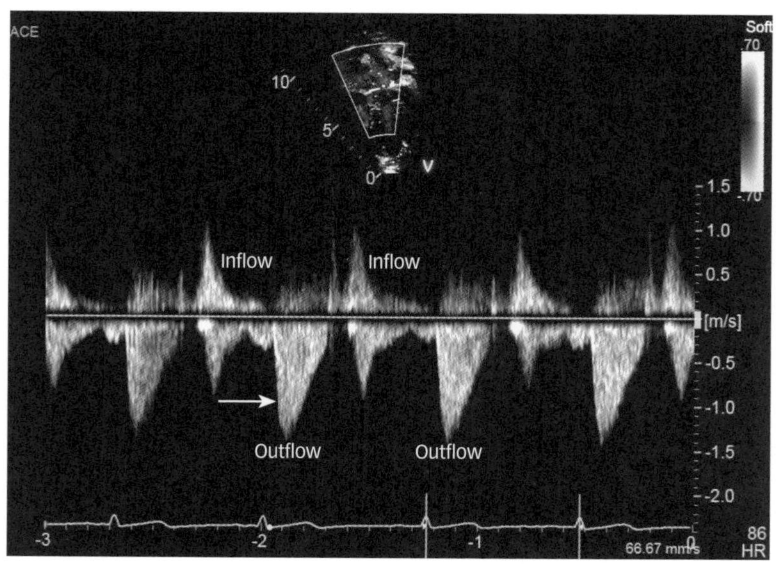

A. Pulmonary valve

B. Tricuspid valve

C. Left pulmonary vein

D. Aortic valve

PART 2

Pathology and Pathophysiology

60. An 11-year-old girl with shortness of breath presents to the emergency department. Echocardiographic M-mode measurements demonstrate a left ventricular (LV) end-diastolic dimension of 55 mm, a Z-score of +5.5, and fractional shortening (FS) of 15%. All other cardiac structures appear normal. Given the findings and this image, what is the most likely diagnosis?

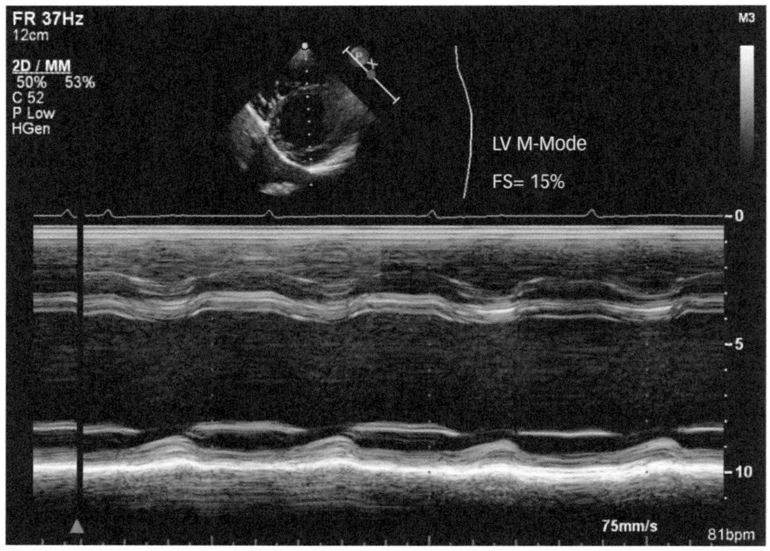

A. Dilated cardiomyopathy
B. Normal heart
C. Hypertrophic cardiomyopathy
D. Pulmonary hypertension

61. Which of the following surgically correctable lesions is the most likely to result in a clinical picture of dilated cardiomyopathy?
A. Right coronary artery to pulmonary artery fistula
B. Juvenile rheumatoid arthritis
C. Anomalous left coronary artery from the pulmonary artery
D. Bacterial myocarditis

62. The most common cause of sudden cardiac death (SCD) in children and young adults is:
A. Ventricular septal defect
B. Bicuspid aortic valve
C. Hypertrophic cardiomyopathy
D. Pericardial effusion

63. What echocardiographic feature helps in the diagnosis of restrictive cardiomyopathy?
    A. Dilated right and left atria
    B. Dilated left ventricle
    C. Respiratory variations in atrioventricular valve inflow
    D. Pericardial effusion

64. This image was obtained from a patient with hypertrophic cardiomyopathy. Which interrogation technique is important to obtain an accurate Doppler flow profile for the left ventricular outflow tract (LVOT)?

See Color Plate 5 on page xxi.

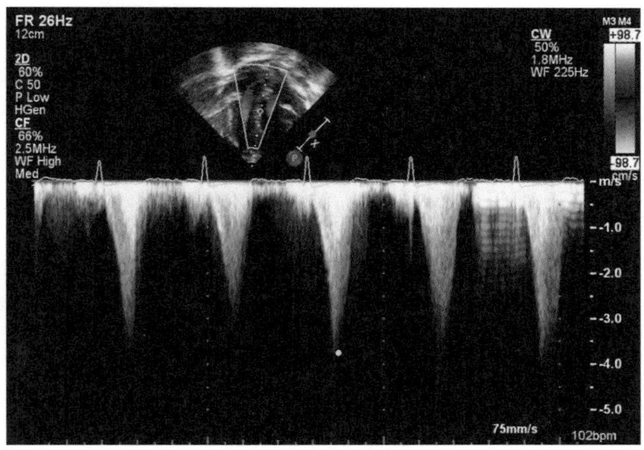

    A. Avoiding mitral valve inflow
    B. Avoiding mitral valve regurgitant flow
    C. Using only pulsed-wave Doppler
    D. Using a parasternal long-axis view to obtain the Doppler flow profile

65. This M-mode image from the parasternal long-axis view demonstrates systolic anterior motion (SAM) of the mitral valve. This echocardiographic feature can be found with what type of cardiac disease?

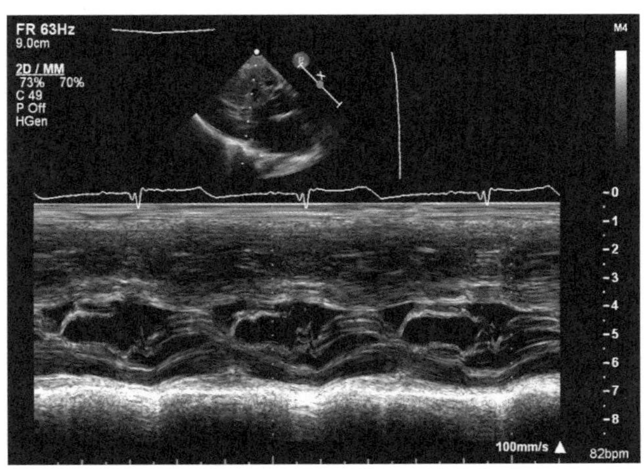

A. Constrictive pericarditis
B. Dilated cardiomyopathy
C. Restrictive cardiomyopathy
D. Hypertrophic cardiomyopathy

66. Which of the following diagnoses is most likely given the findings in this image?

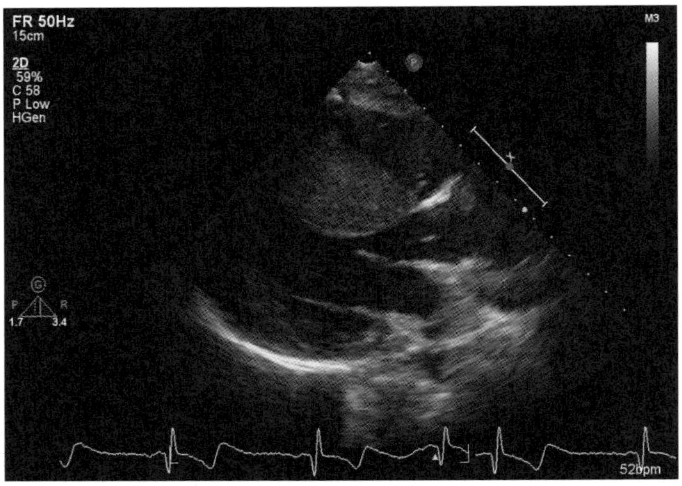

A. Myocarditis
B. Dilated cardiomyopathy
C. Hypertrophic cardiomyopathy
D. Restrictive cardiomyopathy

67. Which of the following is most likely to be present in a 16-year-old patient with restrictive cardiomyopathy?
A. Mitral valve inflow E/A ratio less than 1
B. Mitral valve inflow E-wave deceleration time less than 160 ms
C. E/Ea ratio less than 15
D. Respiratory variation in left ventricular inflow

68. Which of the following is a typical physiologic adaptation seen in sickle cell disease?
A. Increased cardiac output
B. Reduced left ventricular chamber size
C. Decreased stroke volume
D. Decreased heart rate

69. Which of the following diseases is UNLIKELY to be related to secondary hypertrophic cardiomyopathy?
    A. Mitochondrial disease
    B. Noonan syndrome
    C. LEOPARD syndrome
    D. Duchenne muscular dystrophy

70. In restrictive cardiomyopathy, what happens at the end of diastole?
    A. Left ventricular diastolic pressure equals right ventricular diastolic pressure.
    B. Left atrial and left ventricular end-diastolic pressures are normal.
    C. Left atrial end-diastolic pressure is much higher than left ventricular end-diastolic pressure.
    D. Left atrial and left ventricular end-diastolic pressures are both elevated.

71. What is arrhythmogenic right ventricular cardiomyopathy/dysplasia (ARVC/D)?
    A. Parchment heart
    B. Endocardial fibroelastosis
    C. Fatty replacement of the right ventricular myocardium
    D. Metabolic cardiomyopathy

72. A newborn presents at the neonatal intensive care unit with meconium aspiration syndrome. The echocardiogram demonstrates moderate tricuspid valve regurgitation with a peak velocity of 4 m/sec, as well as a flat ventricular septum and decreased right ventricular systolic function. What is the calculated right ventricular pressure?
    A. 64 mmHg
    B. 64 mmHg + right atrial (RA) pressure
    C. 16 mmHg + right atrial (RA) pressure
    D. 16 mmHg

73. A newborn presents with a congenital left diaphragmatic hernia. The ductus arteriosus is closed. Given the findings in images A and B, what is the most likely diagnosis?

A

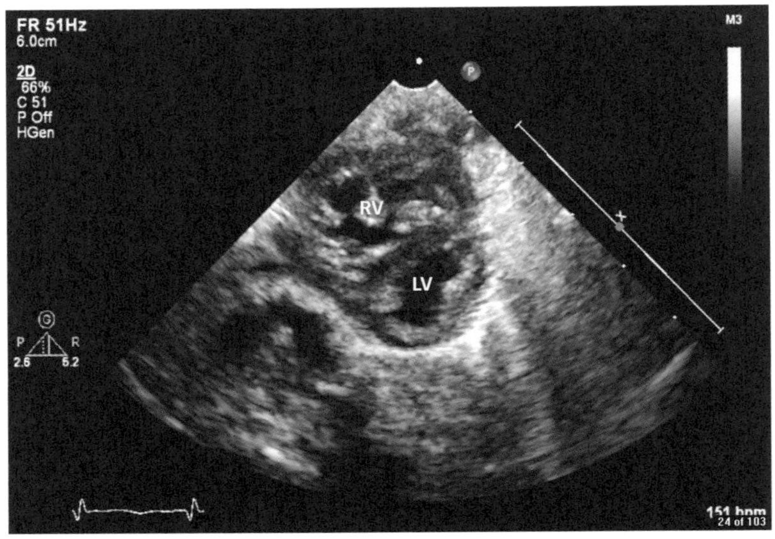

B

See Color Plate 6 on page xxii.

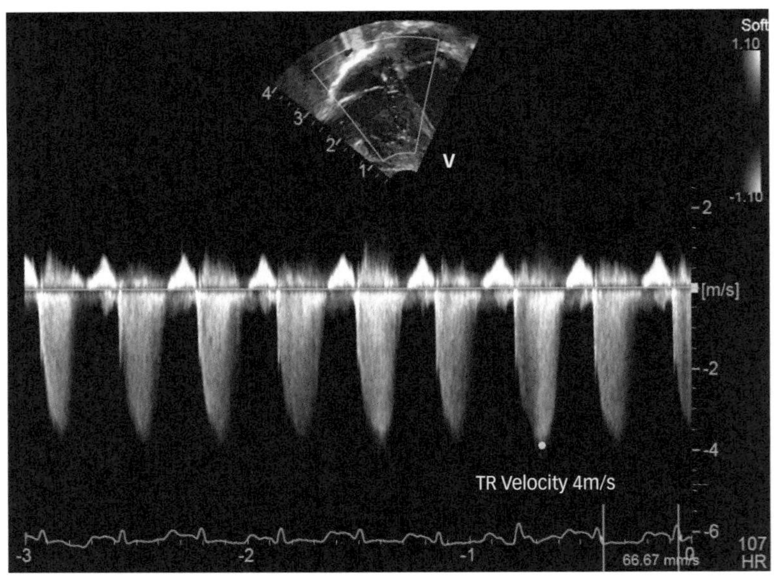

A. Atrial septal defect (ASD)

B. Ventricular septal defect (VSD)

C. Pulmonary hypertension

D. Normal for a newborn

74. Which of these findings suggests pulmonary hypertension?
    A. Mitral valve systolic anterior motion
    B. Aortic valve reopening in late systole
    C. Pulmonary valve motion with an absent A-dip on M-mode
    D. Mitral valve vibration in diastole

75. An infant with a ventricular septal defect (VSD) and no obstruction of the right ventricular outflow tract (RVOT) presents at your echo lab. The infant's blood pressure is 90/60 mmHg. What is the most likely diagnosis based on this history and the findings in this image?

See Color Plate 7 on page xxii.

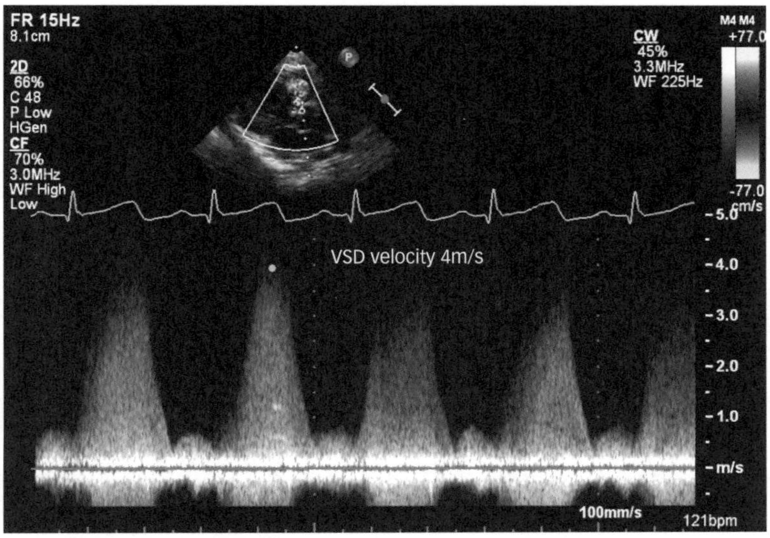

    A. VSD with normal pulmonary artery pressure
    B. VSD with elevated pulmonary artery pressure
    C. VSD with decreased pulmonary artery pressure
    D. VSD with indeterminate pulmonary artery pressure

76. Measurement of which of the following would provide an INDIRECT calculation of pulmonary hypertension by echocardiography?
    A. Tricuspid valve regurgitant jet velocity
    B. Pulmonary valve regurgitant jet velocity
    C. Systemic to pulmonary shunt velocity
    D. Changes in IVC size with respiration

77. Which of the following cardiac defects causes pulmonary arterial hypertension due to unrestricted blood flow into the lungs?
    A. Ventricular septal defect with pulmonary stenosis
    B. Truncus arteriosus
    C. Scimitar syndrome
    D. Mitral valve stenosis

78. The following cardiac defects all produce left-to-right shunting. Which of these defects is most easily missed when pulmonary hypertension is present?
    A. Patent ductus arteriosus
    B. Atrial septal defect
    C. Ventricular septal defect
    D. Aortopulmonary (AP) window

79. A 2-year-old boy is seen in the emergency room with a history of high fever for 10 days. He is noted to have cracked lips and a red, swollen tongue. You obtain an echocardiogram. Based on the findings in this image (arrow) and the clinical findings, what is the most likely diagnosis?

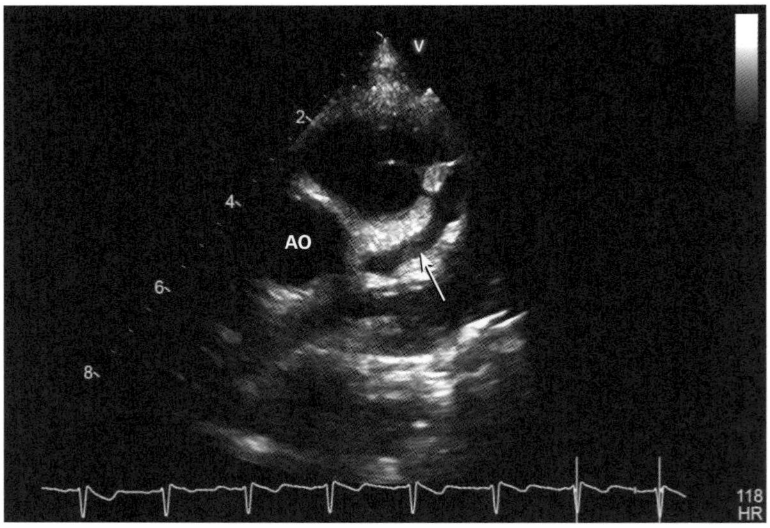

    A. Kawasaki disease
    B. Viral syndrome with fever
    C. Endocarditis
    D. Rheumatic fever

80. Name the coronary artery indicated by the arrow in this image.

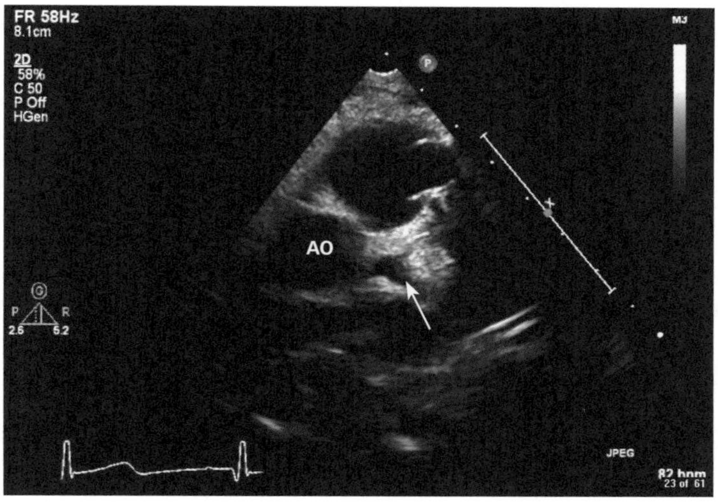

A. Left main coronary artery
B. Left circumflex coronary artery
C. Proximal left anterior descending coronary artery
D. Right coronary artery

AIT—Hotspot

81. Pericardial effusion may lead to cardiac tamponade physiology. Which of the following echocardiographic findings is the best sign of tamponade physiology?
A. Right atrial wall collapse in diastole
B. Large pericardial effusion
C. Respiratory variation of 15% in mitral valve inflow
D. Normal diastolic function

82. Which of the following diagnoses is most likely based on this image?

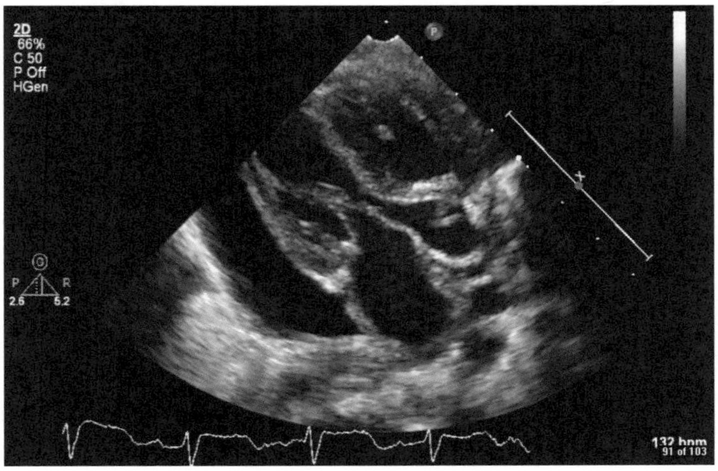

A. Pleural effusion
B. Pericardial effusion
C. Normal heart
D. Ascites

83. Where do early pericardial effusions tend to accumulate?
A. Ventricular apex
B. Right atrium
C. Posterior and inferior wall
D. Right ventricle anterior wall

84. Of the following, which is the most important factor in determining whether a pericardial effusion will cause tamponade physiology?
A. The volume of the effusion
B. The location of the effusion
C. The duration of the effusion
D. The rapidity of the effusion's development

85. When tamponade physiology is present, what happens to mitral valve and tricuspid valve inflow during respiration?
A. During inspiration mitral valve inflow decreases.
B. During inspiration mitral valve inflow increases.
C. During inspiration tricuspid valve inflow decreases.
D. During expiration tricuspid valve inflow increases.

86. What is the first sign of hemodynamic significance with pericardial effusion?
A. Right ventricular free wall collapse in early diastole
B. Right ventricular free wall collapse in early systole
C. Right atrial free wall collapse in late diastole
D. Circumferential effusion

87. Which of the following is the best indication of left ventricular inflow with constrictive pericarditis?
A. E/A ratio less than 1
B. Increased mitral inflow deceleration time
C. Tissue Doppler E/e′ ratio greater than 15
D. Respiratory variation in mitral inflow E-wave velocity greater than 25%

88. Who is at highest risk for infective endocarditis?
    A. Patients undergoing bypass surgery for atrial septal defect repair
    B. Patients with an artificial mitral valve
    C. Patients with a coronary stent
    D. Patients with mild mitral valve prolapse

Refer to video PER-Q89.

89. A patient went to the catheterization laboratory three months ago to have a Melody valve placed in the pulmonary valve position. Today, during a clinic visit, he mentioned that he has been feeling tired for a few weeks. His oral temperature is just over 102° Fahrenheit (39° Celsius). What is the most likely pathology associated with this history and the findings in this video clip from his echocardiogram?
    A. Endocarditis
    B. Thrombus
    C. Tumor
    D. Calcification

90. A young patient is diagnosed with rheumatic fever. What echocardiographic finding would you look for?
    A. Vegetation
    B. Clot
    C. Mitral valve regurgitation
    D. Pulmonary valve stenosis

91. Which of the following is known to cause cardiac toxicity?
    A. Elevated high-density lipoprotein
    B. Brain tumor radiation
    C. Anthracyclines
    D. Dialysis

92. Who is at increased risk for cardiac toxicity?
    A. A patient who received doxorubicin (Adriamycin)
    B. A patient taking atorvastatin (Lipitor)
    C. A patient taking metformin (Glucophage)
    D. A patient taking methimazole (Tapazole)

93. Which echocardiographic finding is considered normal after heart transplantation?
    A. Severe supravalvular pulmonary stenosis
    B. E/A ratio of 16
    C. Echodense ridge at the mid-left atrial level
    D. Increase in mitral valve regurgitation

94. Which of the following parameters is most useful for evaluating early rejection of a transplanted heart?
    A. Measurement of the left ventricular ejection fraction
    B. Measurement of the left ventricular shortening fraction
    C. Measurement of the tricuspid valve regurgitant velocity
    D. Pulsed-wave tissue Doppler evaluation of the lateral mitral annulus

95. Which of the following cardiac defects is the most likely to be found in a patient with Down syndrome?
    A. Double aortic arch
    B. Tricuspid atresia
    C. Transposition of the great arteries
    D. Atrioventricular canal defect

96. Which of the following genetic disorders is most likely associated with the cardiac defect seen in this image?

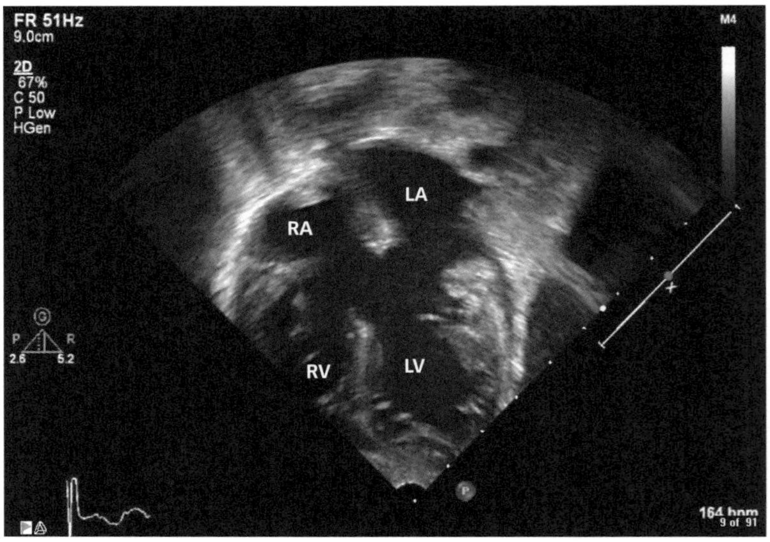

    A. Down syndrome
    B. Noonan syndrome

C. Williams syndrome
D. Shone syndrome

97. Which of the following chromosomal abnormalities is also known as Down syndrome?
A. 22q11 deletion syndrome
B. Trisomy 21
C. Trisomy 18
D. Trisomy 13

98. Which anatomic structure is the arrow in this image pointing to?

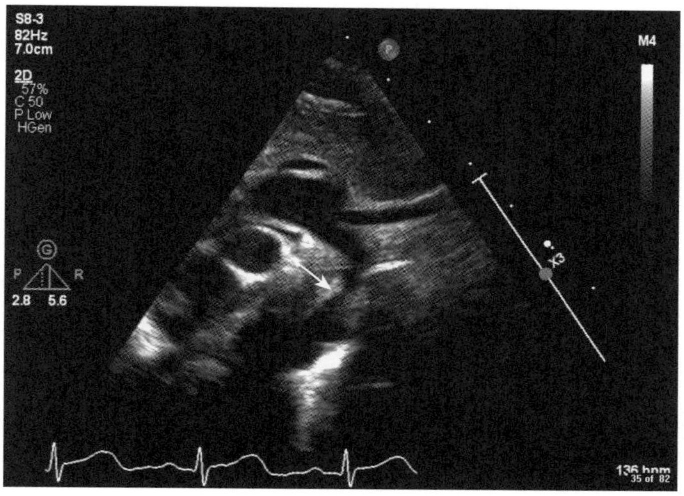

A. Aortic isthmus
B. Left subclavian artery
C. Aberrant left subclavian artery
D. Distal transverse aortic arch

AIT—Hotspot

99. A 5-year-old girl arrives at your echocardiography laboratory. Her mother tells you that she was diagnosed with Turner syndrome. Which of the following cardiac defects is most likely?
A. Primum atrial septal defect
B. Supravalvular aortic stenosis
C. Branch pulmonary artery stenosis
D. Coarctation of the aorta (CoA)

100. DiGeorge syndrome is a chromosomal disorder that results in abnormal development of several organs, including the heart. Which type of cardiac defect is most likely to be found in this condition?
    A. Tetralogy of Fallot
    B. Supramitral valve ring
    C. Pulmonary venous abnormality
    D. Levoatrial cardinal vein

101. A newborn baby is diagnosed with truncus arteriosus by echocardiogram. Which of the following syndromes is associated with this cardiac defect?
    A. Noonan syndrome
    B. DiGeorge syndrome
    C. Ehlers-Danlos syndrome
    D. Holt-Oram syndrome

102. Shone syndrome can be described as a:
    A. Right-sided cardiac lesion
    B. Common arterial trunk defect
    C. Pulmonary venous anomaly
    D. Left-sided cardiac lesion

103. Which of the following chromosomal disorders has the highest incidence of cardiac defects?
    A. Down syndrome
    B. Trisomy 18
    C. Noonan syndrome
    D. Alagille syndrome

104. Which of the following syndromes is associated with this image?

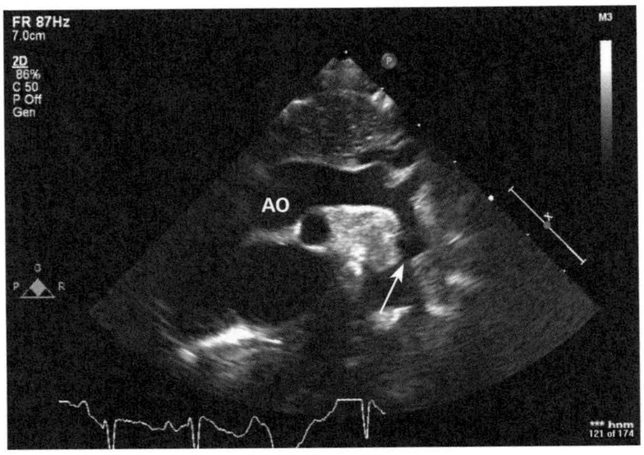

A. Turner syndrome
B. Down syndrome
C. Holt-Oram syndrome
D. Patau syndrome

AIT—Hotspot

105. Which type of interrupted aortic arch (IAA) is most commonly found in DiGeorge syndrome?
   A. IAA type A
   B. IAA type B
   C. IAA type C
   D. IAA types A and C

106. A newborn baby has a chest x-ray consistent with Scimitar syndrome. Which of the following echocardiographic findings do you look for?
   A. Cor triatriatum
   B. Total anomalous pulmonary venous connection
   C. Interrupted inferior vena cava
   D. Partial anomalous pulmonary venous connection

107. Which of the following cardiac defects is often seen with ectopia cordis?
   A. Total anomalous pulmonary venous connection
   B. Tetralogy of Fallot
   C. Atrioventricular canal defect
   D. Ebstein anomaly

108. Which of the following syndromes is associated with partial anomalous pulmonary venous connection?
   A. Turner syndrome
   B. Williams syndrome
   C. Trisomy 21
   D. Alagille syndrome

109. A patient with Marfan syndrome has arrived at the emergency room reporting severe chest pain. Given the history and clinical findings, what abnormality do you expect the echocardiogram will reveal?
   A. Mitral valve regurgitation
   B. Coronary abnormalities

C. Left ventricular wall motion abnormalities

D. Aortic dissection

110. Vascular Ehlers-Danlos syndrome, Loeys-Dietz syndrome, and arterial tortuosity syndrome fall under the category of:

A. Connective tissue disorders

B. Immune system disorders

C. Nervous system disorders

D. Takayasu's syndrome

111. This image most likely represents a long-axis image from a patient with:

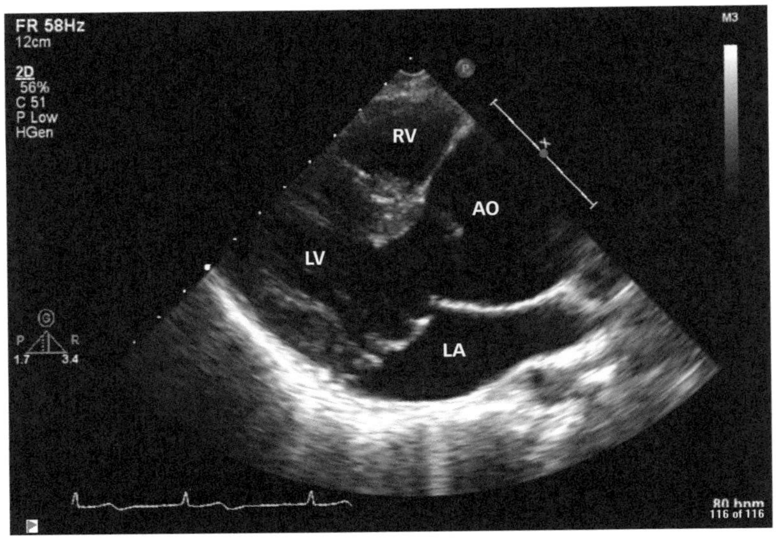

A. Noonan syndrome

B. Marfan syndrome

C. Alagille syndrome

D. Holt-Oram syndrome

112. When a woman with diabetes is pregnant, what is the most likely cardiac abnormality that can affect the newborn baby?

A. Hypertrophic cardiomyopathy

B. Atrial septal defect

C. Patent ductus arteriosus

D. Dilated cardiomyopathy

113. A newborn baby was diagnosed with a cardiac defect by echocardiography, as seen in this apical four-chamber view. This defect may have been caused by maternal exposure during pregnancy to which of the following?

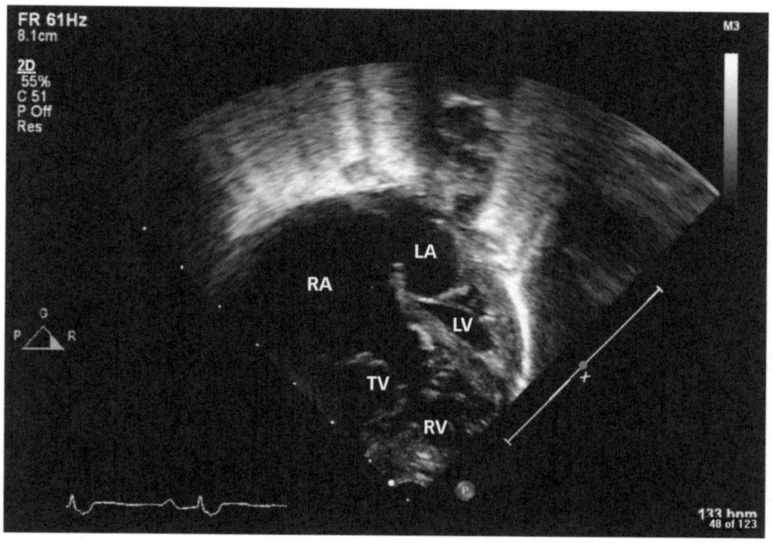

A. Nifedipine
B. Lithium
C. Thalidomide
D. Amphetamine

114. Which of the following is associated with an increased risk of cardiac defects?

A. Gastroschisis
B. Bronchus suis
C. Omphalocele
D. Ogilvie syndrome

115. Which of the following congenital cardiac malformations is most strongly associated with a history of maternal diabetes?

A. Tetralogy of Fallot
B. Sinus venosus atrial septal defects
C. Total anomalous pulmonary venous connection
D. Aortopulmonary window

116. A pregnant woman had a rubella infection during the first trimester of her pregnancy. Which of the following cardiac defects might be found in the child after birth?

A. Coarctation of the aorta

B. Pulmonary valve stenosis

C. Double-outlet right ventricle

D. Tricuspid atresia

117. A 10-year-old boy has high blood pressure noted during a visit to his pediatrician. The physician requests an echocardiogram to determine if a cardiac defect is causing systemic hypertension. What defect should you look for?

A. Hypertrophic cardiomyopathy

B. Mitral valve stenosis

C. Coarctation of the aorta

D. Pulmonary valve stenosis

118. A young adult patient diagnosed with systemic hypertension was referred to cardiology for evaluation. The nurse takes upper and lower extremity blood pressures, obtaining a right arm reading of 145/85 mmHg and a left leg reading of 95/75 mmHg. Which of the following is the most likely diagnosis for this patient?

A. Aortopulmonary window

B. Hypertrophic cardiomyopathy

C. Aortic valve stenosis

D. Coarctation of the aorta

119. What is a typical finding with untreated systemic hypertension?

A. Dilated left ventricle

B. Concentric left ventricular hypertrophy

C. Asymmetric septal hypertrophy

D. Normal diastolic function

120. Which of the following patients are at highest risk for development of systemic venous thrombosis?

A. Patients after a Fontan procedure

B. Patients with a ventricular septal defect

C. Patients with coarctation of the aorta

D. Patients post tetralogy of Fallot repair

121. While skiing, a teenager collided with a large tree and sustained blunt trauma to the chest. He is now in the emergency room and you have been asked to provide an echocardiogram. Which cardiac structure is of greatest concern?

A. Left ventricle

B. Right ventricle

C. Left atrium

D. Right atrium

122. A young patient received chemotherapy for a few months using a central venous line located in the right chest. Recently, the mother has noted that his face appears swollen. What do you evaluate for in an echocardiogram?

A. Vegetation

B. Thrombosis

C. Ventricular function

D. Mass at the inferior vena cava/right atrial junction

Refer to video PER-Q123.

123. Which of the following diagnoses best characterizes the structure (mass) indicated by the arrow in this video clip?

A. Tumor

B. Vegetation in atrium

C. Thrombus

D. Myxoma

AIT—Hotspot

124. Which of the following is commonly associated with asplenia syndrome?

A. Midline liver

B. Intact inferior vena cava

C. Total anomalous pulmonary venous connection

D. All of the above

125. Which of the following is associated with polysplenia syndrome?

A. Interrupted inferior vena cava

B. Dextrocardia

C. Partial anomalous pulmonary venous connection

D. All of the above

See Color Plate 8 on page xxiii.

126. Which of the following is the most likely diagnosis based on the findings in this image?

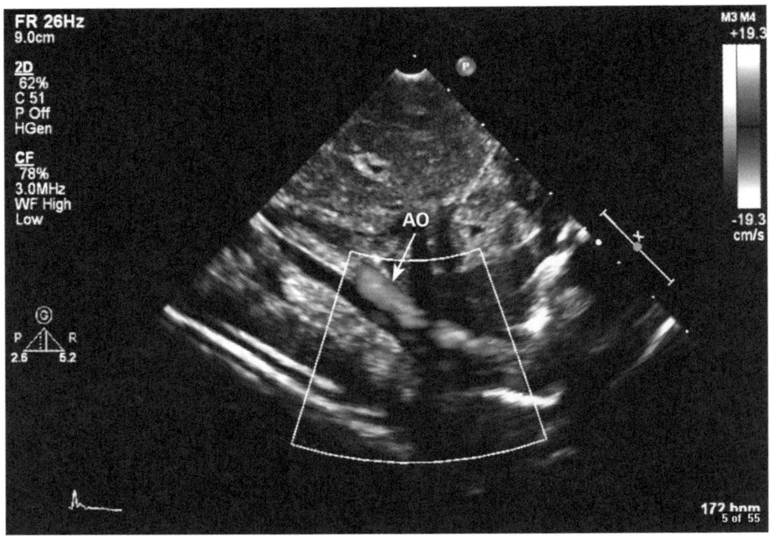

A. Polysplenia

B. Asplenia

C. Intact inferior vena cava

D. Normally related vessels

127. A newborn baby is diagnosed by echocardiography with complex congenital cardiac defects including dextrocardia, double-outlet right ventricle (DORV), unbalanced complete atrioventricular canal (right dominant, with a small left ventricular chamber), common atrium, unroofed coronary sinus, infradiaphragmatic total anomalous pulmonary venous connection (TAPVC), and pulmonary atresia. The liver is noted to be midline. Which of the following is the most likely diagnosis?

A. Loeys-Dietz syndrome

B. Complete atrioventricular block

C. Polysplenia syndrome (left atrial isomerism)

D. Asplenia syndrome (right atrial isomerism)

PART 3

Congenital Anomalies

128. Which of the following correctly describes a type A interrupted left aortic arch?
   A. Interruption between the left common carotid and left subclavian arteries
   B. Interruption between the right and left common carotid arteries
   C. Interruption after the left subclavian artery
   D. Often associated with aberrant origin of the right subclavian artery

129. Which type of interrupted aortic arch (IAA) is the most common?
   A. Type A
   B. Type B
   C. Type C
   D. Type D

130. Which of the following is the correct name of the artery in right arch number 4, as marked in this schematic?

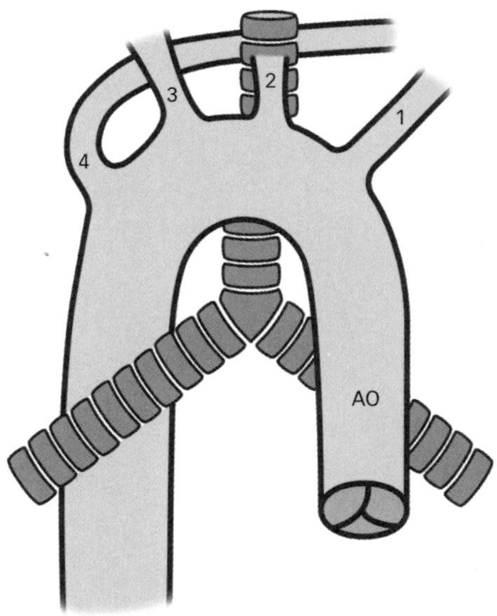

Descending aorta

   A. Aberrant left subclavian artery
   B. Aberrant right subclavian artery
   C. Left carotid artery
   D. Right innominate artery

AIT—Hotspot

131. Which cardiac anomaly is illustrated in this schematic?

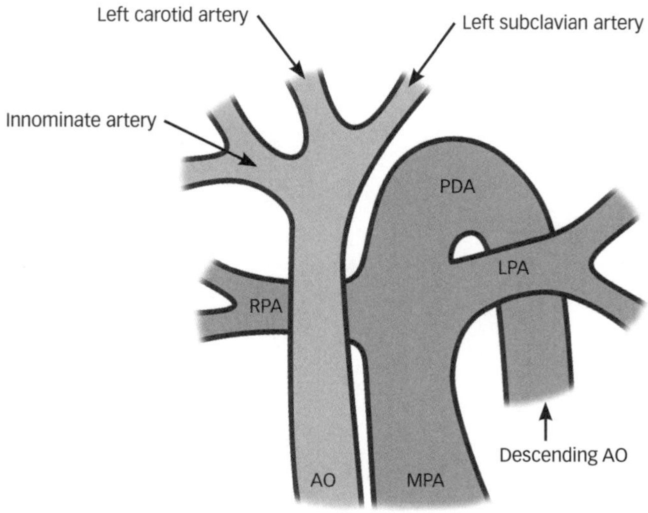

A. Type A interrupted aortic arch (IAA)
B. Type B IAA
C. Type C IAA
D. Double aortic arch

132. Which cardiac anomaly is illustrated in this schematic?

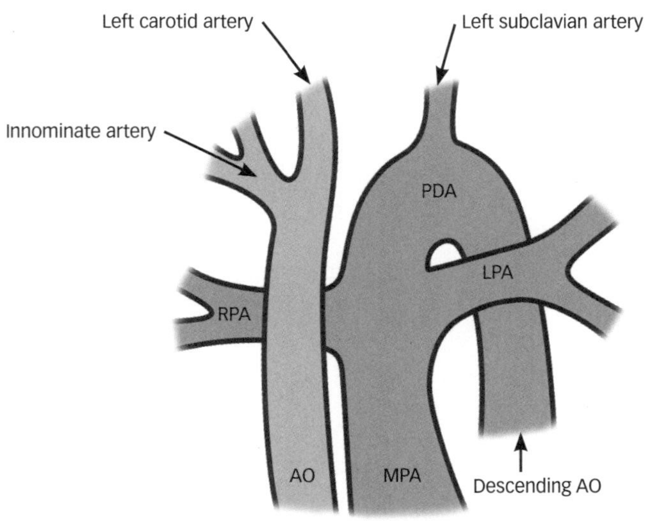

A. Type A interrupted aortic arch (IAA)
B. Type B IAA
C. Type C IAA
D. Coarctation of the aorta

133. Which of the following diagnoses is most consistent with the echocardiographic image seen here?

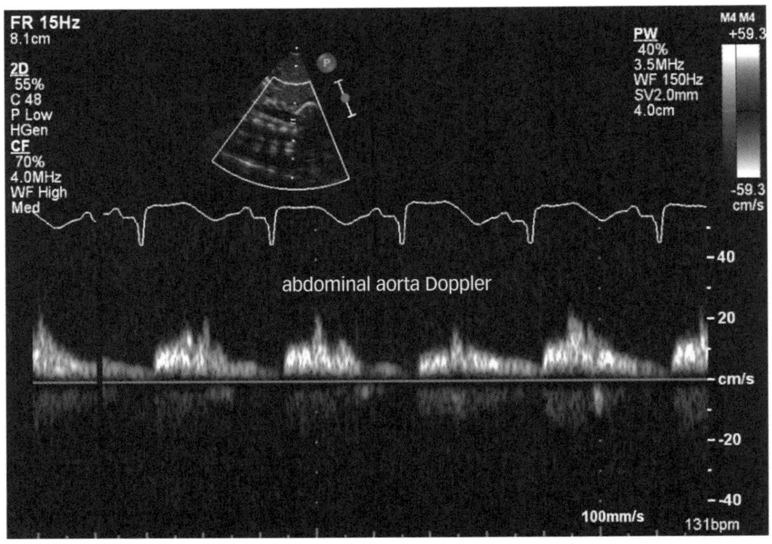

A. Normal flow pattern
B. Coarctation of the aorta (CoA)
C. Large aortopulmonary (AP) collateral
D. Patent ductus arteriosus (PDA)

134. You are examining a patient with severe coarctation of the aorta, pulmonary hypertension, and a patent ductus arteriosus (PDA). Which of these statements best describes the flow pattern through the PDA?
A. PDA flow shunts right to left in systole and left to right in diastole.
B. PDA flow shunts right to left in diastole and left to right in systole.
C. PDA flow shunts left to right in systole only.
D. PDA flow shunts left to right in both systole and diastole.

135. Which anatomic arrangement of the aortic arch produces a vascular ring?
A. Right aortic arch with a retroesophageal left subclavian artery and a left ductal ligament
B. Right aortic arch with mirror-image branching
C. Left aortic arch with an aberrant right subclavian artery
D. Left aortic arch with normal branching and a left ductal ligament

136. Which statement correctly applies to a double aortic arch?
   A. The embryonic right sixth arch persists.
   B. The left aortic arch is generally larger.
   C. The double arch forms the descending aorta close to the diaphragm.
   D. The double aortic arch is a type of vascular ring.

137. An infant with stridor that resembles high-pitched wheezing is in your echocardiography laboratory. Which of the following cardiac defects is most likely to present with this symptom?
   A. Pulmonary valve stenosis
   B. Right aortic arch with mirror-image branching
   C. Abnormal origin of the left pulmonary artery from the right pulmonary artery
   D. Large patent ductus arteriosus

Refer to video PER-Q138.

138. This video clip most likely demonstrates which of the following conditions?
   A. Normal branch of the pulmonary artery
   B. Pulmonary artery sling
   C. Left pulmonary artery stenosis
   D. Patent ductus arteriosus

139. Which of the following aortic arch anatomies can be seen with NO vascular ring?
   A. Right arch with left descending aorta and left ductus arteriosus
   B. Right arch with mirror-image branching and a ductus arteriosus arising anteriorly from the left innominate artery
   C. Right arch with retroesophageal diverticulum of Kommerell and left ductus arteriosus
   D. Double aortic arch

140. A patient has a known anomaly of the left aortic arch. A physical examination reveals that the right-side carotid pulse is stronger than the left-side carotid pulse. Which of the following is the most likely to be found by echocardiography?

A. Double aortic arch
B. Coarctation of the aorta
C. Type B interrupted aortic arch with a closing ductus arteriosus
D. Type C interrupted aortic arch with a closing ductus arteriosus

141. Which of the following aortic arch anomalies will likely need surgical treatment for a vascular ring?
A. Common brachiocephalic trunk
B. Left aortic arch with aberrant right subclavian artery
C. Left aortic arch with right descending aorta and right ductus arteriosus
D. Right arch with mirror-image branching

142. Which of the following anatomic variants of the aortic arch is most commonly encountered?
A. Right aortic arch with anomalous left subclavian artery
B. Left aortic arch with anomalous right subclavian artery
C. Double aortic arch
D. Persistent fifth aortic arch

143. What cardiac anomaly is most likely to be found in patients with coarctation of the aorta?
A. Atrial septal defect
B. Ventricular septal defect
C. Mitral valve stenosis
D. Bicuspid aortic valve

144. In a patient with typical tetralogy of Fallot, which of the following correctly describes the associated ventricular septal defect (VSD)?
A. The conal septum is deviated anteriorly, creating the VSD.
B. The conal septum is deviated posteriorly, creating the VSD.
C. The defect is an inlet VSD.
D. The defect is a subpulmonary VSD.

145. Which of the following would typically be found by echocardiography in a six-month-old patient with tetralogy of Fallot?
    A. Right ventricular dilatation
    B. Patent ductus arteriosus that is required for pulmonary blood flow
    C. Mitral valve to aortic valve fibrous continuity
    D. Ventricular septal defect that produces left-to-right shunting only

146. In what percentage of patients with tetralogy of Fallot are the coronary artery patterns normal?
    A. 88%
    B. 60%
    C. 50%
    D. 25%

147. What is the most common abnormal coronary artery pattern seen with tetralogy of Fallot?
    A. Single left coronary artery
    B. Single right coronary artery
    C. Dual left anterior descending coronary artery
    D. Large conal branch arising from the right coronary artery

148. In a 3-month-old baby with tetralogy of Fallot (TOF), which of the following cardiac defects will most likely be found in addition to the standard features of TOF?
    A. Atrial septal defect
    B. Right aortic arch
    C. Coarctation of the aorta
    D. Abnormal coronary artery

149. Which of the following echocardiographic features will NOT be present in tetralogy of Fallot with an absent pulmonary valve?
    A. Overriding aorta
    B. Aneurysmal pulmonary arteries
    C. Mild right ventricular outflow tract obstruction
    D. Large patent ductus arteriosus

150. These images are from a patient with trisomy 21 (Down syndrome). What is the most likely diagnosis given the findings seen here?

A

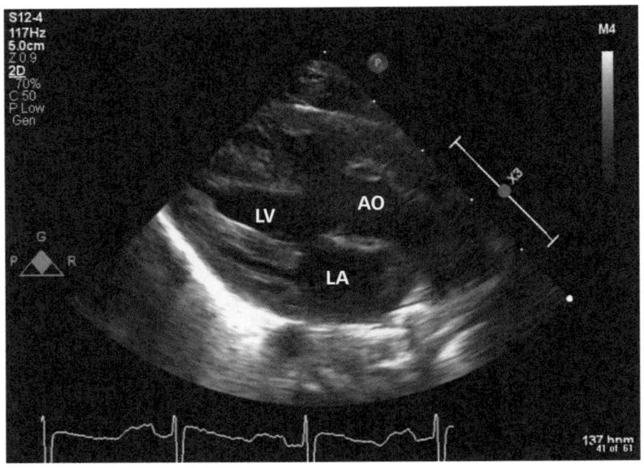

B

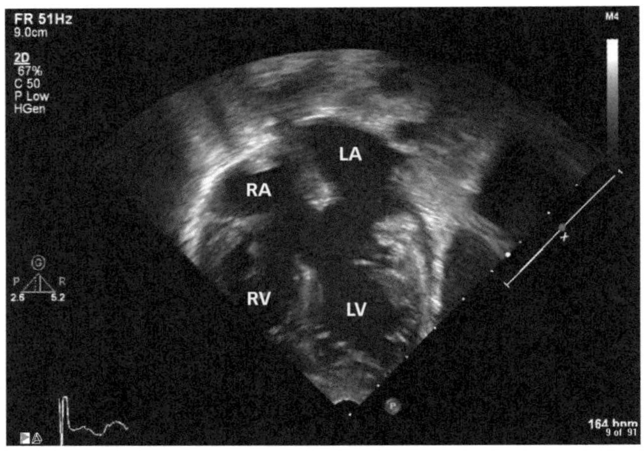

A. Tetralogy of Fallot with pulmonary valve stenosis
B. Tetralogy of Fallot with a common atrioventricular canal defect
C. Transposition of the great arteries
D. More images are required to establish the diagnosis.

151. In a Down syndrome patient, echocardiography demonstrates tetralogy of Fallot (TOF) with a common atrioventricular canal defect (CAVC). Which of the following anatomic variations of a complete common atrioventricular canal defect is the LEAST common?

A. Rastelli type A
B. Rastelli type B

C. Rastelli type C
D. Superior bridging leaflet divided at the level of the ventricular septum

152. What is the most common morphology of the truncal valve in truncus arteriosus?
A. Tricuspid valve
B. Quadricuspid valve
C. Bicuspid valve
D. Unicuspid valve

153. There are two classification schemes for truncus arteriosus (TA): Collett and Edwards' system and Van Praagh's system. While these schemes differ in certain aspects, both use a specific cardiac anatomic feature to segregate truncus arteriosus defects into specific subtypes. What is this anatomic feature?
A. Aortic arch sidedness
B. Number of truncal valve cusps
C. Presence or absence of a ventricular septal defect
D. Origin of the pulmonary arteries

154. In truncus arteriosus, which configuration of the pulmonary arteries is most commonly found?
A. Posterior-left common trunk with a short main pulmonary artery
B. Posterior-left common trunk with separated pulmonary artery origins
C. One pulmonary artery arising from the ascending aorta and the other pulmonary artery arising from the aortic arch
D. Both pulmonary arteries supplied by collaterals

155. What differentiates tetralogy of Fallot with pulmonary atresia from truncus arteriosus?
A. Only one great artery
B. Overriding aorta
C. Pulmonary arteries arising from the arterial trunk
D. Patent ductus arteriosus

156. Using the Van Praagh classification, which type of truncus arteriosus is demonstrated in this image?

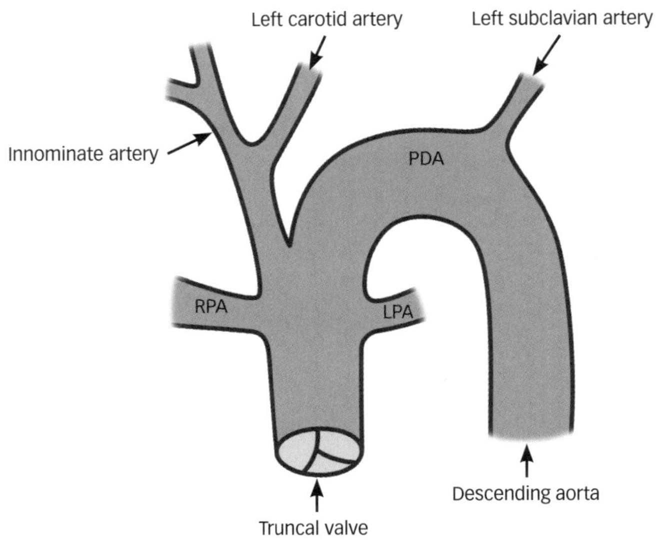

A. Type A1
B. Type A2
C. Type A3
D. Type A4

157. When double-outlet right ventricle (DORV) has an associated ventricular septal defect (VSD), which type of VSD is most common?

A. Subpulmonary VSD
B. Doubly committed VSD
C. Subaortic VSD
D. Noncommitted VSD

158. A newborn baby was diagnosed by echocardiogram with double-outlet right ventricle (DORV). Which of the following great artery relationships is the most likely in DORV?

A. Aorta to the right of the pulmonary artery
B. Aorta directly anterior to the pulmonary artery
C. Aorta leftward and posterior to the pulmonary artery
D. Aorta leftward and anterior to the pulmonary artery

159. Which of the following cardiac defects is associated with leftward juxtaposition of the right atrial appendage?

A. Atrioventricular canal defect
B. Tetralogy of Fallot
C. Hypoplastic left heart syndrome
D. Double-outlet right ventricle

160. What type of ventricular septal defect (VSD) and other associations occur with the Taussig-Bing form of double-outlet right ventricle (DORV)?

A. Subaortic VSD and pulmonary outflow tract obstruction

B. Subpulmonary VSD, side-by-side great arteries, an unobstructed pulmonary outflow tract, and possible subaortic obstruction

C. Subaortic VSD, normally related great arteries, and no outflow tract obstruction to either great artery

D. Doubly committed VSD, aorta anterior and to the right of the pulmonary artery, and no outflow tract obstruction to either great artery

161. In which type of double-outlet right ventricle (DORV) can a patient have an interrupted aortic arch?

A. When the conal septum is deviated toward the subpulmonary outflow tract

B. When the conal septum is deviated toward the subaortic outflow tract

C. With absent subpulmonary conus

D. With absent bilateral conus

162. Your patient was diagnosed with double-outlet right ventricle (DORV). With which of these anatomic variants are you most likely to encounter a straddling mitral valve?

A. DORV with normally related great arteries

B. DORV with a subpulmonary ventricular septal defect (VSD)

C. DORV with a subaortic VSD

D. DORV with no VSD

163. Which of the following is a correct statement about straddling mitral valve (SMV)?

A. SMV is the same as an overriding mitral valve.

B. SMV is abnormal mitral valve chordae attaching to both the right and left ventricles.

C. SMV is straddling chordae attaching to the aortic valve.

D. SMV exists in the absence of a ventricular septal defect.

164. During echocardiography on an infant with congestive heart failure, the examiner's initial impression is that the left ventricle is mildly dilated with normal systolic function and without shunting lesions. However, there is diastolic reversal of flow in the descending aorta that catches the cardiologist's attention, and the cardiologist asks for a rescan of the patient. Which of the following cardiac lesions is causing the cardiologist's concern?
    A. Atrial septal defect
    B. Anomalous left coronary artery from the pulmonary artery
    C. Aortopulmonary window
    D. Transposition of the great arteries

165. Which of the following statements about bicuspid aortic valve is true?
    A. It is more common in males.
    B. It is more common in females.
    C. There is no difference in incidence between males and females.
    D. It is the least common congenital cardiac defect.

Refer to video PER-Q166.

166. Based on the findings in this video clip, what do you also need to evaluate by echocardiography?
    A. Size of ascending aorta
    B. Aortic valve annulus
    C. Right atrium
    D. Left anterior descending artery

167. Which aortic valve cusp would be located closest to a membranous (perimembranous) ventricular septal defect (VSD)?
    A. Left coronary cusp
    B. Right coronary cusp
    C. Noncoronary cusp
    D. All cusps are remote from a membranous VSD.

168. In a patient with a small, restrictive membranous ventricular septal defect (VSD), the color flow Doppler demonstrates left-to-right shunting across the VSD

with a velocity of 4.5 m/sec. The cardiologist requests a follow-up clinic visit with an echocardiogram in 6 months. Of the following choices, what concerns you most besides the VSD?

A. Congestive heart failure

B. Pulmonary hypertension

C. Aortic valve prolapse and regurgitation

D. Endocarditis

169. A newborn baby was diagnosed with critical aortic valve stenosis. Besides evaluating the aortic valve morphology and obtaining the gradient across the aortic valve, what other measurement should you perform that could influence the cardiologist's decision to treat with surgery versus transcatheter therapy?

A. Tricuspid valve annulus size

B. Patent ductus arteriosus size

C. Mitral valve annulus size

D. Main pulmonary artery diameter

170. With rupture of a sinus of Valsalva aneurysm, which heart chamber most commonly receives the left-to-right shunt through the aneurysm?

A. Left ventricle

B. Right ventricle

C. Left atrium

D. Right atrium

171. In the parasternal short-axis view at the level of the great vessels, you see a left-to-right shunt at the 9/10 o'clock position. The right coronary sinus appears mildly dilated. What would help you distinguish a ventricular septal defect (VSD) from a right coronary sinus of Valsalva aneurysm rupture?

A. Visualization of aortic valve prolapse

B. Interrogation with spectral Doppler

C. Visualization of left ventricular dilatation

D. Visualization of a left-to-right shunt into the right ventricle

172. Which of the following cardiac defects is similar in physiology to an aortico–left ventricular tunnel (ALVT)?
   A. Severe mitral valve stenosis
   B. Ventricular septal defect
   C. Severe aortic valve regurgitation
   D. Severe aortic valve stenosis

173. Which of the following cardiac defects is most likely given the findings in this image?

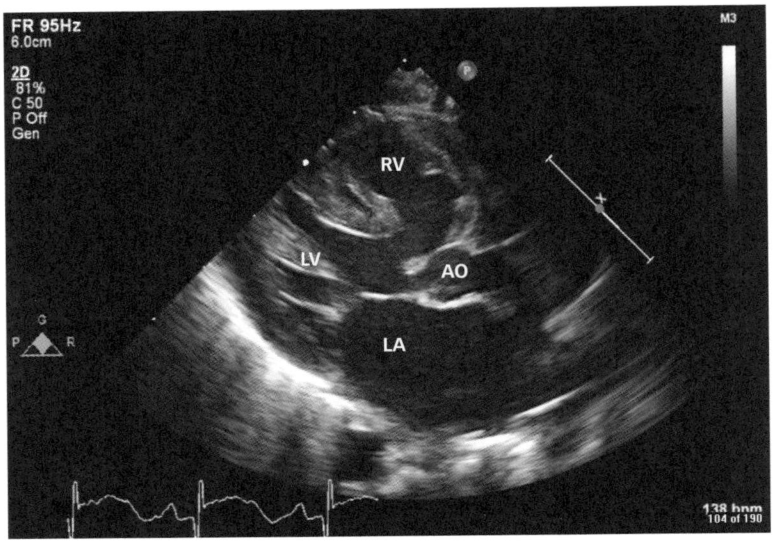

   A. Atrial septal defect
   B. Aortopulmonary window
   C. Muscular ventricular septal defect
   D. Interrupted aortic arch

Refer to video PER-Q174.

174. This patient underwent surgical repair for the lesion that is demonstrated in this video clip. What is the most likely echocardiographic follow-up after surgery?
   A. This is a complete repair; there is no need to perform echocardiographic follow-up.
   B. Echocardiography is required to check for aortic valve stenosis.
   C. Echocardiography is required to determine whether the original lesion has recurred.
   D. Echocardiography is required to check for mitral valve regurgitation.

175. Which type of fibrous continuity is found in 90% of cases of transposition of the great arteries (d-TGA)?
   A. Mitral valve and pulmonary valve fibrous continuity
   B. Mitral valve and tricuspid valve fibrous continuity
   C. Tricuspid valve and aortic valve fibrous continuity
   D. Mitral valve and aortic valve fibrous continuity

176. Which of the following cardiac defects is the most likely to coexist with transposition of the great arteries (d-TGA)?
   A. Coarctation of the aorta
   B. Vascular ring
   C. Total anomalous pulmonary venous connection
   D. Ventricular septal defect

177. What is the <u>second</u> most common coronary artery pattern in transposition of the great arteries (d-TGA)?
   A. Left circumflex from right coronary
   B. Single right coronary
   C. Single left coronary
   D. Intramural left coronary

Refer to video PER-Q178.

178. This video clip was obtained using a parasternal long-axis view. What cardiac defect do you see?
   A. Tetralogy of Fallot
   B. Transposition of the great arteries
   C. Truncus arteriosus
   D. Double-outlet right ventricle

Refer to video PER-Q179.

179. A newborn is diagnosed with the congenital cardiac defect that is demonstrated in this video clip. The patient's oxygen saturation is in the low 60s. What is the most likely reason for the lower oxygen saturation?
   A. Pulmonary valve stenosis
   B. Ventricular septal defect
   C. Restrictive atrial septal defect
   D. Patent ductus arteriosus

180. Which of the following is most likely found in physiologically "corrected" (congenitally corrected) transposition of the great arteries (ccTGA)?

A. Atrial situs solitus

B. Atrial situs inversus

C. Atrial situs ambiguus

D. Atrial ventricular concordance

181. Of the following cardiac defects, which is most often seen in association with physiologically "corrected" (congenitally corrected) transposition of the great arteries (ccTGA)?

A. Partial anomalous pulmonary venous connection

B. Coarctation of the aorta

C. Ventricular septal defect

D. Patent ductus arteriosus

182. Which of the following cardiac defects is most likely to cause pulmonary outflow tract obstruction in physiologically "corrected" (congenitally corrected) transposition of the great arteries (ccTGA)?

A. Double-chambered right ventricle

B. Pulmonary valve stenosis

C. Branch pulmonary artery stenosis

D. Subpulmonary valve stenosis

183. You are scanning a newborn baby with atrial situs inversus and find that the aorta is anterior to and rightward of the pulmonary artery. You use Van Praagh's segmental set notation to describe the anatomy as {I, ____, D}. What should the middle letter be if this patient has a physiologically "corrected" circulation that is a mirror image of congenitally corrected transposition of great arteries {S, L, L}?

A. L

B. D

C. I

D. A

184. An infant was diagnosed with physiologically "corrected" transposition of the great arteries without pulmonary outflow tract obstruction. Echocardiography reveals mild tricuspid valve regurgitation with a velocity of 4.0 m/sec and mild mitral valve regurgitation with a velocity of 3.0 m/sec. What is the pulmonary artery systolic pressure?

A. 64 mmHg + right atrial pressure

B. 16 mmHg + right atrial pressure

C. 18 mmHg + right atrial pressure

D. 36 mmHg + right atrial pressure

185. A 15-year-old boy has a history of congenitally corrected transposition of the great arteries, a very small ventricular septal defect (VSD), and no previous cardiac surgery. He now presents to the emergency room with a loud heart murmur and congestive heart failure. Given this patient's history and symptoms, which of these cardiac malformations is most likely causing his congestive heart failure?

A. Reduced left ventricular function

B. Reduced right ventricular function

C. Mitral valve regurgitation

D. Pulmonary outflow tract obstruction

186. Which of the following ECG findings will most likely be seen in a patient with congenitally corrected transposition of the great arteries?

A. Complete heart block

B. Sinus tachycardia

C. Premature ventricular beats

D. Supraventricular tachycardia

187. Which of the following imaging views would you choose to evaluate the superior vena cava (SVC) pathway obstruction after a Mustard procedure?

A. Apical four-chamber view

B. Parasternal short-axis view

C. Apical five-chamber view

D. Suprasternal notch view

188. If you were the cardiac surgeon, which procedure could you perform to convert a congenitally corrected transposition of the great arteries into an anatomic correction?
   A. Mustard procedure
   B. Arterial switch operation
   C. Senning repair
   D. Double switch procedure

189. Which of these imaging windows is the best to evaluate the atrial septum?
   A. Parasternal short-axis view
   B. Apical four-chamber view
   C. Subxiphoid long-axis view
   D. High right parasternal view

Refer to video PER-Q190.

190. Which type of shunt is demonstrated in this video clip?
   A. Left-to-right shunt
   B. Right-to-left shunt
   C. Bidirectional shunt
   D. The type of shunt cannot be identified based on this video clip.

191. Which imaging window is the best to diagnose a sinus venosus atrial septal defect?
   A. Apical four-chamber view
   B. Parasternal short-axis view
   C. Subxiphoid coronal (long-axis) view
   D. Subxiphoid sagittal (short-axis) view

Refer to video PER-Q192.

192. Which of the following cardiac anomalies will be associated with the defect seen in this video clip?
   A. Pulmonary stenosis
   B. Partial anomalous pulmonary venous connection
   C. Ventricular septal defect
   D. Cleft mitral valve

193. Which of the following cardiac anomalies is most frequently associated with the cardiac defect seen in this image?

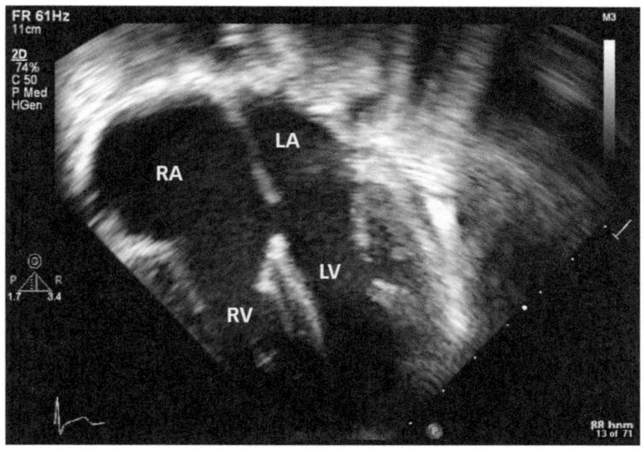

A. Cleft mitral valve

B. Ventricular septal defect

C. Transposition of the great arteries

D. Interrupted aortic arch

194. You are examining a toddler with a moderate-sized secundum atrial septal defect (ASD). Color Doppler demonstrates a left-to-right shunt across the ASD. Which cardiac structure will you see dilated first?

A. Left atrium

B. Left ventricle

C. Right ventricle

D. Coronary sinus

195. In which of the following cardiac defects is device closure currently contraindicated?

A. Secundum atrial septal defect (ASD)

B. Sinus venosus ASD

C. Patent foramen ovale

D. Perimembranous ventricular septal defect

196. Which of the following would you expect to see in a 5-year-old boy with an atrial septal defect?

A. Dilated right atrium and right ventricle due to volume overload

B. Dilated right atrium and right ventricle due to increased pulmonary artery pressure

C. Ventricular septum manifesting paradoxical movement due to pulmonary hypertension

D. Right-to-left shunt

197. You are imaging from the parasternal short-axis view at the mid-left ventricle level. Color flow Doppler demonstrates a ventricular septal defect (VSD) at the 9 o'clock position. Which of the following VSD locations is correct?

A. Posterior muscular VSD

B. Mid-muscular VSD

C. Anterior muscular VSD

D. Apical muscular VSD

Refer to video PER-Q198.

198. Which of the following diagnoses is most likely given the findings in this video clip?

A. Posterior muscular ventricular septal defect (VSD)

B. Mid-muscular VSD

C. Anterior muscular VSD

D. Apical muscular VSD

Refer to video PER-Q199.

199. Which of the following diagnoses is most likely given the findings in this video clip?

A. Perimembranous ventricular septal defect (VSD)

B. Inlet VSD

C. Muscular VSD

D. Supracristal VSD

200. Which type of ventricular septal defect (VSD) is associated with a mitral valve cleft?

A. Perimembranous VSD

B. Atrioventricular canal type VSD

C. Outlet VSD

D. Supracristal VSD

Refer to video PER-Q201.

201. Which of the following ventricular septal defects (VSDs) is most likely given the findings in this video clip?

A. Inlet VSD

B. Malalignment VSD

C. Supracristal VSD

D. Apical muscular VSD

202. Which type of ventricular septal defect (VSD) might produce prolapse of the right coronary cusp of the aortic valve?

A. Doubly committed VSD

B. Intramural VSD

C. Inlet VSD

D. Anterior muscular VSD

203. Which of the following cardiac findings is caused by a subpulmonary ventricular septal defect (VSD)?

A. Pulmonary valve stenosis

B. Aortic valve regurgitation

C. Mitral valve prolapse

D. Mitral valve stenosis

204. A teenage boy comes to the cardiology clinic because of a heart murmur. Echocardiography demonstrates a small perimembranous ventricular septal defect (VSD) with left-to-right shunting and a peak velocity of 2.5 m/sec. The patient's systemic blood pressure is 110/70 mmHg and his chest x-ray appears normal. What cardiac malformation is most commonly associated with the clinical and echocardiographic findings for this patient?

A. Pulmonary valve stenosis

B. Double-chambered right ventricle

C. Supravalvular aortic stenosis

D. Mitral valve stenosis

205. A sinus venosus atrial septal defect (ASD) is often associated with anomalous pulmonary venous return. Which of the following pulmonary veins is typically involved in such cases?

A. Right lower pulmonary vein

B. Right middle pulmonary vein

C. Right upper pulmonary vein

D. Right side pulmonary veins

206. An echocardiogram demonstrates a complete atrioventricular canal defect (AVCD), with the anterior-superior bridging leaflet partially divided and inserting into a papillary muscle in the right ventricle. What type of AVCD would this be?

A. Rastelli A

B. Rastelli B

C. Rastelli C

D. Rastelli D

207. Which of the following diagnoses is most likely, given the findings in this image?

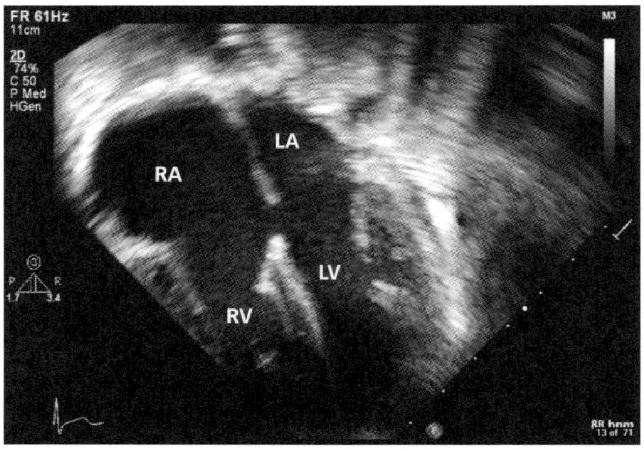

A. Complete atrioventricular canal defect (AVCD)

B. Transitional AVCD

C. Partial AVCD

D. Dilated coronary sinus

208. How many atrioventricular valve leaflets are there in a Rastelli type C complete atrioventricular canal defect?

A. 2

B. 3

C. 4

D. 5

209. How would you describe the typical left ventricular papillary muscle anatomy in a complete atrioventricular canal defect?

A. Normal

B. Rotated counterclockwise

C. Rotated clockwise

D. Having only one papillary muscle

210. An 18-year-old male had an atrioventricular canal defect repair when he was 6 months old. Besides left AV valve regurgitation, which of the following complications is most likely to be progressive and might need another operation in the future?

A. Small residual atrial septal defect
B. Small residual ventricular septal defect
C. Aortic valve stenosis
D. Left ventricular outflow tract obstruction

211. While performing a high parasternal short-axis scan you visualize a venous structure posterior to the left pulmonary artery and draining superiorly to the innominate (brachiocephalic) vein. What is this structure?

A. Vertical vein
B. Axillary vein
C. Azygos vein
D. Phrenic vein

212. The most common type of total anomalous pulmonary venous connection (TAPVC) is:

A. Infradiaphragmatic
B. Cardiac
C. Supracardiac
D. Mixed

213. Which of the following conditions is most likely to appear on echocardiography as a larger than usual amount of blood flow returning from the superior vena cava to the right atrium?

A. Supracardiac total anomalous pulmonary venous connection
B. Large atrial septal defect
C. Tetralogy of Fallot
D. Truncus arteriosus

Refer to video PER-Q214.

214. While performing the sweep seen in this video clip, you visualize an extra vascular structure between the inferior vena cava and the abdominal aorta. This vascular structure most likely represents:

A. Higher gastric vein
B. Azygos vein

C. Vertical vein

D. Hemiazygos vein

Refer to video PER-Q215.

215. While scanning in an apical four-chamber view, you note significant leftward malalignment of the atrial septum. This video clip is representative of this scenario. Which of the following forms of congenital heart disease does the video demonstrate?

A. Supramitral ring

B. Intracardiac total anomalous pulmonary venous drainage

C. Cor triatriatum sinister

D. Mitral valve arcade

216. Total anomalous pulmonary venous connection (TAPVC) is best explained by which embryologic mechanism listed below?

A. Secondary heart field migration abnormality

B. Failure of the common pulmonary vein–left atrial connection

C. Primary heart field abnormality

D. Persistence of the right anterior cardinal vein

217. Which form of total anomalous pulmonary venous connection (TAPVC) is seen in this image?

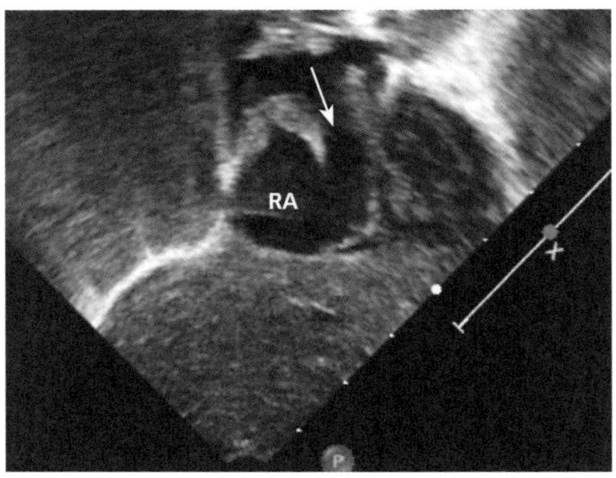

A. Infradiaphragmatic TAPVC

B. Supracardiac TAPVC

C. Mixed TAPVC

D. Intracardiac TAPVC

Refer to video PER-Q218.

218. Which anomaly does this video clip best demonstrate?
    A. Interruption of the inferior vena cava with hemiazygos continuation
    B. Vascular sling
    C. Supracardiac total anomalous pulmonary venous connection
    D. Interruption of the inferior vena cava with azygos continuation

219. While performing a subcostal short-axis scan, you find a dilated right superior vena cava (SVC) with increased flow and left-to-right atrial-level shunting. What is the most likely reason for the dilatation of the SVC?
    A. Partial anomalous pulmonary venous connection
    B. Left SVC shunting to the left atrium
    C. Left SVC shunting to the coronary sinus
    D. Total anomalous pulmonary venous connection

220. What statement is most likely to be true of a vertical vein coursing between the left pulmonary artery and left mainstem bronchus in total anomalous pulmonary venous connection?
    A. The vein is not obstructed.
    B. The vein is obstructed.
    C. The vertical vein is not clinically significant.
    D. Vertical veins do not course between the left pulmonary artery and left mainstream bronchus.

221. Which of the following is NOT usually seen with a partial anomalous pulmonary venous connection?
    A. Intact atrial septum
    B. Atrial septal defect
    C. Left ventricular enlargement
    D. Right ventricular enlargement

222. You are scanning a newborn in the neonatal intensive care unit, and your echocardiographic findings are heart dextroposition, no atrial-level shunting, right pulmonary veins to the inferior vena cava, and a small right pulmonary artery. What best explains the dextroposition of the heart?
   A. Increase in left lung volume to accommodate for oxygenation
   B. Left ventricular enlargement
   C. Right-to-left atrial-level shunting
   D. Right lung hypoplasia

223. Which of the following best describes the flow pattern in this spectral Doppler image of a pulmonary vein?

See Color Plate 9 on page xxiii.

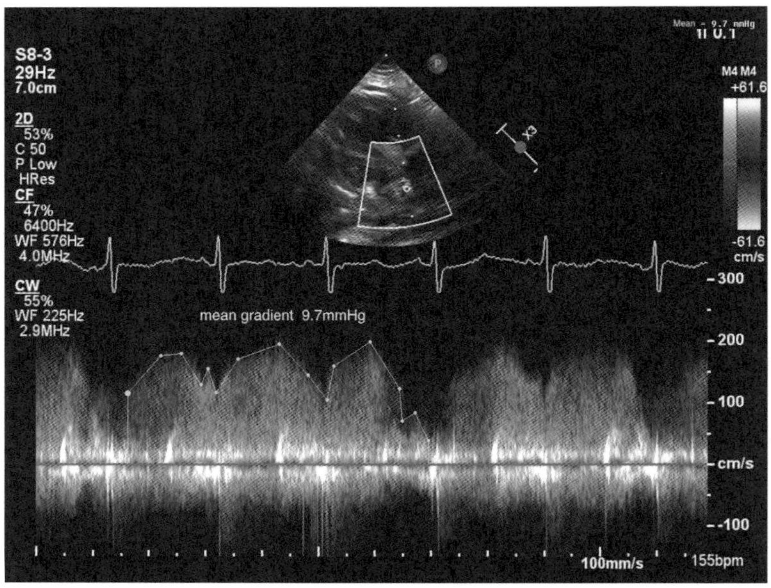

   A. Prominent A-wave reversal
   B. Phasic laminar flow
   C. Normal mean gradient
   D. Diminished phasic flow

224. Which of the following options is LEAST likely to be associated with pulmonary vein stenosis?
   A. Biatrial enlargement
   B. Dilated right ventricle
   C. Right atrial enlargement
   D. Dilated main pulmonary artery

225. Name the anatomic structure the arrow is pointing to in this image:

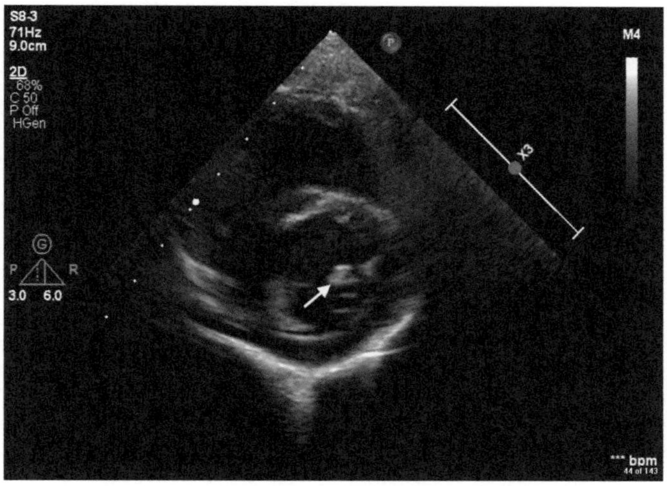

A. Left ventricular posteromedial papillary muscle

B. Left ventricular inferior wall

C. Left ventricular anterolateral papillary muscle

D. Small left ventricular diverticulum

AIT—Hotspot

226. While scanning a newborn in the neonatal intensive care unit, you perform your subcostal short-axis sweep and find the chordae tendineae returning to only one group of papillary muscles in the left ventricle. Offline analysis provides a mitral annulus Z-score of −3.0. This most likely represents:

A. Ebstein anomaly

B. Increased likelihood of a double orifice mitral valve

C. Parachute mitral valve

D. Straddling mitral valve

227. While looking at a parasternal short-axis view of the left ventricle, you find two papillary muscles that are at the 5 and 6 o'clock positions. What other morphologic feature are you most likely to find in this ventricle?

A. Chordae tendineae tethering

B. Infundibulum

C. Increased interchordal spacing

D. Chordal attachments of the atrioventricular valve to the interventricular septum

228. A myxomatous mitral valve is best described as a:
    A. Normal mitral valve
    B. Mitral valve with redundant leaflets and a thickened appearance
    C. Mitral valve with normal histologic findings
    D. Nonexistent mitral valve disease

229. A cleft mitral valve is:
    A. Synonymous with Ebstein anomaly
    B. Generally not seen with an ostium primum atrial septal defect
    C. Always incompetent
    D. A possible finding with no other cardiac defects

230. Cor triatriatum is best characterized as:
    A. A ridge of tissue subdividing the left atrium that is located below the left atrial appendage
    B. A ridge of tissue subdividing the left atrium that is located above the left atrial appendage
    C. A ridge of tissue that is often associated with pulmonary vein atresia
    D. A ridge of tissue that is always associated with mitral valve regurgitation

231. Which choice below best describes the setting in which you would see a straddling mitral valve?
    A. Ventricular septal defect
    B. Patent foramen ovale
    C. Atrial septal defect
    D. Transposition of the great arteries (d-TGA) with intact ventricular septum

232. You are scanning a 1-week-old patient. The echocardiographic findings include a unicuspid pulmonary valve with a small annulus, a flattened interventricular septum during systole, mild pulmonary regurgitation, a moderate-sized patent ductus arteriosus (PDA), and a peak pulmonary valve velocity of 1.8 m/sec. Which best explains why the velocity through the pulmonary valve is 1.8 m/sec?

A. Normal pulmonary vascular resistance
B. Muscular VSD
C. Increased pulmonary vascular resistance and a PDA
D. Atrial septal defect

Refer to video PER-Q233.

233. This video clip corresponds to normally related great arteries. Which type of ventricular septal defect (VSD) is most commonly associated with the pulmonary stenosis seen in this clip?
A. Posteriorly malaligned VSD
B. Anteriorly malaligned VSD
C. Mid-muscular VSD
D. Apical VSD

234. While performing presurgical echocardiography on a patient who was diagnosed with moderate pulmonary stenosis, you find that the peak pulmonary valve gradient is 15 mmHg. The pulmonary valve appears dysplastic with a pulmonary annulus Z-score of −3.3. Which factor below best explains the low peak pulmonary gradient?
A. Right ventricular hypertrophy
B. Right ventricular dilatation
C. Mitral valve regurgitation
D. Depressed right ventricular systolic function

Refer to video PER-Q235.

235. What type of pulmonary valve (PV) is seen in this video clip?
A. Dome-shaped PV
B. Bicuspid PV
C. Normal PV
D. Trileaflet PV

236. Diastolic flow reversal in the branch pulmonary arteries is most likely associated with:
A. Mild pulmonary valve insufficiency
B. Moderate pulmonary valve stenosis
C. Severe pulmonary valve insufficiency
D. Nothing related to pulmonary valve pathology

Refer to video PER-Q237.

237. Identify the most likely form of congenital heart disease seen in this video clip:
    A. Doming pulmonary valve
    B. Tetralogy of Fallot with pulmonary atresia
    C. Pulmonary atresia with intact ventricular septum
    D. Tetralogy of Fallot with absent pulmonary valve syndrome

238. Which of the following is normally NOT associated with subpulmonary valve stenosis?
    A. Anteriorly malaligned ventricular septal defect (VSD)
    B. Double-chambered right ventricle
    C. Absorption of the subaortic conus
    D. Perimembranous VSD

239. Which of these views is best for evaluating double-chambered right ventricle with spectral Doppler, color Doppler flow imaging, and 2D imaging?
    A. Parasternal long-axis with leftward angulation toward the pulmonary valve
    B. Apical four-chamber with superior and anterior angulation toward the pulmonary valve
    C. Parasternal short-axis at the papillary muscle level
    D. Subcostal short-axis with angulation toward the right ventricular outflow tract/pulmonary valve

240. In double-chambered right ventricle, where is the subdivision of the right ventricle?
    A. Between the sinus and inflow segments of the right ventricle
    B. Between the left ventricular sinus and the right ventricular sinus
    C. Between the sinus and infundibulum segments of the right ventricle
    D. Between the proximal and distal portions of the conal septum

241. The higher-pressure chamber in double-chambered right ventricle is considered to be the:
    A. Right ventricular sinus
    B. Infundibulum

C. Conus arteriosus
D. Main pulmonary artery

242. The most common form of ventricular septal defect (VSD) associated with double-chambered right ventricle is:
A. Inlet VSD
B. Mid-muscular VSD
C. Perimembranous VSD
D. Anterior malalignment VSD

243. While reviewing a patient's chart before performing echocardiography, you learn that the patient tested positive for Alagille syndrome. What is the most likely form of congenital heart disease that you will encounter?
A. Interrupted aortic arch type B
B. Supravalvular pulmonary stenosis
C. Rhabdomyoma
D. Atrioventricular septal defect

244. In which population will you find physiologic peripheral pulmonary branch stenosis?
A. Infants
B. Teenagers
C. Young adults
D. Middle-aged adults

245. In the setting of tetralogy of Fallot (TOF) with absent pulmonary valve syndrome, what anomaly of the pulmonary branch arteries are you most likely to find?
A. Absent right pulmonary artery
B. Aneurysmal branch pulmonary arteries
C. Right pulmonary artery from the ascending aorta
D. Discontinuous branch pulmonary arteries with bilateral ductus arteriosus

246. In which of these genetic syndromes are you most likely to see pulmonary valve stenosis?
A. Holt-Oram syndrome
B. Trisomy 21
C. Turner syndrome
D. Noonan syndrome

247. Right ventricle–dependent coronary circulation (RVDCC) in pulmonary atresia with intact ventricular septum (PA/IVS) is best explained by which of the following?
   A. Coronary dilatation
   B. Coronary artery obstruction
   C. Anomalous left coronary artery from the pulmonary artery
   D. Anomalous right coronary artery from the pulmonary artery

Refer to video PER-Q248.

248. What does this video clip demonstrate?
   A. Anomalous left coronary artery from the pulmonary artery
   B. Kawasaki disease
   C. Coronary-cameral fistula
   D. Coronary artery obstruction

249. What is the most common location of the terminal end of a coronary-cameral fistula?
   A. Right ventricle
   B. Coronary sinus
   C. Left ventricle
   D. Left atrium

250. Which of the following is most likely to be associated with a coronary-cameral fistula?
   A. Atrioventricular septal defect
   B. Tetralogy of Fallot with pulmonary stenosis
   C. Common atrioventricular canal
   D. Pulmonary atresia with intact ventricular septum

251. In the setting of pulmonary atresia with intact ventricular septum (PA/IVS), the right ventricular outflow tract can be opened to establish antegrade flow through the right ventricle into the pulmonary artery, potentially encouraging right ventricular growth. This can be achieved by surgery (pulmonary valvotomy) or heart catheterization (pulmonary valve perforation and dilatation). This is also known as right ventricular decompression, because right

ventricular pressure falls dramatically after the outflow tract is opened. Which of the following is a contraindication to decompressing the right ventricle?

A. Pulmonary annulus Z-score of −1.2

B. Right ventricle–dependent coronary circulation

C. Severe tricuspid regurgitation

D. Moderate tricuspid regurgitation

252. Which pulmonary valve morphology is most commonly found in tetralogy of Fallot?

A. Trileaflet

B. Unicuspid

C. Bicuspid

D. Absent

253. You are in the intensive care unit scanning a patient with pulmonary atresia with intact ventricular septum (PA/IVS). In order to obtain offline measurements, you obtain clear images of the pulmonary valve annulus, main pulmonary artery, pulmonary artery branches, and tricuspid valve. Which of these dimensions correlates best with right ventricular size?

A. Pulmonary valve annulus diameter

B. Main pulmonary artery diameter

C. Tricuspid valve annulus diameter

D. Branch pulmonary artery diameters

254. Which of these options best describes the atrial-level shunting pattern seen in a newborn with pulmonary atresia with intact ventricular septum (PA/IVS)?

A. Restrictive left-to-right shunting

B. Right-to-left atrial-level shunting

C. Left-to-right atrial-level shunting

D. No shunting, with an intact atrial septum

255. While on call, you are asked to perform repeat echocardiography on a neonate that earlier had an echocardiogram showing a thickened pulmonary valve with limited motion. The resident advises you that the patient previously was receiving an intravenous

infusion of prostaglandin (PGE1), but it was turned off based on the prior echocardiographic report. Systemic arterial oxygen saturations (which were in the 90s) have now dropped to the low 60s. When you perform the echocardiogram, which of these tasks should you complete first?

A. Acquire good apical views to estimate the left ventricular ejection fraction.
B. Acquire a ductal view to visualize the patency of the ductus arteriosus.
C. Measure tricuspid regurgitation to estimate right ventricular systolic pressure.
D. Evaluate atrial-level shunting.

256. While scanning a 1-week-old patient in the emergency department, you visualize tricuspid atresia with transposition of the great arteries (d-TGA). What atrial-level shunting pattern would you most likely see?

A. Bidirectional atrial-level shunting
B. A morphologic left atrial to morphologic right atrial shunt
C. A morphologic right atrial to morphologic left atrial shunt
D. No atrial level shunting by color flow Doppler

257. While scanning a patient in the intensive care unit, you discover that the patient has tricuspid atresia with d-malposed great arteries and normal visceroatrial situs. What atrial appendage abnormality is most likely associated with this type of tricuspid atresia?

A. Bilateral left atrial appendages
B. Right-sided juxtaposition of the atrial appendages
C. Bilateral right atrial appendages
D. Left-sided juxtaposition of the atrial appendages

Refer to video PER-Q258.

258. Which situs of the abdominal viscera does this video clip demonstrate?

A. Abdominal visceral situs inversus
B. Abdominal visceral situs solitus
C. Abdominal visceral situs ambiguus
D. Left-sided stomach

Refer to video PER-Q259.

259. Given the findings in this video clip, what form of congenital heart disease is most likely present?
    A. Unbalanced common atrioventricular canal
    B. Muscular tricuspid atresia
    C. Hypoplastic left heart syndrome
    D. Pulmonary atresia with intact ventricular septum

260. You are asked to perform echocardiography on a patient with tricuspid atresia and transposition of the great arteries (d-TGA). The cardiology fellow notifies you that the reason for the echocardiogram is that the chest and abdominal x-ray as well as the physical examination demonstrated hepatomegaly. Which option best describes what you might find on the echocardiogram?
    A. Restrictive ventricular septal defect
    B. Restrictive atrial-level shunting
    C. Large patent ductus arteriosus
    D. Common atrium

261. Which of the following options is seen in up to 25% of patients with tetralogy of Fallot (TOF)?
    A. Persistence of the fifth aortic arch
    B. Left aortic arch with aberrant right subclavian artery
    C. Double aortic arch
    D. Right aortic arch

262. While scanning a patient with tetralogy of Fallot (TOF), you find that the left pulmonary artery is completely supplied by a left-sided patent ductus arteriosus arising from the base of the left innominate (brachiocephalic) artery, and the right pulmonary artery has its usual origin from the pulmonary trunk. Which of these options below best fits this scenario?
    A. Prostaglandin E1 (PGE1) is contraindicated.
    B. This is TOF with absent pulmonary valve.
    C. The pulmonary arteries are discontinuous.
    D. The pulmonary arteries are confluent.

Refer to video PER-Q263.

263. What is the most likely condition demonstrated in this video clip?
   A. Large patent ductus arteriosus
   B. Pulmonary artery sling
   C. Hemitruncus
   D. Aortopulmonary window

Refer to video PER-Q264.

264. What view was used to obtain this video clip?
   A. Suprasternal notch of the pulmonary veins, "crab view"
   B. High right parasternal view of the inferior vena cava, atrial septum, and superior vena cava
   C. Parasternal long-axis view of the right ventricular inflow tract
   D. High left parasternal, ductal view

265. This spectral Doppler image of a patent ductus arteriosus (PDA) is most likely to be seen in which of these settings?

See Color Plate 10 on page xxiv.

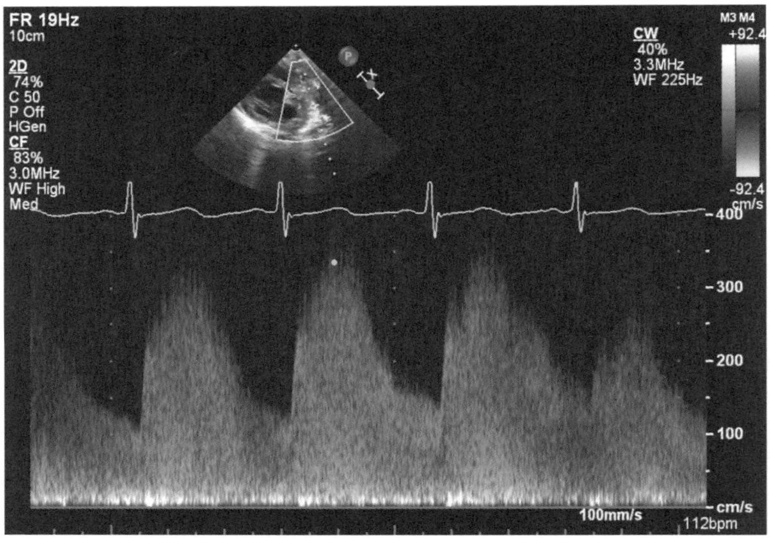

   A. Pulmonary hypertension
   B. Normal pulmonary vascular resistance (PVR)
   C. Left-to-right shunt with high velocity, indicating a large PDA
   D. Interrupted aortic arch type B

Refer to video PER-Q266.

266. Which of these choices best describes what is seen in this video clip?
   A. Mesocardia
   B. Dextrocardia

C. Dextroposition
D. Levocardia

Refer to video PER-Q267.

267. The findings seen in this video clip suggest which of these congenital heart defects?
A. Aortopulmonary window
B. Anomalous left coronary artery from the pulmonary artery
C. Coronary artery ectasia
D. Coronary artery ostial atresia

268. What causes myocardial ischemia in anomalous left coronary artery from the pulmonary artery?
A. Deoxygenated blood from the pulmonary artery
B. Coronary artery steal
C. High pulmonary vascular resistance
D. Severe mitral regurgitation

Refer to video PER-Q269.

269. This video clip is a parasternal short-axis view and most likely demonstrates which of these conditions?
A. Coronary fistula
B. Anomalous right coronary artery from the pulmonary artery
C. Intramural right coronary artery
D. Normal coronary flow

270. Which of the following best describes an intramural course of the left main coronary artery (LMCA)?
A. The LMCA courses between the two great vessels, partially within the walls of the aorta.
B. The LMCA courses through the infundibulum and emerges to the left of the aorta.
C. The LMCA courses between the aorta and the pulmonary artery.
D. It is a normal path of the LMCA.

271. Aortopulmonary collateral vessels (APCs) are most likely to originate from which of the following?
A. Descending aorta
B. Azygos vein
C. Left pulmonary artery
D. Hemiazygos vein

272. Which of these congenital heart conditions is most likely to be associated with aortopulmonary collateral vessels?
   A. Severe aortic coarctation
   B. Tetralogy of Fallot with pulmonary atresia
   C. Van Praagh type A1 truncus arteriosus
   D. Hypoplastic left heart syndrome with mitral atresia and aortic atresia

273. Which of these options is most useful in identifying aortopulmonary collaterals arising from the abdominal aorta?
   A. 2D imaging
   B. Color flow Doppler
   C. M-mode imaging
   D. Speckle tracking echocardiography

274. Supravalvular aortic stenosis is most often associated with which of the following?
   A. Down syndrome
   B. Holt-Oram syndrome
   C. Williams-Beuren syndrome
   D. Char syndrome

275. Supravalvular aortic stenosis usually occurs in which of these aortic segments?
   A. Proximal transverse aortic arch
   B. Sinotubular junction
   C. Distal transverse aortic arch
   D. Ascending aorta

276. The most common coronary artery abnormality associated with supravalvular aortic stenosis is:
   A. Anomalous left coronary artery from the pulmonary artery
   B. Anomalous right coronary artery from the pulmonary artery
   C. Coronary-cameral fistula
   D. Coronary ostial stenosis

277. Which letter in this image is positioned at the sinotubular junction?

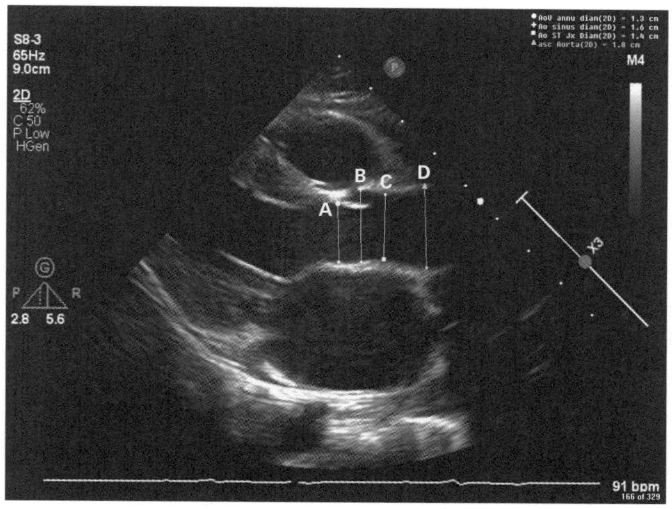

A. A

B. B

C. C

D. D

AIT—Hotspot

278. The superior vena cava is a remnant of which embryologic system?

A. Right anterior cardinal vein

B. Left anterior cardinal vein

C. Vitelline system

D. Splanchnic system

279. Which statement is most often true of the morphologic right atrium?

A. It receives the superior vena cava.

B. It receives the inferior vena cava.

C. It is connected to a tricuspid valve.

D. It contains the limbus of the fossa ovalis.

280. An interrupted inferior vena cava is usually associated with which of the following?

A. Dilated azygos vein

B. Dilated innominate vein

C. Left-sided superior vena cava

D. Anomalous pulmonary venous drainage

281. A 1-month-old infant is noted to have multiple echogenicities in the left ventricular myocardium and the interventricular septum. These appear smaller when he returns for a follow-up exam in 6 months. These echogenicities most likely represent:

A. Fibromas

B. Rhabdomyomas

C. Teratomas

D. Myxomas

282. Rhabdomyomas are commonly associated with which condition?

A. Tuberous sclerosis

B. Down syndrome

C. Turner syndrome

D. DiGeorge syndrome

Refer to video PER-Q283.

283. This video clip demonstrates a mass that is most likely a:

A. Fibroma

B. Rhabdomyoma

C. Teratoma

D. Myxoma

284. What results when the common pulmonary venous plexus does not become incorporated into the left atrium?

A. Partial anomalous pulmonary venous connection

B. Cor triatriatum

C. Total anomalous pulmonary venous connection

D. Supravalvular mitral ring

285. When the common pulmonary vein becomes only partially incorporated into the left atrium, what anomaly results?

A. Cor triatriatum

B. Partial anomalous pulmonary venous connection

C. Total anomalous pulmonary venous connection

D. Supravalvular mitral ring

286. The left superior vena cava is a remnant of which primitive structure?
 A. Horns of the sinus venosus
 B. Left anterior cardinal system
 C. Umbilicovitelline system
 D. Splanchnic system

287. Which anatomic structure or structures should you visualize to distinguish between cor triatriatum and a supravalvular mitral ring?
 A. Left atrial appendage
 B. Right pulmonary veins
 C. Fossa ovalis
 D. Coronary sinus

Refer to video PER-Q288.

288. What is most likely demonstrated in this video clip?
 A. Fibroma
 B. Rhabdomyoma
 C. Extension of Wilms tumor
 D. Myxoma

289. In cor triatriatum, which structure has failed to be fully incorporated into the left atrium?
 A. Common pulmonary vein
 B. Left cardinal vein
 C. Azygos vein
 D. Crista terminalis

Refer to video PER-Q290.

290. What structure is seen in this video clip obtained from the suprasternal notch view?
 A. Azygos vein
 B. Interrupted inferior vena cava
 C. Retroaortic innominate vein
 D. Left pulmonary vein

291. A left-sided superior vena cava (SVC) usually drains to the:
 A. Left pulmonary vein
 B. Coronary sinus
 C. Left atrium
 D. Coronary artery

292. What structure is the arrow in this image pointing to?

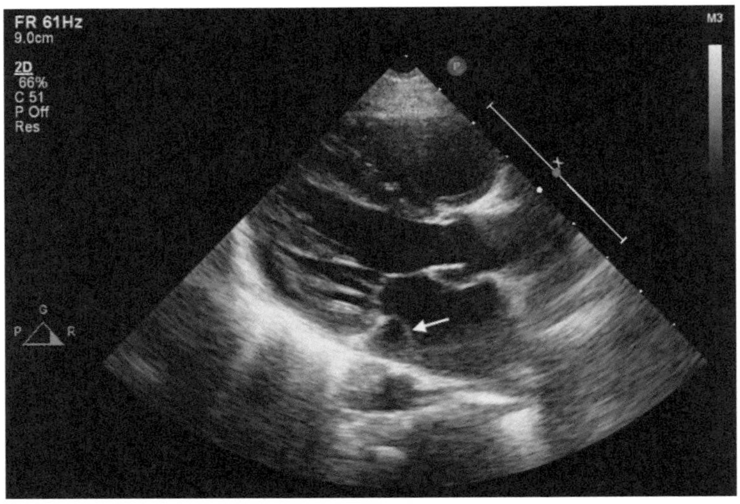

A. Descending aorta
B. Left atrium
C. Supramitral valve ring
D. Dilated coronary sinus

AIT—Hotspot

293. The finding in question 292 is suggestive of:
A. Left-sided superior vena cava
B. Cor triatriatum
C. Supracardiac total anomalous pulmonary venous connection
D. Interrupted inferior vena cava

294. A pericardial effusion is often seen with a:
A. Left atrial myxoma
B. Rhabdomyoma
C. Teratoma
D. Fibroma

295. When scanning a patient with a left-sided congenital diaphragmatic hernia, you notice that you need to move the transducer more rightward to obtain your apical and subcostal views, and the apex of the heart still appears leftward. This is an example of which of the following:
A. Dextrocardia
B. Dextroposition
C. Dextroversion
D. Dextromethorphan

296. You are scanning a patient with Kartagener syndrome. What do you expect to find with regard to cardiac positioning?
   A. Levocardia
   B. Dextroposition
   C. Dextrocardia
   D. Dextroversion

297. In the case of Kartagener syndrome presented in question 296, what would you expect the atrial situs to be?
   A. Situs inversus
   B. Situs solitus
   C. Situs ambiguus
   D. Bronchus suis

298. You are interrogating the innominate (brachiocephalic) vein and note a structure toward the left that is draining up from below into the innominate vein with a low-velocity phasic flow pattern. What structure could this be?
   A. Left-sided superior vena cava
   B. Anomalous pulmonary vein
   C. Azygos vein
   D. Arteriovenous malformation

Refer to video PER-Q299.

299. Which type of surgical procedure is seen in this video clip?
   A. Fontan completion
   B. LeCompte with arterial switch operation
   C. Bilateral bidirectional Glenn
   D. Norwood with Sano

300. You are interrogating a neonatal heart using a parasternal long-axis view and note that the right ventricle is dilated. Which of the following defects can cause this finding in a neonate?
   A. Patent foramen ovale
   B. Patent ductus arteriosus
   C. Tricuspid atresia
   D. Total anomalous pulmonary venous drainage

301. As you are scanning in the high parasternal view with color Doppler, you notice a vascular structure that drains superiorly. With spectral Doppler, there is a venous flow pattern. Which of these vascular structures are you visualizing?
   A. Left-sided superior vena cava
   B. Vertical vein with supracardiac total anomalous pulmonary venous connection
   C. Vertical vein with infracardiac total anomalous pulmonary venous connection
   D. Retroaortic innominate vein

302. During an echocardiography exam you note a structure in the right atrium that appears membranous with a wind-sock appearance. The structure is directed toward the tricuspid valve. What is the most likely diagnosis?
   A. Cor triatriatum sinister
   B. Cor triatriatum dextrum
   C. Atrial myxoma
   D. Ebstein anomaly

303. Which of the following findings is most likely in a patient with an interrupted inferior vena cava?
   A. Dilated superior vena cava
   B. Dilated coronary sinus
   C. Dilated hepatic veins
   D. Dilated innominate vein

304. You are conducting an exam of a patient with dextrocardia. When imaging from the apical or subcostal view, you should:
   A. Flip the transducer 180° so that the apex points leftward
   B. Maintain normal positioning of the transducer but flip the image R–L 180°
   C. Maintain normal positioning of the transducer and do nothing different
   D. Ask the patient to lie on her left side

305. When you are imaging a patient with suspected heterotaxy, which of the following is true?
   A. The inferior vena cava (IVC) and hepatic veins always drain to the same atrium.

B. The IVC and hepatic veins always drain to the right atrium.
C. The IVC and hepatic veins always drain to separate atria.
D. The IVC and hepatic veins can have various connections.

306. When scanning in the subcostal sagittal view, you notice a structure below the diaphragm that runs parallel along the descending aorta with a venous flow pattern coursing superiorly. What is this patient likely to have?
A. Infracardiac total anomalous pulmonary venous connection
B. Interrupted inferior vena cava
C. Fontan completion
D. Hepatic arteriovenous malformations

307. A female patient with Turner syndrome in the neonatal intensive care unit is scheduled for an echocardiogram. Which duct-dependent lesion listed below is most likely to be found?
A. Tetralogy of Fallot
B. Interrupted aortic arch with a posterior malalignment ventricular septal defect
C. Hypoplastic left heart syndrome
D. Pulmonary atresia with intact ventricular septum

308. A 1-week-old patient comes into the emergency room and is diagnosed with hypoplastic left heart syndrome. In this patient, the atrial-level shunting pattern is most likely:
A. Bidirectional
B. Right to left
C. Not present
D. Left to right

309. In hypoplastic left heart syndrome with mitral atresia and aortic atresia, cerebral perfusion is most likely:
A. Retrograde from the patent ductus arteriosus
B. Antegrade from the ascending aorta
C. Right to left from atrial-level shunting
D. Derived from a levoatrial cardinal artery

Refer to video PER-Q310.

310. What condition is seen in this video clip?
   A. Unguarded mitral valve orifice
   B. Hypoplastic left heart syndrome
   C. Ebstein anomaly of the tricuspid valve
   D. None of the above

Refer to video PER-Q311.

311. This video clip was taken immediately after a patient with hypoplastic left heart syndrome (HLHS) was transferred into the cardiac intensive care unit. What does this clip reveal about the atrial septum?
   A. Atrial-level shunting is from the right atrium to the left atrium.
   B. The atrial septal defect is very large, flow is laminar, and these findings are not unusual in the presence of HLHS
   C. Atrial-level shunting appears restrictive (left-to-right shunt), but further investigation is needed.
   D. No atrial-level shunting is seen.

Refer to video PER-Q312.

312. This video clip is taken from a patient with pulmonary atresia with intact ventricular septum. Which statement below best describes the atrial-level shunt?
   A. Morphologic left-to-right atrial shunt
   B. Morphologic right-to-left atrial shunt
   C. Septum primum atrial septal defect
   D. Superior sinus venosus atrial septal defect

Refer to video PER-Q313.

313. This video clip is most consistent with:
   A. Aortic valve atresia in the setting of hypoplastic left heart syndrome
   B. Double aortic arch
   C. Total anomalous pulmonary venous connection
   D. Small right-sided superior vena cava

Refer to video PER-Q314.

314. Which of the following congenital heart anomalies is seen in this video clip?
   A. Transitional atrioventricular canal
   B. Redundant mitral valve chordae tendineae in the setting of L-looped ventricles
   C. Ebstein anomaly of the tricuspid valve
   D. Muscular tricuspid atresia

PART 4

Postoperative Anatomy

315. You are examining a newborn who has undergone a transannular patch repair of tetralogy of Fallot without complication. What is the expected course for this patient?

A. There are no anticipated future cardiac interventions; the patient is "repaired" and being monitored by the cardiologist.

B. The patient will need a pulmonary valve replacement, most likely before 18 years of age, to address progressive pulmonary valve insufficiency with right heart dilatation.

C. The patient may develop secondary aortic regurgitation due to a size discrepancy when the aorta and pulmonary artery were moved during surgery.

D. A vascular ring may develop during this patient's adolescence.

316. All of the following are expected findings in a postoperative tetralogy of Fallot patient EXCEPT:

A. Residual shunting across the ventricular septal defect

B. Pulmonary valve insufficiency

C. Mild right ventricular outflow/pulmonary valve stenosis

D. Patent left ventricular outflow tract

317. A 16-year-old girl presents for an echocardiogram. She is obese and has a history of tetralogy of Fallot repair. The pulmonologist referred her for an echocardiogram because of possible obstructive sleep apnea and requests an estimation of pulmonary systolic pressure to evaluate for pulmonary hypertension. The following measurements were obtained:

- Systolic blood pressure = 115 mmHg
- Tricuspid regurgitant jet = 4.5 m/sec (peak gradient = 81 mmHg)
- Pulmonary valve velocity = 5 m/sec
- Right pulmonary artery velocity = 2.3 m/sec
- Left pulmonary artery velocity = 2 m/sec

What is the estimated pulmonary artery pressure?

A. Approximately 81 mmHg (elevated)

B. Approximately 86–90 mmHg (elevated)

C. Approximately 40 mmHg (within normal limits)

D. The pulmonary artery pressure cannot be determined.

318. A 4-year-old girl with DiGeorge syndrome undergoes an echocardiography exam that demonstrates a velocity of 2 m/sec across the pulmonary valve, with nearly continuous diastolic pulmonary regurgitation. She has significant dilatation of the right ventricle and an abnormal tricuspid annular plane systolic excursion (TAPSE) measurement. Her pulmonary valve insufficiency is most likely graded as:

A. Trivial

B. Mild

C. Moderate

D. Severe

319. Your patient is an 8-year-old girl with a history of tetralogy of Fallot (TOF). Her complete history is unknown, but she has a surgical scar indicating that she had a cardiac surgical repair. On the echocardiogram, a portion of the septum near the base of the heart appears echobright with hypokinesis. In a short-axis view, there is mild flattening of the septum. What does this finding suggest?

A. Pulmonary hypertension is present.

B. A conal branch from the right coronary artery was ligated at the time of surgery.

C. The finding is common and expected post TOF repair.

D. The finding is concerning and you should immediately contact the cardiologist to review the echocardiogram.

320. For patients with a history of surgically repaired tetralogy of Fallot, you should obtain all of the following measurements EXCEPT:

A. Left pulmonary artery diameter

B. Left upper pulmonary vein diameter

C. Velocity across the pulmonary valve using pulsed-wave Doppler

D. Velocity across the pulmonary valve using continuous-wave Doppler

321. Displacement or upward "tilting" of the tricuspid valve annulus may be seen in older pediatric patients with tetralogy of Fallot. This occurs secondary to:
   A. Left ventricular dysfunction
   B. Tricuspid valve insufficiency
   C. Ebstein anomaly
   D. Right ventricular dilatation

322. A 12-year-old patient presents to you with a history of a transannular patch repair of tetralogy of Fallot during infancy and placement of a Contegra conduit pulmonary valve replacement at 11 years of age. The conduit will be seen connecting what cardiac structures?
   A. Right atrium to right ventricle
   B. Aorta to right pulmonary artery
   C. Aorta to main pulmonary artery
   D. Right ventricle to pulmonary artery

323. You are examining a 4-year-old patient with tetralogy of Fallot who is status post transannular patch repair during infancy. Echo findings include normal left ventricular systolic function, mild right ventricular dilatation with normal systolic function, mild septal flattening with a small ventricular septal defect seen, a peak velocity of 5 m/sec across the defect, mild pulmonary insufficiency, and a peak velocity across the pulmonary valve (by both pulsed-wave and continuous-wave Doppler) of 2 m/sec. There is no residual right ventricular outflow tract obstruction. This patient has:
   A. Typical findings post transannular patch repair
   B. Pulmonary hypertension
   C. Concerning findings that will likely require surgical intervention within the year
   D. Possible pulmonary hypertension requiring evaluation of tricuspid valve regurgitant jet velocity

324. When examining a patient with a history of coarctation of the aorta, it is important to perform Doppler evaluation of which cardiac structures?
   A. Isthmus and descending aorta
   B. Abdominal aorta

C. Aortic valve

D. All of the above

325. A 3-year-old boy presents with a history of aortic stenosis and coarctation of the aorta status post coarctation repair during infancy. The velocity across the isthmus of the aorta is 4 m/sec. What is the best estimation of the re-coarctation peak gradient?

A. 16 mmHg

B. 64 mmHg

C. 64 mmHg plus aortic valve velocity

D. More information is needed to make this calculation.

326. A 5-year-old patient presents for an echocardiogram. His mother states that he had a coarctation of the aorta that was repaired when he was 1 year old. He has no midline thoracotomy or subscapular scar. He most likely underwent:

A. Stent placement in the region of the coarctation

B. Robotic surgery for coarctation repair

C. Balloon aortoplasty for coarctation of the aorta

D. Serial direct dilatation with an aortic dilator

327. When examining a patient with a history of coarctation of the aorta status post repair, you obtain V_1 and V_2 velocities when evaluating the aortic arch. What do V_1 and V_2 represent?

A. V_1 represents the velocity at the mitral valve and V_2 the velocity in the descending aorta.

B. V_1 represents the velocity in the subvalvular aortic region and V_2 the velocity in the descending aorta.

C. V_1 represents the velocity in the left subclavian artery and V_2 the velocity in the descending aorta.

D. V_1 represents the velocity in the ascending aorta and V_2 the velocity in the descending aorta.

328. A 6-year-old patient presents for an echocardiogram with a history of a surgically repaired coarctation of the aorta. What other cardiac lesions commonly associated with coarctation of the aorta might be seen on this patient's echocardiogram?

A. Bicuspid aortic valve and ventricular septal defect

B. Ebstein anomaly of the tricuspid valve

C. Supravalvular pulmonary stenosis
D. Anomalous left coronary artery from the pulmonary artery

329. A 5-year-old girl underwent balloon aortoplasty for coarctation of the aorta at 3 years of age. During the echocardiography exam she is very fearful and refuses suprasternal notch imaging. Where could alternate imaging be obtained to determine if she might have a significant re-coarctation?
A. Parasternal long-axis
B. Parasternal short-axis
C. Subcostal views
D. High right parasternal views

330. You are performing echocardiography on a postoperative coarctation patient with a re-coarctation. If you place the Doppler cursor in the descending aorta, what Doppler waveform would you expect to see?
A. Late-peaking dagger-shaped Doppler waveform
B. Double envelope Doppler waveform
C. Rounded Doppler envelope
D. Early-peaking Doppler or reverse dagger

331. A 1-month-old infant presents for evaluation after repair of coarctation of the aorta. The aortic arch appears widely patent by 2D imaging, with no significant turbulence seen by color flow Doppler. Spectral Doppler evaluation is performed in the suprasternal notch view. There is a normal velocity by pulsed-wave Doppler in the region of repair. Continuous-wave Doppler yields a 3.6 m/sec velocity. There is normal pulsatility of the abdominal aorta confirmed by Doppler. What is the most likely reason for the increased velocity seen by continuous-wave Doppler?
A. There is a re-coarctation of the aorta.
B. Patent ductus arteriosus flow is being sampled.
C. There is a dynamic coarctation that is seen only intermittently.
D. The cursor is not well aligned and there is peripheral branch pulmonary stenosis.

332. A 12-year-old patient underwent coarctation repair via balloon aortoplasty as a toddler. There is no residual coarctation. What additional finding would be expected on an echocardiogram?

A. Widening of the distance between the left subclavian and left carotid arteries

B. Bovine arch

C. Aberrant right subclavian artery

D. Diastolic flow continuation on Doppler obtained in the abdominal aorta

333. A 17-year-old girl with a history of coarctation of the aorta undergoes echocardiography. She was repaired at 2 years of age in another country. The pediatrician is concerned because she has no detectable pulse in her left arm. Her left arm is also slightly shorter than her right arm. On echocardiogram, she will most likely have:

A. A severely stenotic left subclavian artery because a clot likely developed in the artery as a complication during coarctation repair

B. An absent left subclavian artery because of recoarctation

C. An absent left subclavian artery because it was used for a subclavian flap coarctation repair

D. An aneurysm of the left subclavian artery, a common complication of older surgical techniques for coarctation repair

334. Which cardiac structure is NOT frequently affected in a patient with a history of critical aortic stenosis?

A. Aortic arch

B. Pulmonary valve

C. Mitral valve

D. Left ventricle

335. You are performing a stat bedside echocardiogram in the intensive care unit on a 10-year-old patient who has undergone aortic valve repair secondary to aortic stenosis. The pulsed-wave Doppler velocity across the aortic valve is 1.3 m/sec. There is trivial aortic insufficiency.

The fractional shortening is 10%. The cardiologist asks you for your assessment of the echocardiogram. What do you tell her?

A. There may be significant residual aortic stenosis in the setting of poor cardiac output.

B. There is poor left ventricular systolic function with no aortic stenosis.

C. There is depressed left ventricular systolic function and mild aortic stenosis based on the velocity obtained.

D. There is subaortic stenosis.

336. An infant presents for an echocardiogram. The patient underwent repair of a coarctation of the aorta and resection of a subaortic membrane as well as resection of a supravalvular mitral ring with a mitral valvuloplasty. There is a parachute mitral valve. This patient has findings consistent with:

A. Patau syndrome (trisomy 13)

B. Shone syndrome

C. DiGeorge syndrome

D. Down syndrome (trisomy 21)

337. An infant presents for an echocardiogram. The patient underwent resection of a supravalvular mitral ring with a mitral valvuloplasty. There is a parachute mitral valve. The mitral valve gradient is measured appropriately with a value of 6 mmHg. Which of the following describes this finding?

A. A mean gradient consistent with mild stenosis

B. A peak gradient consistent with moderate stenosis

C. A mean gradient consistent with moderate stenosis

D. A mean gradient consistent with severe stenosis

338. An 11-year-old boy with a history of mechanical aortic valve replacement undergoes echocardiography. Leaflet movement is seen and the mean gradient across the valve is 25 mmHg by Doppler. What is the degree of aortic stenosis (AS)?

A. AS cannot be determined without knowing the baseline gradient obtained early after valve implantation.

B. The Doppler gradient is consistent with moderate stenosis.

C. AS can be determined only in adult patients.
D. This is trivial AS in the setting of a mechanical valve.

339. What would you expect to find in a child after pulmonary balloon valvuloplasty for critical pulmonary stenosis?
A. Mild pulmonary stenosis
B. Mild pulmonary insufficiency
C. Moderate pulmonary insufficiency
D. Both A and B

340. The Starnes procedure, performed in patients with severe forms of Ebstein anomaly of the tricuspid valve, consists of:
A. Closing the tricuspid valve with a fenestrated patch, thereby excluding the right ventricle
B. Tricuspid valve replacement using a specific type of suturing technique
C. Moving the tricuspid valve annulus to the normal position
D. Suturing the septal and posterior leaflets together to create a competent valve

341. A 3-year-old patient presents for an echocardiogram. She underwent a balloon valvuloplasty during infancy for critical aortic valve stenosis. This alleviated her aortic valve stenosis, and she had a normal velocity across her aortic valve following the procedure, but she developed aortic regurgitation after the valvuloplasty. Today's echocardiogram again demonstrates aortic regurgitation. There is flow reversal in the descending aorta. How would you characterize the degree of aortic insufficiency?
A. Mild
B. Mild to moderate
C. Moderate to severe
D. Indeterminable

342. A 12-year-old obese patient presents for an echocardiogram. Her mother says she is concerned because her daughter snores at night and worries this could strain her heart. An echocardiogram demonstrates a velocity of 3.5 m/sec across the pulmonary valve. The tricuspid

regurgitant jet has a velocity of 3.7 m/sec. This patient's findings are consistent with:

A. Mild pulmonary stenosis only

B. Moderate pulmonary stenosis only

C. Both pulmonary hypertension and mild pulmonary stenosis

D. Both pulmonary hypertension and moderate pulmonary stenosis

343. A 15-year-old girl has a history of a Ross procedure performed for aortic stenosis at 10 years of age. The echocardiogram will most likely demonstrate:

A. Mild to moderate subvalvular pulmonary stenosis

B. Mild to moderate subvalvular aortic stenosis

C. Mild to moderate aortic valve insufficiency

D. Mild to moderate pulmonary valve insufficiency

344. An infant with hypoplastic left heart syndrome with mitral and aortic atresia has undergone a Norwood operation. The infant now has reduced ventricular systolic function. In this setting which of the following would be the important focus of an echocardiography exam?

A. Patency of the source of pulmonary blood flow

B. Patency of Norwood anastomosis

C. Assessment of the atrial septum

D. Assessment of tricuspid valve function

345. A 1-month-old infant with hypoplastic left heart syndrome status post Norwood presents with progressive cyanosis and oxygen saturations in the 60s without oxygen supplementation. The right ventricle–to–pulmonary artery conduit (known as a Sano conduit) is well seen with a peak systolic velocity of 2 m/sec, without evidence of stenosis. What should be the initial focus of the echocardiographic exam after establishing adequacy of pulmonary blood flow to both branch pulmonary arteries?

A. Patency of the Norwood anastomosis

B. Assessment of tricuspid valve stenosis

C. Assessment of the atrial septum

D. Patency of the superior vena cava

346. This color Doppler image, obtained from a suprasternal coronal image, most likely represents flow through a:

See Color Plate 11 on page xxiv.

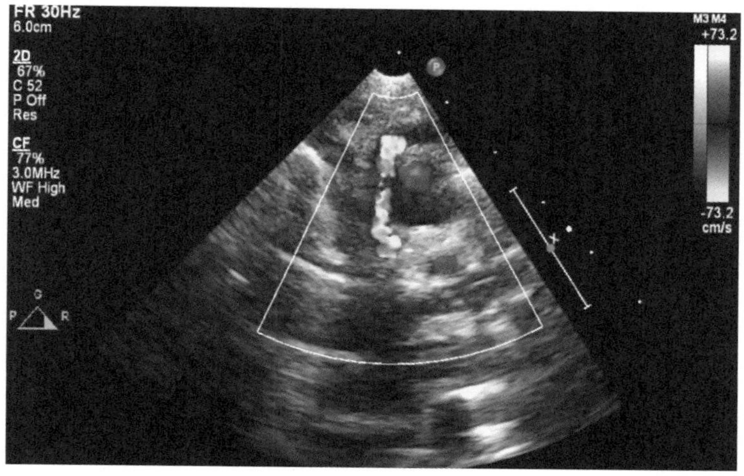

A. Modified Blalock-Taussig shunt
B. Right ventricle–pulmonary artery (Sano) conduit
C. Norwood anastomosis
D. Hybrid palliation

347. This Doppler image demonstrates blood flow in the descending aortic arch after Norwood palliation. The waveform pattern is:

See Color Plate 12 on page xxv.

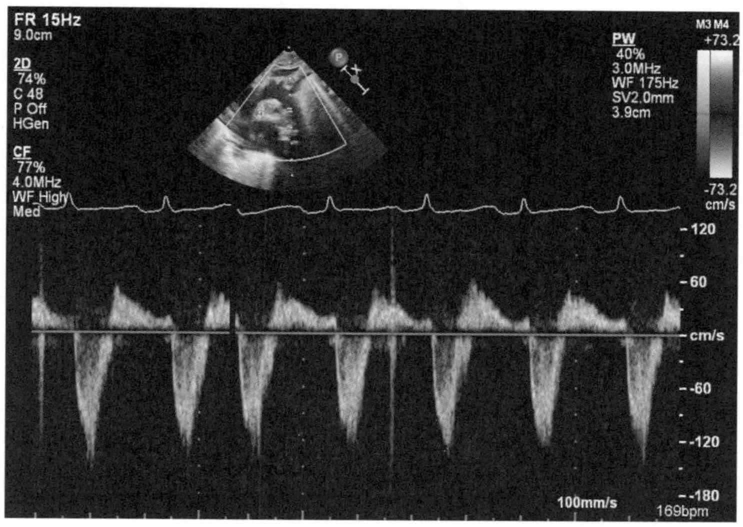

A. Normal for Norwood, with a right ventricle-to-pulmonary artery (Sano) shunt
B. Normal for Norwood, with a Blalock-Taussig (systemic-to-pulmonary artery) shunt
C. Suggestive of a coarctation
D. Suggestive of severe tricuspid insufficiency

348. You are about to scan a patient who has undergone a Norwood procedure with a modified Blalock-Taussig shunt (BTS). The BTS is anastomosed to the:
   A. Right ventricle
   B. Left ventricle
   C. Pulmonary artery
   D. Inferior vena cava

349. After a nonfenestrated Fontan procedure, which is the only systemic venous return that continues to drain to the right atrium?
   A. Hepatic veins
   B. Hemiazygos vein
   C. Azygos vein
   D. Coronary sinus

350. You are scanning a new patient with a history of bilateral bidirectional Glenn surgery. What do you need to look for regarding the Glenn surgery?
   A. Patent inferior vena cava to pulmonary artery connection
   B. Patent aortopulmonary connection
   C. Patent right-sided superior vena cava (SVC) to right pulmonary artery connection
   D. Patent right-sided SVC to right pulmonary artery and patent left-sided SVC to left-sided pulmonary artery connections

351. Which structure listed below is sewn to an extracardiac Fontan conduit?
   A. Abdominal aorta
   B. Celiac artery
   C. Inferior vena cava
   D. Superior vena cava

352. This spectral Doppler signal is obtained in a well-appearing infant with oxygen saturation of 85% after stage I Norwood palliation. Of the following, which spectral profile does this image most likely represent?

See Color Plate 13 on page xxv.

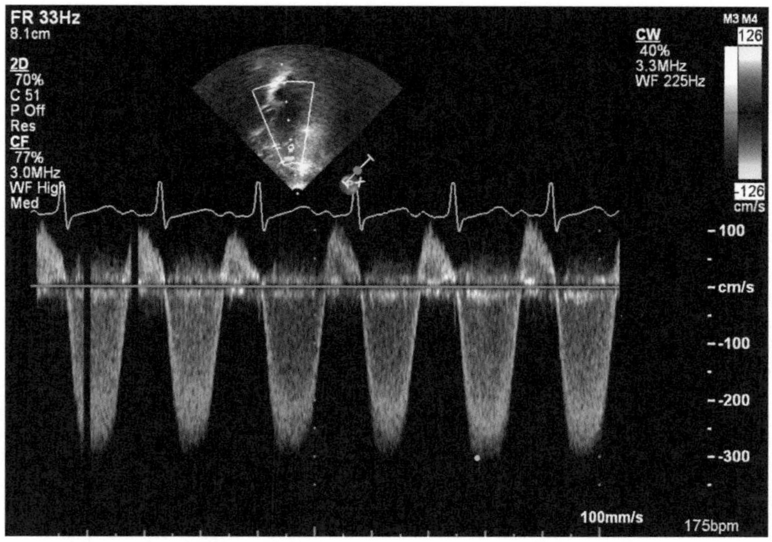

A. Flow through a modified Blalock-Taussig shunt
B. Flow through a pulmonary artery band
C. Flow through the tricuspid valve
D. Flow through a right ventricle–to–pulmonary artery conduit

353. Which structure listed below is sewn to the right pulmonary artery in a bidirectional Glenn shunt?
A. Innominate artery
B. Superior vena cava
C. Hemiazygos vein
D. Left subclavian artery

Refer to video PER-Q354.

354. A 3-month-old with a double-outlet right ventricle with subvalvular and valvular pulmonary stenosis has undergone a surgical intervention to augment pulmonary blood flow. She presents with significant cyanosis. This video clip suggests that the cyanosis is due to:
A. Obstructed bidirectional Glenn anastomosis
B. Obstructed modified Blalock-Taussig shunt
C. Pulmonary edema from excessive pulmonary blood flow
D. Branch pulmonary artery stenosis

355. A patient with a single ventricle has undergone a Norwood procedure with a modified Blalock-Taussig shunt. Following the procedure, spectral Doppler of the descending aorta cannot be used to assess coarctation of the aorta reliably. Why not?

A. There is diastolic runoff in the Norwood anastomosis.

B. There is diastolic runoff through the shunt.

C. Cyanotic children develop aortopulmonary collaterals.

D. Patch material is used for the aortic arch repair.

356. This image was obtained from a suprasternal coronal window and most likely represents:

See Color Plate 14 on page xxvi.

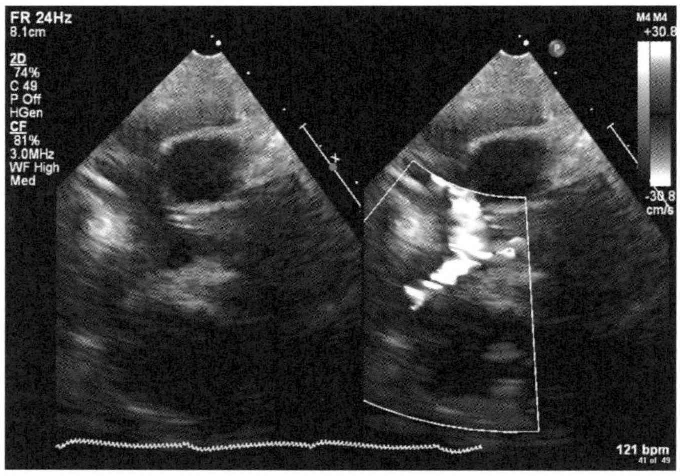

A. Bidirectional Glenn anastomosis

B. Norwood anastomosis

C. Extracardiac Fontan conduit

D. Lateral tunnel Fontan conduit

357. A Kawashima Glenn procedure is performed in the setting of heterotaxy with:

A. Isolated left superior vena cava (SVC)

B. Total anomalous pulmonary venous connection to a right SVC

C. Interrupted inferior vena cava (IVC) with azygos or hemiazygos continuation to the SVC

D. Mixed anomalous pulmonary venous drainage

358. For the echocardiographic exam that follows an arterial switch operation with a LeCompte maneuver to correct transposition of the great arteries (d-TGA), which view best demonstrates the pulmonary arteries?

A. Parasternal long-axis view
B. Parasternal short-axis view
C. Apical four-chamber view
D. Suprasternal coronal view

359. What is the most common early complication after an arterial switch operation?
A. Supravalvular neopulmonary stenosis
B. Supravalvular neoaortic stenosis
C. Coronary artery obstruction
D. Coarctation of the aorta

360. The most common complication after the atrial switch operation (Mustard or Senning) for transposition of the great arteries (d-TGA) is:
A. Superior vena cava pathway obstruction
B. Inferior vena cava pathway obstruction
C. Supravalvular neopulmonary stenosis
D. Subaortic obstruction

361. This image demonstrates the aortic and pulmonary artery relationship in which condition?

See Color Plate 15 on page xxvi.

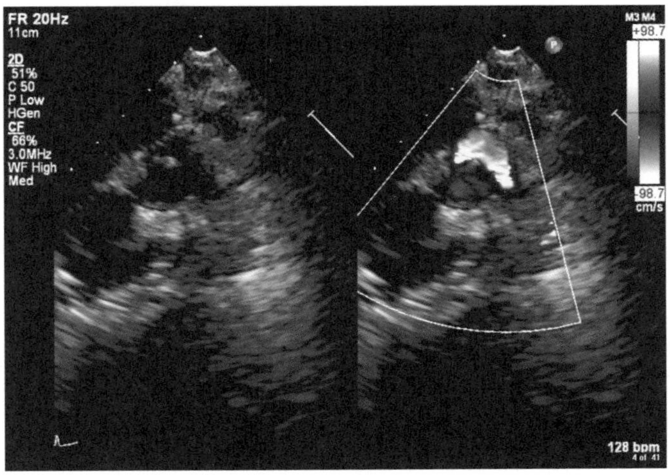

A. Congenitally corrected transposition of the great arteries
B. Preoperative transposition of the great arteries (d-TGA)
C. Transposition of the great arteries (d-TGA) following an arterial switch operation
D. Truncus arteriosus type I

Refer to video PER-Q362.

362. A 3-year-old male with single-ventricle anatomy is status post bidirectional Glenn procedure and a subsequent extracardiac nonfenestrated Fontan procedure. An echocardiogram of the patient, performed in the cardiothoracic intensive care unit, is shown below. This video clip demonstrates:
    A. Fontan anastomosis obstruction
    B. Fontan thrombus
    C. Bidirectional Glenn thrombus
    D. Systemic arterial obstruction

Refer to video PER-Q363.

363. This video clip is of a 1-month-old infant after palliation of hypoplastic left heart syndrome. What is seen in this clip?
    A. Unobstructed Norwood anastomosis
    B. Reconstructed aortic arch
    C. Free aortic insufficiency
    D. Hybrid palliation

364. Continuous flow in the branch pulmonary arteries after hybrid palliation is supplied by:
    A. A modified Blalock-Taussig shunt
    B. A right ventricle–to–pulmonary artery conduit
    C. Antegrade systolic pulmonary artery flow and retrograde diastolic flow via a ductal stent
    D. Antegrade flow only

365. Your patient is 9 months old with tricuspid atresia status post bidirectional Glenn procedure. He now presents with cyanosis. You are asked to perform a contrast injection with agitated saline in an intravenous line located in the right lower extremity. An apical four-chamber view will most likely demonstrate evidence of:
    A. Venovenous collaterals
    B. Arteriovenous malformations
    C. Aortopulmonary collaterals
    D. Normal systemic venous return

366. A 9-month-old patient with pulmonary atresia with intact ventricular septum (PA/IVS), status post bidirectional Glenn procedure, presents with cyanosis. Two-dimensional echocardiography with color Doppler demonstrates narrowing of the Glenn anastomosis, with a 2 mmHg mean gradient. Injection of agitated saline in the right upper extremity will most likely demonstrate evidence of:

   A. Venovenous collaterals
   B. Arteriovenous malformations
   C. Aortopulmonary collaterals
   D. No contrast return to the heart

367. Your patient is the infant in question 366. Where should you focus the echocardiographic evaluation to assess the return of contrast?

   A. Atria
   B. Distal branch pulmonary arteries
   C. Aorta
   D. Superior vena cava

368. An infant with hypoplastic left heart syndrome was palliated with a Norwood procedure with a modified Blalock-Taussig (BT) shunt. Initial postoperative oxygen saturation was 75%, and echocardiography was performed while the patient was on inotropic support and mechanical ventilation was demonstrating a peak velocity across the BT shunt of 2.3 m/sec. Two weeks later, following clinical improvement of the patient that included extubation and cessation of inotropic support, pulse oximetry demonstrates an oxygen saturation of 85% and a routine echocardiogram demonstrates a modified BT shunt velocity of 3.5 m/sec. What is the most likely cause of this difference?

   A. BT shunt obstruction
   B. Coarctation of the distal Norwood anastomosis
   C. Reduction in pulmonary vascular resistance
   D. Aortopulmonary collateral flow

369. A 7-year-old child with pulmonary atresia and an intact ventricular septum presents for routine evaluation. His pulse oximetry reveals an oxygen saturation of 86%. Given these images, his desaturation is most likely due to which of the following?

A

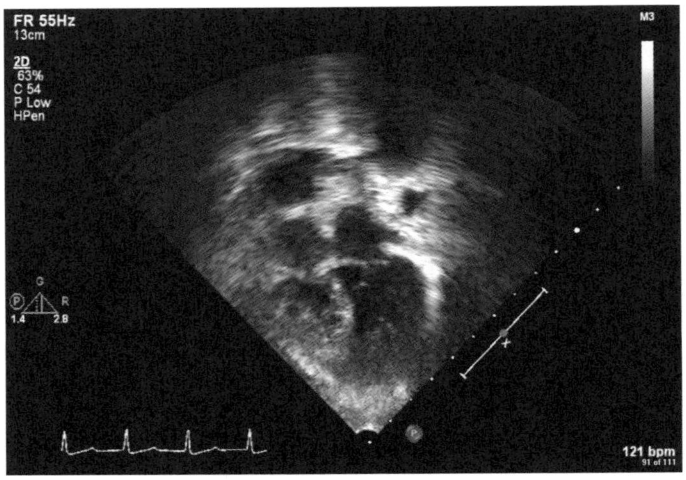

B

See Color Plate 16 on page xxvii.

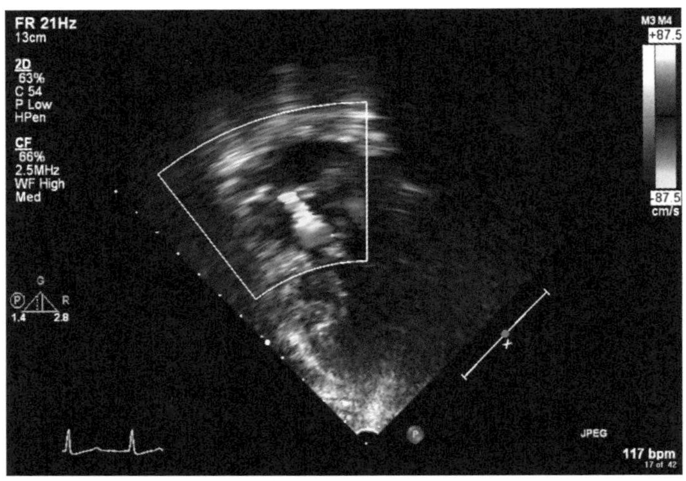

A. He has had a bidirectional Glenn but not a Fontan palliation.
B. He has had a fenestrated Fontan procedure with right-to-left shunting.
C. There are arteriovenous malformations.
D. There are venovenous collaterals.

370. A 7-year-old male with a history of transposition of the great arteries (d-TGA), which was treated in infancy with an arterial switch procedure, presents for evaluation of syncope with exertion. Echocardiography

demonstrated depressed ventricular septal and left ventricular apical wall motion; coronary origins were not well seen. The most likely source of the depressed wall motion in this patient is:

A. Compression from the LeCompte position of the pulmonary arteries

B. Dilatation of the mitral valve annulus from chronic mitral insufficiency

C. Kinking of the left main coronary artery branch point between the circumflex and left anterior descending arteries

D. Occlusion of an isolated left anterior descending coronary artery

371. A 1-year-old female with congenitally corrected transposition of the great arteries (ccTGA) with a restrictive perimembranous ventricular septal defect (VSD) underwent an anatomic repair—a double switch operation—that included VSD closure at 3 months of age. During a routine follow-up assessment you note a bradycardic rhythm for the patient's age. Wall motion is normal and there is no evidence of a ventricular patch or other baffle leak; she was previously in a normal sinus rhythm following the double switch procedure. The most likely etiology of the bradycardia is:

A. Spontaneous complete heart block

B. Complete heart block related to VSD closure

C. Complete heart block from coronary hypoperfusion of the atrioventricular node

D. Atrial fibrillation with slow ventricular response

372. Which of the following has the potential for biventricular circulation, without the need for Fontan palliation?

A. Hypoplastic left heart syndrome with mitral atresia

B. Tricuspid atresia, nonrestrictive ventricular septal defect, and normally related great arteries

C. Pulmonary atresia with intact ventricular septum and mild tricuspid valve/right ventricular hypoplasia

D. Double-outlet right ventricle (DORV) with mitral atresia

373. Many institutions routinely perform fenestration of the Fontan pathway/conduit when performing a Fontan completion. However, some institutions do not routinely fenestrate every Fontan patient, instead reserving fenestration for selected high-risk situations. In those institutions that perform selective fenestrations, indications for fenestration could include all of the following EXCEPT:

    A. Poor ventricular function
    B. Evidence of pulmonary hypertension
    C. Significant atrioventricular valve regurgitation
    D. Significant preoperative cyanosis

374. Which subset of patients are at highest risk of mortality?

    A. Patients with d-TGA with no ventricular septal defect (VSD)
    B. Patients with d-TGA with a large subpulmonary VSD
    C. Patients with d-TGA with a large VSD and left ventricular outflow tract obstruction
    D. Patients with double-outlet right ventricle, a subpulmonary VSD, and right ventricular outflow tract obstruction

375. Which anomaly is repaired by the Rastelli operation?

    A. Tetralogy of Fallot
    B. Transposition of the great arteries (d-TGA) with ventricular septal defect (VSD) and right ventricular outflow tract (RVOT) obstruction
    C. D-TGA with VSD and left ventricular outflow tract (LVOT) obstruction
    D. Congenitally corrected TGA with VSD

376. A 15-year-old male is undergoing routine evaluation after an arterial switch operation for transposition of the great arteries (d-TGA) with an intact ventricular septum, performed when he was a neonate. He has had an uncomplicated clinical course. His echocardiogram demonstrates no regional wall motion abnormalities, normal biventricular function, and mild supravalvular pulmonary stenosis. A cardiac magnetic resonance imaging study is being arranged. Why?

A. To evaluate for early underlying coronary artery plaque formation
B. To assess for atrioventricular valve dysfunction
C. To assess for pulmonary vascular disease
D. To evaluate for proximal coronary artery obstruction

377. You are reviewing the operative report for a patient with transposition of the great arteries (d-TGA) who has undergone an arterial switch operation. Specifically, you want to assess the child's potential risk for increased morbidity. There are a number of important coronary artery variations in patients with d-TGA. Of these, which of the following coronary patterns poses the highest risk of complications and mortality?
A. Circumflex from the right coronary artery
B. Intramural left coronary artery
C. Inverted pattern
D. Single right coronary artery

378. For pediatric patients with severe aortic valve disease, there are several possible surgical interventions, including the Ross procedure. What happens during this procedure?
A. Replacement of the aortic valve with the native pulmonary valve
B. Subaortic resection and aortic valvuloplasty
C. Aortic valve replacement using a bioprosthetic valve
D. Aortic valve replacement using a homograft conduit

379. In the pediatric population there are several important benefits to performing the Ross procedure as opposed to using mechanical valve replacement. What is the main *disadvantage* of performing the Ross procedure?
A. The neoaortic valve does not grow with the patient.
B. There is a need for ongoing postoperative anticoagulation therapy.
C. The neoaortic valve needs to be replaced within a year.
D. It is a surgery that replaces two valves instead of one.

380. In pediatric patients who have undergone the Ross procedure for aortic valve disease, what is the most common postoperative finding involving the neoaortic valve?
   A. Neoaortic stenosis
   B. Neoaortic valve insufficiency
   C. Supravalvular aortic stenosis
   D. Subaortic stenosis

381. After a Ross procedure, which vascular structure is most at risk for progressive dilatation over time and requires serial measurement by echocardiography?
   A. Right ventricle–to–pulmonary artery conduit (allograft)
   B. Descending aorta
   C. Neoaortic root (pulmonary autograft)
   D. Main pulmonary artery

382. While mortality for pediatric patients who undergo a Ross procedure is low, there is a significant risk for post-procedure complications that require reintervention. Serial echocardiography follow-up is therefore important to determine the need for surgical reintervention. Which anatomic component of the heart is most likely to require earlier reoperation at follow-up?
   A. Right ventricle–to–pulmonary artery conduit
   B. Aortic arch
   C. Neoaortic valve (autograft)
   D. Coronary arteries

383. Another concern for pediatric patients who undergo a Ross procedure is the postoperative risk of subaortic stenosis developing over time. In follow-up, echocardiography is very important to evaluate for the recurrence of subaortic stenosis and the possible need for surgical reintervention. What additional cardiac finding is most often seen in association with subaortic stenosis and might indicate a need for reintervention?
   A. Right ventricle–to–pulmonary artery conduit (allograft) stenosis
   B. New or worsening neoaortic valve insufficiency
   C. Right ventricle–to–pulmonary artery conduit (allograft) insufficiency
   D. Neoaortic valve stenosis

384. Total anomalous pulmonary venous connection (TAPVC) is an embryonic failure of the pulmonary venous buds to connect directly to the posterior aspect of the developing left atrium, resulting in pulmonary venous return to the right atrium via alternate pulmonary-to-systemic venous connections. TAPVC may also present with obstruction in the anomalous draining veins and can be associated with more complex cardiac anomalies. Regardless of the site of the pulmonary-to-systemic venous connection, the goal of surgical repair is the same—to reestablish a normal connection of the pulmonary veins to the left atrium. Which of the following choices is the most common reason for early postoperative instability after TAPVC repair?

A. Pulmonary hypertension

B. Aortic arch obstruction

C. Patent ductus arteriosus

D. Atrioventricular valve regurgitation

385. A 6-month-old male infant with a history of total anomalous pulmonary venous connection (TAPVC) repaired at birth presents to the emergency room in respiratory distress with hypoxia. A chest x-ray is performed and shows bilateral white-out of the lungs, and a presumptive diagnosis of pneumonia is made. Antibiotics are given, but due to the patient's history of TAPVC an echocardiogram is also ordered. What is the most common late postoperative complication after surgical repair of TAPVC?

A. Depressed cardiac function

B. Residual atrial septal defect

C. Pulmonary venous anastomosis obstruction

D. Aortic arch obstruction

386. A 2-year-old patient is being seen in the cardiology clinic for follow-up after repair of total anomalous pulmonary venous connection (TAPVC). He has a recent history of worsening exercise tolerance and increased work of breathing. The echocardiogram shows evidence of pulmonary hypertension, including an elevated tricuspid regurgitant jet peak systolic velocity greater than 4 m/sec (64 mmHg). With this clinical history what must you evaluate in this patient?

A. Atrial septum
B. Aortic arch
C. Ventricular septum
D. Pulmonary venous anastomosis

387. A 5-year-old patient is being seen in the cardiology clinic for follow-up of a sinus venosus atrial septal defect (ASD) with partial anomalous pulmonary venous connection (PAPVC) to the superior vena cava (SVC). The surgery entailed baffling of the right upper PAPVC to the SVC–right atrial junction with closure of the sinus venosus ASD. The patient has a recent history of headaches and intermittent facial swelling. A pulsed-wave Doppler signal is obtained across the lower aspect of the SVC and is compared to the prior year's study. In these images what does the pulsed-wave Doppler pattern on the more recent echocardiogram suggest?

A

See Color Plate 18 on page xxvii.

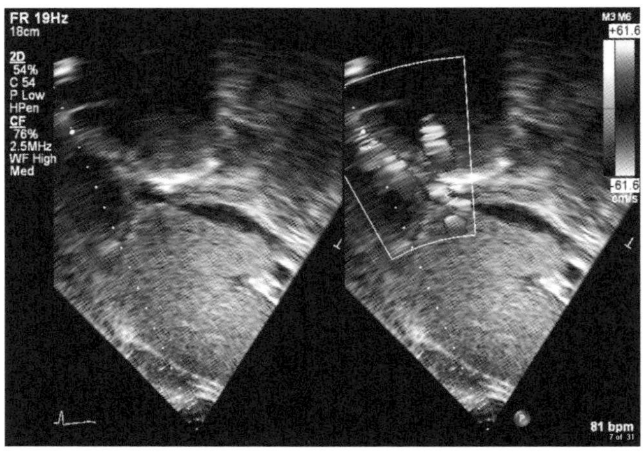

B

See Color Plate 19 on page xxviii.

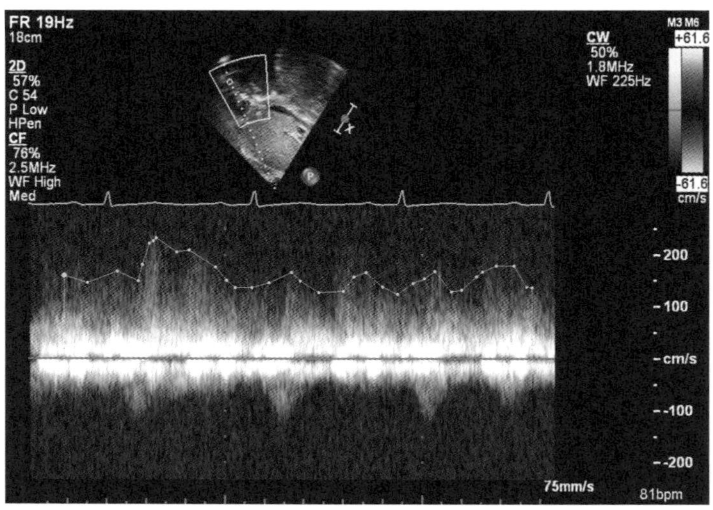

A. Diastolic cardiac dysfunction

B. Elevated left atrial filling pressure

C. SVC baffle stenosis

D. Pulmonary venous obstruction

388. A 2-year-old patient is being seen in the cardiology clinic for follow-up after repair of a sinus venosus atrial septal defect (ASD) and right-sided partial anomalous pulmonary venous connection (PAPVC), which drained to the superior vena cava (SVC) with a baffle closure to the left atrium. The parents are concerned that he has a decreased energy level and is fatigued all the time. A pulsed-wave Doppler signal is obtained across the right pulmonary veins as they enter the left atrium across the baffle. What does this image suggest?

See Color Plate 20 on page xxviii.

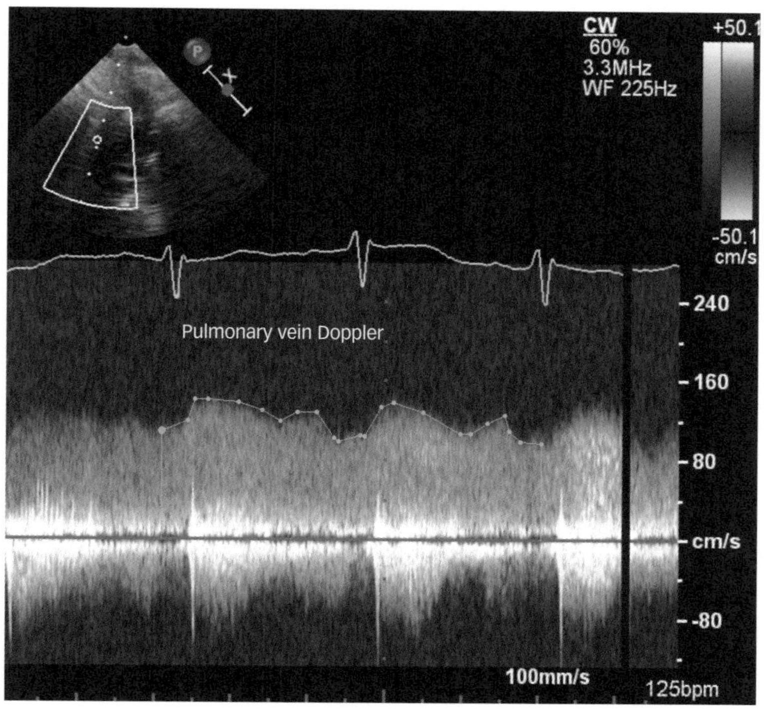

A. Diastolic cardiac dysfunction

B. Pulmonary venous baffle obstruction

C. Elevated left atrial filling pressure

D. Decreased left atrial filling pressure

389. Pulmonary artery (PA) banding surgery for congenital heart disease is often used to restrict excessive pulmonary blood flow, increase systemic perfusion, and protect the pulmonary vascular bed from pathologic changes

due to prolonged pulmonary hypertension until a more definitive repair or palliation can be performed safely. PA banding is NOT used for which of these conditions?

A. Single ventricle with unguarded pulmonary blood flow
B. Tetralogy of Fallot
C. Double-outlet right ventricle
D. Multiple ventricular septal defects

390. Pulmonary artery (PA) banding surgery can also be used in cases of unrepaired transposition of the great arteries (d-TGA) in preparation for an arterial switch operation. The goal of the PA band in this scenario is to train the left ventricle (LV) so that the LV will not fail after the arterial switch operation. The PA band accomplishes this by:

A. Increasing LV wall thickness and LV mass
B. Decreasing LV afterload
C. Improving LV diastolic function
D. Increasing cardiac output

391. During an assessment of pulmonary artery (PA) band placement in follow-up echocardiographic evaluation, it is important to look for common postoperative complications such as proximal PA dilatation, pulmonary valve injury, and pulmonary valve insufficiency. Which of the following is also very important to assess in association with PA band placement?

A. Pulmonary venous return
B. Proximal aortic artery dilatation
C. Aortic valve insufficiency
D. Compromised branch pulmonary artery flow

392. Your patient is a 6-month-old infant who has had pulmonary artery (PA) banding to address multiple large muscular ventricular septal defects (VSDs) and now presents with worsening cyanosis. The echocardiogram reveals the PA band in good position between the pulmonary valve and branch pulmonary arteries, with an increased peak systolic Doppler gradient across the PA band of 100 mmHg compared to 60 mmHg at the prior visit. What do you suspect is the primary problem?

A. Slipped PA band causing branch pulmonary artery stenosis
B. Pulmonary hypertension
C. Pulmonary valve insufficiency
D. PA band that is too tight

393. You are called to the cardiac ward to assess a post-operative patient after pulmonary artery (PA) banding. Clinical findings include persistent difficulties feeding, increased work of breathing, and an inability to wean to room air, with increased pulmonary vascular markings and edema on chest x-ray. An echocardiogram has been ordered to evaluate multiple large ventricular septal defects (VSDs). Your findings include a peak systolic gradient of 30 mmHg across the PA band, which is located just above the pulmonary valve prior to the bifurcation of the branch pulmonary arteries. The echocardiogram also shows a dilated left atrium and left ventricle, normal systolic function, and only left-to-right shunting at the VSDs. What do you suspect is the primary problem?

A. Slipped PA band, causing branch pulmonary artery stenosis
B. Pulmonary hypertension
C. PA band that is too loose
D. Pulmonary valve insufficiency

394. You are performing follow-up echocardiography on a patient with a diagnosis of double-outlet right ventricle (DORV) after pulmonary artery (PA) banding. You are unable to see flow into the right pulmonary artery (RPA). There is an elevated Doppler peak systolic velocity across the PA band, and the left pulmonary artery (LPA) appears to have increased flow velocity. The patient was also noted to have lower oxygen saturations than she had during the prior visit. What should you be concerned about?

A. PA band migration with compromised RPA flow
B. Pulmonary valve insufficiency
C. PA band being too tight
D. PA band being too loose

395. Which of the following procedures is most appropriate to repair transposition of the great arteries (d-TGA), ventricular septal defect (VSD), and subpulmonary stenosis due to the difficulty of repairing left ventricular outflow tract (LVOT) obstruction?

A. Arterial switch

B. Rastelli

C. Norwood

D. Fontan

396. Which of the following describes a Rastelli surgical repair?

A. Placement of an intraventricular baffle and an RV-to-PA conduit

B. VSD patch closure and right ventricular outflow patch repair

C. Arterial switch operation and subaortic stenosis resection

D. Replacement of the aortic valve with the native pulmonary valve

397. After Rastelli repair, percutaneous intervention with or without stent placement or repeat heart surgery may be required in the presence of certain complications. Which of the following complications most commonly requires such postoperative intervention?

A. Right ventricle–to–pulmonary artery conduit stenosis

B. Atrioventricular valve regurgitation

C. Right ventricle–to–pulmonary artery conduit insufficiency

D. Decreased left ventricular systolic function

398. Which postoperative complication after Rastelli repair requires reoperation and increases the risk for heart block?

A. Right ventricle–to–pulmonary artery conduit stenosis

B. Atrioventricular valve regurgitation

C. Right ventricle–to–pulmonary artery conduit insufficiency

D. Left ventricular outflow tract obstruction

399. A 10-year-old male with acute fulminant myocarditis in severe congestive heart failure needed to be emergently placed on extracorporeal membrane oxygenation (ECMO). The surgeons would like you to check that the placement of the ECMO cannula is correct, using transthoracic echocardiography (TTE). How do you demonstrate correct cannula placement using TTE?
   A. The venous cannula position should be in the right atrium.
   B. The venous cannula position should be in the right ventricle.
   C. The aortic cannula position should be in the left ventricle.
   D. The aortic cannula position should be down the descending aorta.

400. A 10-year-old male with dilated cardiomyopathy (DCM) presented with severe congestive heart failure exacerbation and was placed on a ventricular assist device (VAD). After several weeks on the VAD he is noted to have an acute neurologic change and seizures. The surgeons would like the patient evaluated by transthoracic echocardiography. What do you think you might find?
   A. Worsening systolic heart function
   B. Intracavitary thrombus
   C. Elevated atrial filling pressure
   D. Worsening diastolic heart function

401. A 3-month-old born prematurely at 24 weeks has a history of multiple echocardiograms to check for closure of a patent ductus arteriosus (PDA) and assess heart function. The infant has a history of a long-standing indwelling central venous line (CVL) in the superior vena cava. What potential complication of a long-standing CVL should be evaluated?
   A. Thrombus
   B. Heart function
   C. Systolic cardiac dysfunction
   D. Decreased left atrial filling pressure

402. Last year, your patient with tetralogy of Fallot (TOF) had a pulmonary artery stent placed to correct stenosis in the left pulmonary artery (LPA). On today's follow-up exam the LPA stent is not well seen on echocardiography, and no flow can be demonstrated in the LPA. Also, the right pulmonary artery (RPA) appears larger, with increased flow noted at a peak velocity of 2 m/sec. What are you looking for on the echocardiogram?
   A. Cardiac dysfunction
   B. Residual ventricular septal defect
   C. LPA stent obstruction
   D. RPA stenosis

403. A 5-year-old female is being assessed for possible transcatheter device closure for a large atrial septal defect (ASD). What finding on the echocardiogram evaluation would prevent placement of an ASD device closure?
   A. Dilated right atrium and right ventricle
   B. Large inferior ASD rim
   C. Atrioventricular valve regurgitation
   D. Sinus venosus ASD with partial anomalous pulmonary venous connection (PAPVC)

404. A 5-year-old female underwent transcatheter device closure of a large secundum atrial septal defect (ASD) one day ago, without complication. She was kept overnight for observation, and prior to her discharge home you are asked to perform an echocardiogram to evaluate the device. What finding on echocardiographic evaluation would you immediately report to the treating cardiologist?
   A. Dilated right atrium and right ventricle
   B. Small residual ASD
   C. Device embolization
   D. Mild atrioventricular valve regurgitation

405. A patient needs a follow-up echocardiographic assessment after device closure of an atrial septal defect (ASD). The physician asks you to evaluate right pulmonary venous flow because she suspects:
   A. Right pulmonary vein obstruction
   B. Partial anomalous pulmonary venous drainage

C. Pulmonary hypertension

D. Pulmonary regurgitation

406. After transcatheter occlusion of a patent ductus arteriosus (PDA), which structure should be evaluated by echocardiography?

A. Aortic valve

B. Right pulmonary artery

C. Left pulmonary artery

D. Tricuspid valve

407. You perform an echocardiogram on a patient with patent ductus arteriosus (PDA) device closure. You notice the patient has differential blood pressures between the upper and lower extremities, based on noninvasive assessment. What do you think this patient might have?

A. Coarctation

B. Residual PDA

C. Poor left ventricular function

D. This is a normal finding.

408. You are performing follow-up echocardiography on a 3-year-old girl who is status post ventricular septal defect (VSD) closure. There appears to be tricuspid valve regurgitation (TR) with a peak velocity of 4 m/sec, but the ventricular septum does not have a flat contour, suggesting a low right ventricular and pulmonary artery pressure. What explanation can you give for the high TR velocity?

A. The patient has pulmonary hypertension.

B. The high-velocity jet represents a possible residual VSD with left ventricle–to–right ventricle shunting.

C. A high TR velocity is a normal finding after VSD surgery.

D. The high-velocity jet represents a possible residual VSD with left ventricle–to–right atrial shunting.

409. What is the most common complication after repair of an isolated ventricular septal defect (VSD)?

A. Pericardial effusion

B. Residual VSD

C. Tricuspid valve regurgitation

D. Decreased left ventricular systolic function

410. You are performing echocardiography on a 12-year-old patient with a history of an arterial switch operation. You want to evaluate the right ventricular outflow tract. Which view would be the most useful?
   A. Parasternal long-axis view
   B. Parasternal short-axis view
   C. Apical four-chamber view
   D. Subcostal sagittal view

411. Obstruction of the right ventricular outflow tract (RVOT) is a common complication following the arterial switch operation (ASO). What other long-term abnormalities should you focus on during a post-ASO echocardiographic examination?
   A. Neoaortic valve regurgitation
   B. Neoaortic valve stenosis
   C. Coarctation
   D. Development of pulmonary hypertension

412. Which of the following cardiac defects needs an arterial switch operation?
   A. Tricuspid atresia
   B. Ebstein anomaly
   C. Transposition of the great arteries (d-TGA)
   D. Double aortic arch

413. A newborn baby with hypoplastic left heart syndrome has undergone stage I palliation. Which of the following is an integral part of this surgery?
   A. Repair of the mitral valve
   B. Placement of a pulmonary artery band
   C. Placement of a stent in the superior vena cava
   D. Placement of a systemic–to–pulmonary artery shunt

414. A stat echocardiogram is requested in the cardiac intensive care unit. The physician has told you that the patient has a hypoplastic left heart and just underwent a Norwood procedure with modified Blalock-Taussig (BT) shunt, but he cannot hear a heart murmur. Based on this physical finding, what is the critical focus of your study?

A. Possible pericardial effusion
B. Possible BT shunt obstruction
C. Ruling out coarctation of the aorta
D. Possible restrictive atrial shunt

415. What is the typical spectral Doppler profile of a modified Blalock-Taussig (BT) shunt?
A. Low velocity
B. High velocity in systole and low velocity in diastole
C. High velocity through systole with continuation into diastole
D. Low velocity like venous flow

416. What is stage II of hypoplastic left heart palliation?
A. Connecting the superior vena cava directly to the right pulmonary artery
B. Connecting the inferior vena cava to the right pulmonary artery
C. Creating a shunt from a systemic artery to a pulmonary artery
D. Creating a shunt from the right ventricle to the main pulmonary artery

417. What is stage III of hypoplastic left heart palliation?
A. Complete bilateral superior vena cava connection to the pulmonary arteries
B. Redirection of inferior vena cava blood directly to the pulmonary arteries
C. Reconstruction of the atrial septum
D. Reconstruction of the aortic arch

418. What is the fenestration that is performed as part of a fenestrated Fontan procedure?
A. An opening made in the atrial septum
B. A small hole created between the Fontan pathway/conduit and the atrium, providing a left-to-right shunt
C. A small hole created between the Fontan pathway/conduit and the atrium, providing a right-to-left shunt
D. An unusual "fenestration flow pattern" across the atrioventricular valve(s)

419. A patient had a Fontan procedure (extracardiac conduit) at 3 years of age. Recently she was noted to have significant elevation in systemic venous pressure due to high pulmonary vascular resistance. Her cardiologist decided to create a fenestration of the Fontan conduit in the catheterization lab. You perform an echocardiogram after the procedure. How do you interpret the flow across the fenestration?

A. If the flow across the fenestration is high-velocity, it means that the pulmonary vascular resistance is high.

B. No matter whether the flow velocity across the fenestration is high or low, it is difficult to determine pulmonary vascular resistance.

C. Absence of visible flow across the fenestration from a standard apical four-chamber view means that the fenestration is no longer patent.

D. Because there is a right-to-left shunt across the fenestration, the color Doppler of the fenestration jet should be in blue from the apical four-chamber view.

420. Which of the following operations is an atrial switch procedure?

A. Norwood procedure

B. Ross procedure

C. Rastelli procedure

D. Mustard procedure

421. Which of the following cardiac defects will require a Fontan procedure?

A. Balanced atrioventricular septal defect

B. Double-inlet left ventricle

C. Tetralogy of Fallot

D. Truncus arteriosus

422. Which of the following statements about a rocking prosthetic mitral valve (PMV) is true?

A. A rocking PMV is normal in the setting of size mismatch between the patient and the PMV.

B. PMV rocking is seen with washing regurgitation jets in normally operating PMVs.

C. A rocking PMV is indicative of valve dehiscence.

D. PMV rocking is often seen in pediatric prosthetic valve placement.

423. An abscess visualized in the area of bioprosthetic valve implantation is:
   A. Echolucent
   B. Best evaluated with 2D imaging only
   C. Best evaluated with speckle tracking echocardiography (STE)
   D. Usually not considered a complication of bioprosthetic valve, but instead of a mechanical valve

424. You are performing echocardiography on a patient with a mechanical mitral valve and note small jets between the ring sutures and disks. What is your assessment?
   A. Jets seen around the sewing ring (perivalvular jets) are normal.
   B. Jets seen with mechanical mitral valves are an early sign of thrombus.
   C. Jets are considered an early sign of valve dehiscence.
   D. Jets seen between the sewing ring and discs are normal.

Refer to video PER-Q425.

425. What does this video clip demonstrate?
   A. Prosthetic valve with normal function
   B. Washing jets and normal valve function
   C. Perivalvular leak
   D. Rocking mechanical mitral valve

Refer to video PER-Q426.

426. This video clip most likely demonstrates:
   A. Restricted mechanical mitral leaflet motion
   B. Normal mechanical mitral valve leaflet motion
   C. Dehiscence of the mechanical mitral valve
   D. Thrombus formation on the base of the mechanical valve sewing ring

427. Which statement best describes why it is so important to obtain an echocardiogram of a prosthetic valve immediately post implantation?
   A. Gradients recorded soon after implantation are the highest that will be recorded during the lifetime of the valve and can be used as a baseline.
   B. Early post-implantation echocardiography provides baselines for many aspects of valve function, including (and not limited to) gradients, regurgitation, and leaflet motion.

C. Early post-implantation echocardiography can exclude perivalvular leaks; a perivalvular leak that manifests later in the postoperative period would then be considered a normal finding.

D. The first echocardiographic exam will document bioprosthetic valve clicks with spectral Doppler.

428. Spectral Doppler examination of a normally functioning mechanical heart valve will demonstrate:

A. Moderate regurgitation

B. Absence of valve clicks

C. Increased gradients compared to native normal valves

D. Decreased gradients compared to normal native valves

429. How many flow orifices does a bileaflet tilting disk valve have?

A. One

B. Two

C. Three

D. Four

430. Compared with a native valve, how likely is a prosthetic heart valve (PHV) to be associated with pannus?

A. More likely

B. Less likely

C. Equally likely

D. Pannus formation has no association with PHVs.

431. Which of the following is the best description of the Alfieri procedure?

A. Procedure used to relieve mitral valve stenosis

B. Repair of a bicuspid aortic valve

C. Transplantation of the pulmonary valve to the aortic valve position and implantation of an allograft in the pulmonary position

D. Suture repair of the mitral valve regurgitation that may resemble a double orifice

432. The view of the left atrium is most obscured in which of the following scan planes?

A. Mid-esophageal four-chamber view with a prosthetic mitral valve closed, using transesophageal echocardiography

B. Mid-esophageal two-chamber view with a prosthetic mitral valve open, using transesophageal echocardiography

C. Parasternal long-axis view in the presence of mechanical aortic and mitral valves, using transthoracic echocardiography

D. Parasternal long-axis view with a closed bioprosthetic mitral valve in the presence of a normal aortic valve, using transthoracic echocardiography

Refer to video PER-Q433.

433. Describe the leaflet motion in this video clip.

A. Normal leaflet motion of a caged-ball prosthetic mitral valve

B. Restrictive motion of the anterior mitral leaflet, with reverberation artifact seen in the left atrium

C. 2D imaging of normal mitral leaflet motion of a bileaflet tilting disk valve

D. Normal leaflet motion of a native mitral valve

434. Your patient has a prosthetic mitral valve. What does this spectral Doppler image most likely represent?

See Color Plate 21 on page xxix.

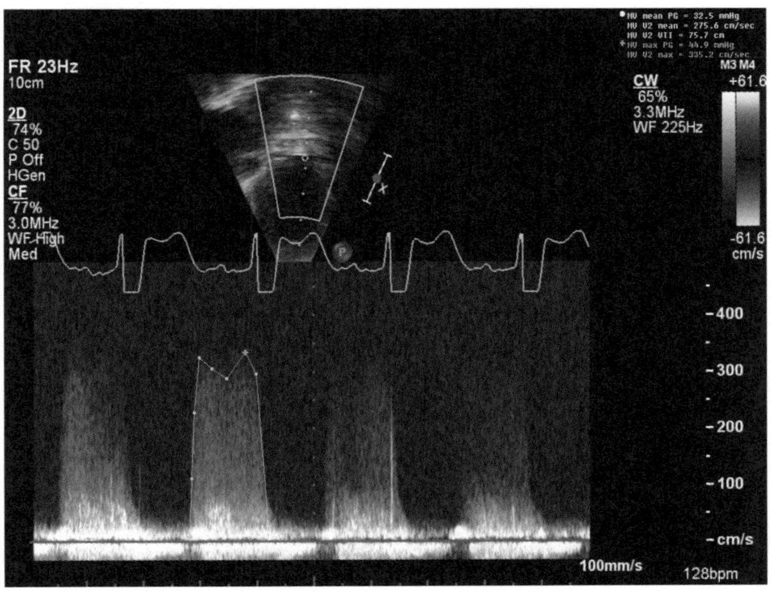

A. Normal leaflet motion with an increased valve gradient, which is normal in prosthetic valves
B. Normal leaflet motion with significant valve regurgitation, as suggested by flow above the baseline
C. Obstruction of the valve leaflet, as indicated by the increased valve gradient and the diminished valve clicks
D. This image is not diagnostic, and no information about the prosthetic valve can be assessed.

435. Which of the following is demonstrated in this image?

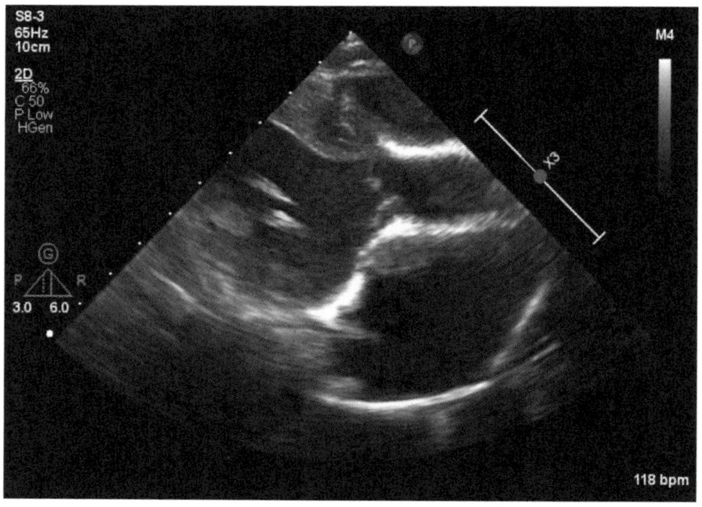

A. Conduit surrounding the ascending aorta, most likely implanted to alleviate dilatation
B. Dehiscence of the prosthetic aortic valve
C. Echodense area below the native aortic valve, which represents clot
D. Echolucent area below the native aortic valve, which represents an abscess

436. Which of the following is NOT found to cause superior vena cava syndrome (SVC syndrome)?
A. Thrombosis in the innominate vein
B. Glenn anastomosis obstruction
C. Right middle lobe pneumonia
D. Mediastinal mass near the SVC

PART 5

Clinical Standards and Guidelines

437. Your patient is a neonate who weighs about 6.5 pounds (3 kilograms) with mild hypoplasia of the left-sided structures. A biventricular repair is being contemplated. You have been asked to measure the aortic valve, aortic root, and ascending aortic diameters, all of which will be critical to deciding whether this intervention is feasible. In the parasternal long-axis view, which of the following transducers would be the most appropriate for obtaining these measurements?

A. 5 MHz curvilinear array

B. 5 MHz phased array

C. 15 MHz linear (sequential) array

D. 12 MHz phased array

438. In a newborn baby with coarctation of the aorta, which transducer would you use to obtain the best 2D image of the aortic arch?

A. 12 MHz

B. 8 MHz

C. 5 MHz

D. 3D matrix

439. A blind continuous-wave (CW) Doppler probe, also known as a pencil probe, is most appropriate to evaluate which of the following cardiac defects, from which echocardiographic window?

A. Aortic valve stenosis, from the suprasternal notch window

B. Shunting across an atrial septal defect, from the subcostal window

C. Coarctation of the aorta, from an apical window

D. Unobstructed total anomalous pulmonary venous connection to the coronary sinus, from the suprasternal notch window

440. Which statement about continuous-wave (CW) Doppler is TRUE?

A. CW Doppler has range resolution.

B. CW Doppler has no range ambiguity.

C. CW Doppler can measure high velocities.

D. CW Doppler is more subject to aliasing than pulsed-wave Doppler.

441. In a 2-year-old boy with coarctation of the aorta, you use an 8 MHz transducer for the entire study, but you cannot obtain an ideal Doppler signal. What is your next step?

A. Change to a 12 MHz transducer.

B. Use the same transducer but increase the gain by 50%.

C. Use a 3D matrix transducer.

D. Change to a 5 MHz transducer.

442. You are performing an echocardiographic evaluation of a 7-year-old patient with coarctation of the aorta. While 2D imaging of the aortic arch is very good, the color flow Doppler signal of aortic arch flow and flow through the coarctation are not well seen. How might you improve the color flow Doppler image quality in this patient?

A. Decrease the overall 2D imaging gain.

B. Use a lower-frequency transducer.

C. Decrease the Nyquist limit (pulse repetition frequency) for the color flow signal.

D. Narrow the sector width.

443. A 5 MHz curvilinear array transducer is best suited for which of these tasks?

A. Obstetric/fetal imaging

B. Vascular imaging

C. Neonatal imaging

D. Imaging of an adult with a limited transthoracic window

444. Which type of transducer should be used for 3D/4D imaging?

A. Annular array probe

B. Multifrequency phased array probe

C. High-resolution 12 MHz single-crystal phased array probe

D. Matrix array probe

445. You are performing an echocardiographic study and wish to increase the image contrast so that you can visualize the coronary arteries more clearly. Which control will you use?

A. Persistence

B. Transmit power

C. Dynamic range/compression

D. Line density

AIT—SIC*

446. Your patient is a small baby, born prematurely. Which of the following transducers would you choose to examine this infant?

A. A high-frequency transducer for all views, because the focal zone is larger.

B. A high-frequency transducer for the suprasternal view, because it provides better lateral resolution.

C. A low-frequency transducer for the subcostal view, because it provides a higher axial resolution.

D. A low-frequency transducer for the subcostal view, because it provides better temporal resolution.

447. All of the following maneuvers can improve temporal resolution (resulting in a higher frame rate) EXCEPT:

A. Narrowing the sector width

B. Imaging in 2D only, without color

C. Decreasing the depth

D. Decreasing transducer frequency

AIT—SIC

---

*Questions marked ***AIT—SIC*** are similar to ARDMS Advanced Item Type (AIT) questions called "Semi-Interactive Console" items. These require you to use your cursor to adjust controls on an onscreen console to correct a problem with the image presented. The console is "semi-interactive" because only some of the controls can be "adjusted." AIT—SIC items are currently limited to the Sonography Principles and Instrumentation (SPI) examination and as of this printing do not appear on the Pediatric Echocardiography exam, but as a bonus feature we have identified similar items in this mock exam.

448. You are imaging a patient with total anomalous pulmonary venous connection, and you are trying to use color flow Doppler to visualize flow in the individual veins returning to the pulmonary venous confluence. What maneuver is most helpful for improving visualization of the pulmonary veins?

A. Increasing color flow Doppler gain

B. Decreasing 2D imaging gains

C. Reducing the color flow Doppler scale

D. Changing from brightness to variance mode

AIT—SIC

449. Tissue harmonic imaging is best suited to which of these objectives?

A. Enhancing color Doppler imaging

B. Improving endocardial border definition

C. Improving spectral Doppler signal detection

D. Enhancing M-mode imaging

AIT—SIC

450. What is the purpose of adjusting the time gain compensation?

A. Narrow the image sector to increase the frame rate

B. Assign Doppler color values to compensate for aliasing during low-flow visualization

C. Increase dynamic range to improve visualization of weaker returning ultrasound signals

D. Compensate for attenuation by boosting signal amplitudes at different depths

AIT—SIC

451. How do you improve temporal resolution in pediatric echocardiography?

A. Change focus.

B. Change to a higher-frequency transducer.

C. Change gain range.

D. Reduce image sector size.

AIT—SIC

452. What is the problem with this spectral Doppler tracing?

See Color Plate 22 on page xxix.

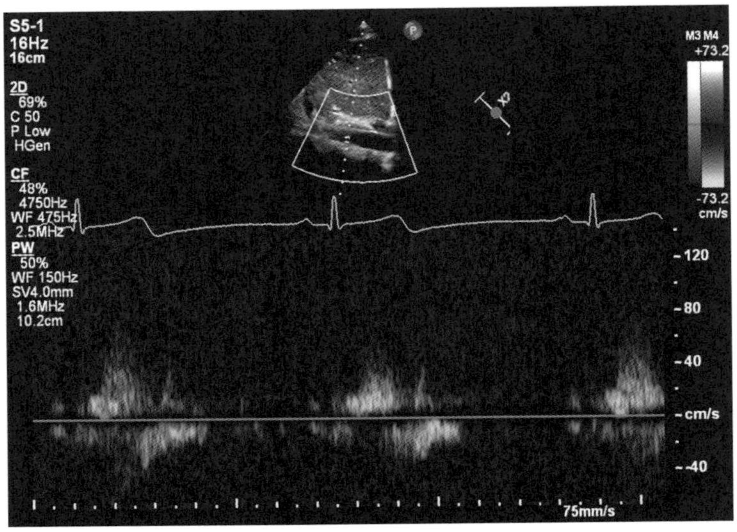

A. Poor angle of insonation

B. Doppler gain not high enough

C. Abnormal Doppler baseline

D. Continuous-wave Doppler should be used instead of pulsed-wave Doppler.

453. What type of artifact is associated with the atrial septum seen in this image?

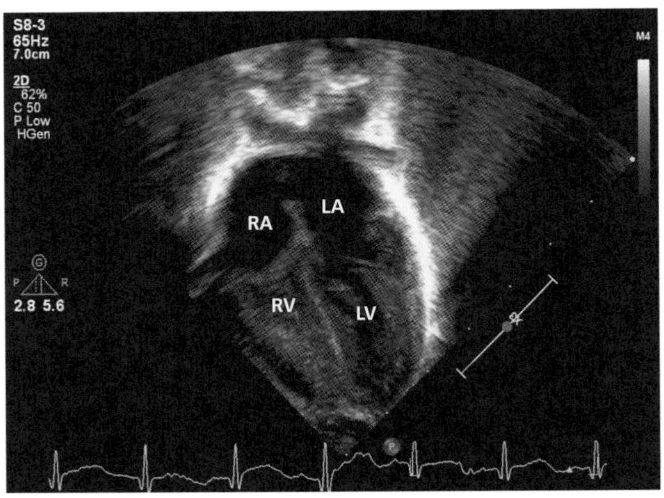

A. Side lobe artifact

B. Image dropout artifact

C. Slice-thickness artifact

D. There is no artifact; there is a secundum atrial septal defect.

454. When are mirror-image artifacts most likely to be seen?

A. When you are focusing the beam near two structures of similar tissue types
B. When the focal point is located at a fluid-tissue interface
C. When the object you are interrogating is located in lung tissue
D. When a strong reflector is located behind an object along the path of the primary ultrasound beam

455. What does this spectral Doppler tracing demonstrate?

See Color Plate 23 on page xxx.

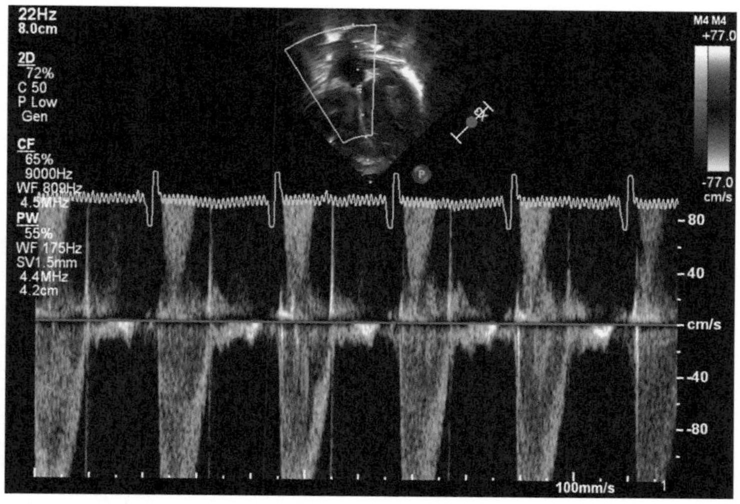

A. Aliasing
B. Excessive gain
C. Typical venous spectral Doppler flow pattern
D. Flow across the mitral valve

456. The arrow in this image is pointing to an artifact. Why does this artifact occur?

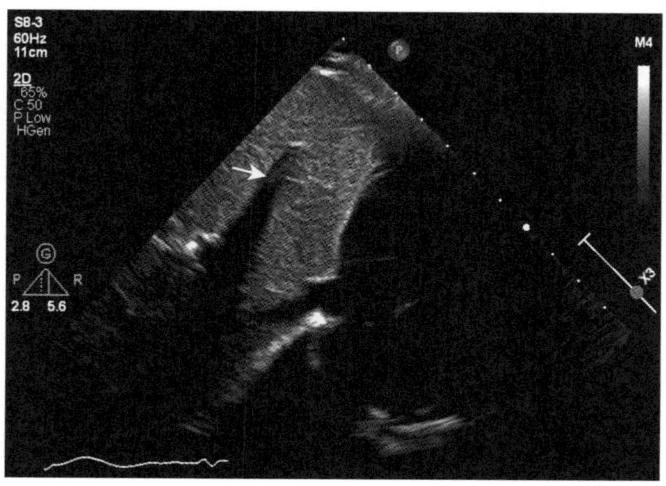

A. Improper selection of transducer frequency
B. Excessive speckling of the tissue
C. Suboptimal angle of insonation
D. Large acoustic impedance mismatch between two structures

457. What is true about mirror-image artifacts?
A. Incorrect time gain compensation produces mirror-image artifacts.
B. A mechanical mitral valve can cause a mirror-image artifact.
C. The real structure appears deeper than the artifact.
D. The artifact appears deeper than the real structure.

458. How would you correct the artifact seen in this image?

See Color Plate 24 on page xxx.

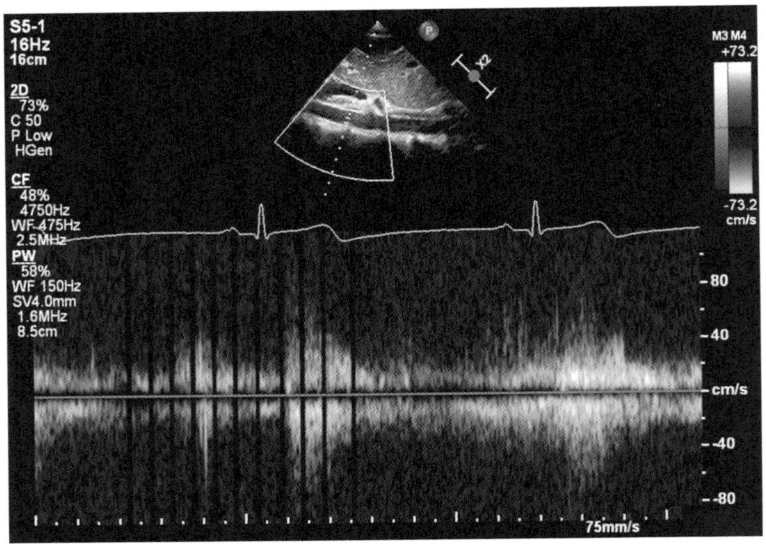

A. Change to a lower-frequency transducer.
B. Angle the sound beam so it is more parallel to the direction of flow.
C. Change the spectral Doppler baseline.
D. Increase the spectral Doppler scale.

AIT—SIC

459. Which of the following standard imaging views is best to evaluate the individual pulmonary veins?
A. Suprasternal coronal view
B. Subcostal long-axis view
C. Apical four-chamber view
D. Parasternal long-axis view

460. The best echocardiographic view to evaluate visceroatrial situs is the subcostal long-axis (transverse) sweep, beginning below the diaphragm. All of the following seen in this sweep are useful for the determination of situs EXCEPT:

A. Position of the azygos and hemiazygos veins
B. Position of the liver
C. Position of the hepatic segment of the inferior vena cava
D. Morphology of the atrial appendage

461. What should be done to correct this image to make it acceptable for pediatric echocardiography?

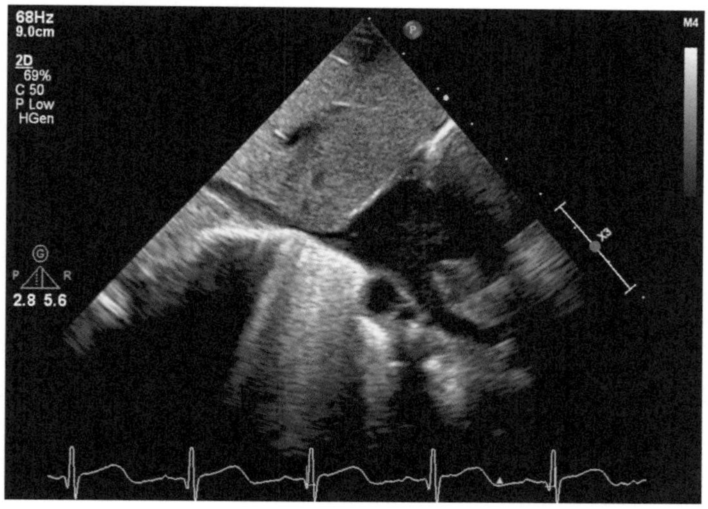

A. Nothing; the image is acceptable as is.
B. Rotate the transducer notch 180°.
C. Invert the image and rotate the transducer notch to 6 o'clock.
D. Invert the image and rotate the transducer notch to 3 o'clock.

AIT—SIC

Refer to video PER-Q462.

462. This video clip was obtained from a subcostal short-axis sweep. From this sweep, what can be determined regarding visceroatrial situs and cardiac position in this patient?

A. Situs solitus with levocardia
B. Situs inversus with dextrocardia
C. Situs ambiguus with mesocardia
D. Nothing, based on this sweep

463. The subcostal sweeps provide excellent anatomic and physiologic information in pediatric patients with many different types of congenital heart disease (CHD). For which of the following CHDs are the subcostal views most useful?

A. Supracardiac total anomalous pulmonary venous connection (TAPVC)
B. Infradiaphragmatic TAPVC
C. Coarctation of the aorta
D. Double aortic arch

464. You are asked to perform an echocardiogram on a patient whose heart, on chest x-ray, was noted to be located in the right chest (dextrocardia). There is a question as to whether the patient has congenital heart disease. Which of the following represents the best initial echocardiographic approach?

A. Subcostal long-axis sweep
B. Subcostal short-axis sweep
C. Parasternal long-axis sweep
D. Parasternal short-axis sweep

Refer to video PER-Q465.

465. What echocardiographic view was used for this video clip, and what cardiac structure are the arrows pointing to?

A. Parasternal short-axis view; left ventricular outflow tract
B. Apical three-chamber view; left ventricular outflow tract
C. Subcostal short-axis view; right ventricular outflow tract
D. Subcostal long-axis view; right ventricular inflow tract

AIT—Hotspot

Refer to video PER-Q466.

466. In this video clip what structure is marked by the arrows?

A. Right pulmonary artery
B. Right upper pulmonary vein
C. Right aortic arch
D. Innominate vein

AIT—Hotspot

467. In this subcostal short-axis image, not all cardiac information is visible. What maneuver should the operator perform to improve the imaging?

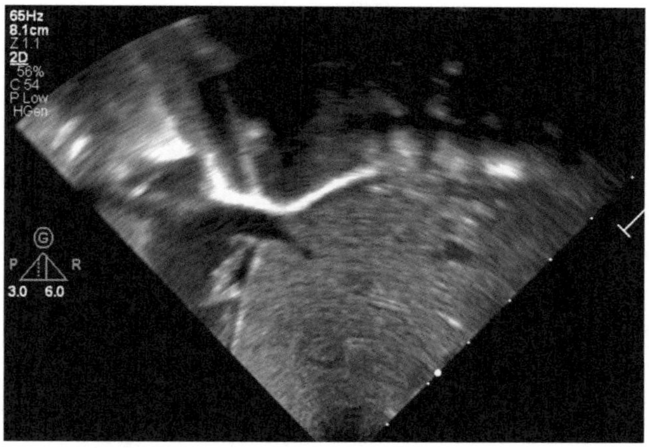

A. Rotate the transducer clockwise.
B. Rotate the transducer counterclockwise.
C. Move the "tail" of the transducer toward the feet (more inferiorly).
D. Move the tail of the transducer toward the head (more superiorly).

468. Using the subcostal long-axis sweep, more superior angulation of the transducer is most useful to evaluate which of the following?
A. Right and left ventricular outflow tracts
B. Individual pulmonary veins
C. Anatomy of the ductus arteriosus
D. Semilunar valve morphology

469. How should the apical four-chamber view be displayed for a pediatric echocardiogram?
A. Apex up, transducer notch/dot at 9 o'clock
B. Apex down, transducer notch/dot at 3 o'clock
C. Apex down, transducer notch/dot at 6 o'clock
D. Apex up, transducer notch/dot at 3 o'clock

470. The apical four-chamber and apical five-chamber views provide excellent diagnostic imaging of all of the following cardiac structures EXCEPT the:
A. Atrial septum
B. Tricuspid valve

C. Mitral valve
D. Left ventricular outflow tract

471. The apical four-chamber view is NOT useful for obtaining which parameter of systolic function?
   A. Left ventricular ejection fraction by single-plane modified Simpson's method
   B. Right ventricular fractional area change
   C. Left ventricular circumferential strain
   D. Tricuspid annular plane systolic excursion

472. You are scanning a patient with mirror-image dextrocardia. Your transducer is on the chest, positioned for the parasternal long-axis view that you just obtained. From this position, how do you rotate the transducer to obtain a parasternal short-axis view, and where will the transducer marker be pointed?
   A. Clockwise rotation; transducer marker pointing to the patient's left hip
   B. Counterclockwise rotation; transducer marker pointing to the patient's right hip
   C. Counterclockwise rotation; transducer marker pointing to the patient's right shoulder
   D. Clockwise rotation; transducer marker pointing to the patient's left shoulder

473. From the apical four-chamber view, what maneuver was performed to obtain the following image?

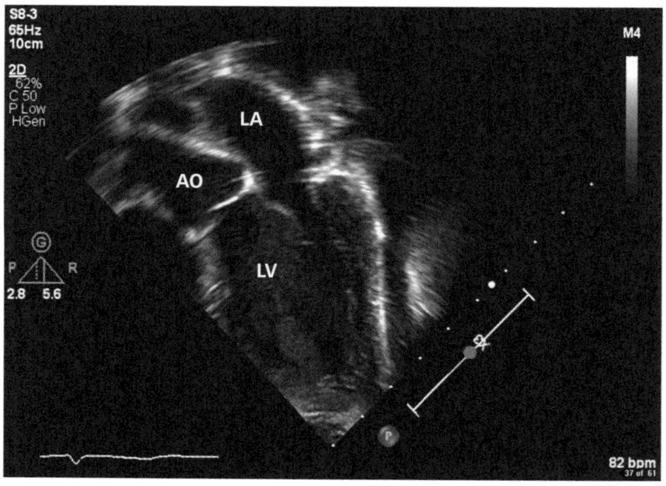

   A. Posterior angulation of the transducer
   B. Anterior angulation of the transducer

C. Rotation of the transducer counterclockwise with the notch/dot at 12–1 o'clock

D. Rotation of the transducer clockwise with the notch/dot at 4 o'clock

474. From the apical four-chamber view, what maneuver would you perform to obtain the following image?

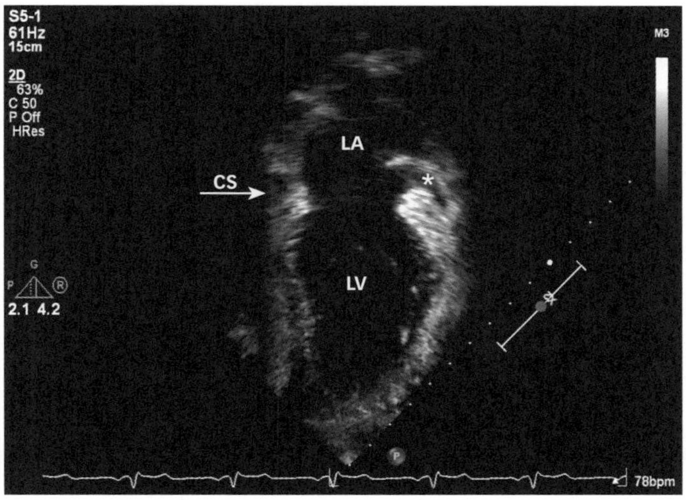

A. Rotate the transducer clockwise with the notch/dot at 6–7 o'clock.

B. Rotate the transducer counterclockwise with the notch/dot at 12–1 o'clock.

C. Angle the transducer to the right.

D. Angle the transducer to the left.

Refer to video PER-Q475.

475. This video clip is from the parasternal long-axis view. What transducer maneuver was performed?

A. Angulation to patient's right, then left

B. Angulation superiorly, then inferiorly

C. Rotation clockwise, then counterclockwise

D. Movement toward the right side of the patient's sternum, then toward the patient's left axilla

476. From the parasternal long-axis view, with rightward angulation of the transducer, all of the following additional cardiac structures can be imaged EXCEPT:

A. The coronary sinus

B. The mid to distal right coronary artery and posterior descending coronary artery

C. The right upper pulmonary vein

D. The right atrial appendage

Refer to video PER-Q477.

477. You want to obtain a standard parasternal long-axis view of your patient's heart and start with the view seen in this video clip. What is the next step?
   A. Rotate the transducer clockwise.
   B. Angle the transducer to the right.
   C. Move the transducer superiorly toward the right shoulder.
   D. Begin recording the images; this is a standard parasternal long-axis view.

478. Which view is the best to demonstrate the azygos vein draining into the superior vena cava?
   A. Subcostal sagittal view
   B. Subcostal coronal view
   C. Suprasternal coronal view
   D. Suprasternal sagittal view

Refer to video PER-Q479.

479. This video clip was obtained from what scan plane?
   A. High right parasternal parasagittal
   B. Suprasternal coronal
   C. Suprasternal sagittal
   D. Parasternal long-axis with rightward angulation

480. Which of the following echocardiographic views is the best to demonstrate a left superior vena cava?
   A. Parasternal long-axis view
   B. Parasternal short-axis view
   C. Apical four-chamber view
   D. Suprasternal coronal view

481. Which view best visualizes the origins and proximal courses for the right and left coronary arteries?
   A. High right parasternal parasagittal view at the level of the ascending aorta
   B. Parasternal short-axis view at the level of the aortic valve
   C. Apical four-chamber view with anterior angulation to visualize the aortic valve
   D. Subcostal short-axis en face view of the aortic valve

Refer to video PER-Q482.

482. What scan plane or window was used to obtain this video clip?
    A. Suprasternal notch coronal view
    B. Standard parasternal long-axis view with leftward angulation
    C. Left supraclavicular coronal view
    D. High left parasternal parasagittal view

483. You are attempting to evaluate the aortic arch in a patient with suspected coarctation of the aorta, but you are unable to visualize the distal aortic arch clearly by standard suprasternal imaging. What might your next step be?
    A. Move the transducer to a lower parasternal position to visualize the aortic arch.
    B. Place the patient in a left lateral decubitus position and try to reimage from the suprasternal window.
    C. Place a pillow under the patient's neck and shoulders and try to reimage from the suprasternal window.
    D. Move the transducer to the right supraclavicular position and attempt to reimage.

484. What is the best transducer position and maneuver to optimize visualization of the innominate (brachiocephalic) vein?
    A. Suprasternal sagittal view with the transducer notch/dot at 1–2 o'clock; axis from the left should point to the patient's right hip.
    B. Suprasternal coronal view with the transducer notch/dot at 3 o'clock; transducer should be angled anteriorly.
    C. High left parasternal view with the transducer notch/dot at 3 o'clock; transducer should be angled superiorly.
    D. High right parasternal parasagittal view with the transducer notch/dot at 12 o'clock; transducer should be angled to the patient's right side.

Refer to video PER-Q485.

485. This video clip is taken from a suprasternal coronal view. What is the structure indicated by the arrow?
   A. Left lower pulmonary vein
   B. Left pulmonary artery
   C. Coronary sinus
   D. Left atrial appendage

AIT—Hotspot

Refer to video PER-Q486.

486. The sweep in this video demonstrates which of the following?
   A. Left aortic arch, normal head and neck artery branching pattern
   B. Right aortic arch, mirror-image head and neck artery branching pattern
   C. Double aortic arch
   D. Aortic arch with indeterminate sidedness

487. You have obtained a suprasternal sagittal view of the aortic arch and want to use this view to determine aortic arch sidedness. Which of the following CANNOT be used to help determine aortic arch sidedness?
   A. Angulation of the transducer and transducer notch/dot setting
   B. Position of the aortic arch in relation to the trachea
   C. Appearance of the aortic arch
   D. Displaying the branching of the first head and neck arteries

PART 6

Measurement Techniques and Quantification

488. Which number marks the structure that is being used to measure the aortic isthmus?

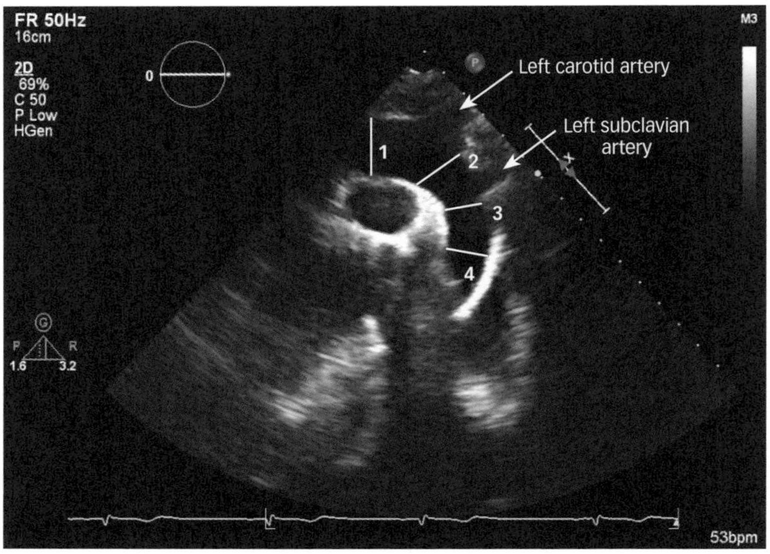

A. 1

B. 2

C. 3

D. 4

AIT—Hotspot

489. If the ascending aortic diameter is 12 mm, what measurement for the proximal aortic arch is considered hypoplastic?

A. 7 mm

B. 8 mm

C. 9 mm

D. 10 mm

490. The ascending aorta velocity is 2 m/sec, and aortic isthmus velocity is 4 m/sec. What is the true peak gradient across the aortic isthmus?

A. 16 mmHg

B. 36 mmHg

C. 48 mmHg

D. 64 mmHg

491. Which of the following cardiac defects has the spectral Doppler profile shown in this image?

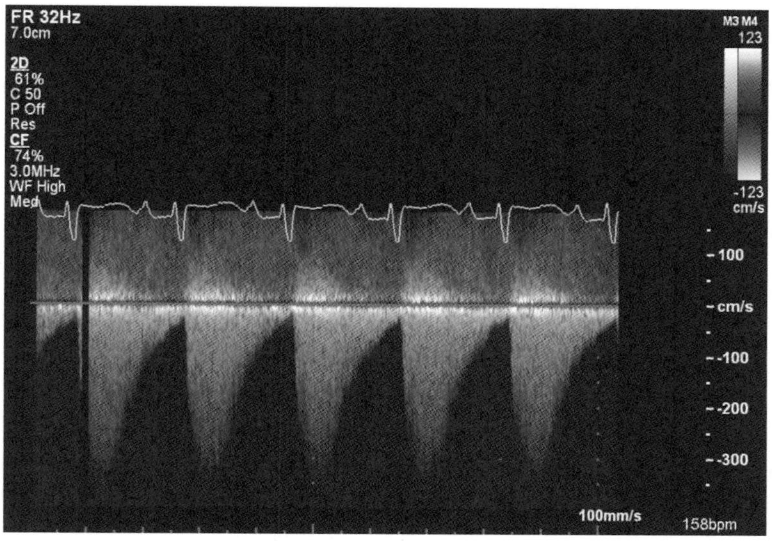

A. Aortic valve stenosis

B. Subaortic stenosis

C. Severe pulmonary valve stenosis

D. Coarctation of the aorta

492. You may use the simplified Bernoulli equation to calculate a pressure gradient that would be considered accurate in a patient who has:

A. Subaortic and aortic valve stenosis

B. Pulmonary valve stenosis

C. A supramitral valve ring and mitral valve stenosis

D. Long-segment coarctation

493. All of the following conditions will affect accurate assessment of aortic valve stenosis EXCEPT:

A. A large patent ductus arteriosus

B. Anemia

C. Mild pulmonary valve stenosis

D. A dilated left ventricle with a shortening fraction of 20% and an ejection fraction of 40%

Refer to video PER-Q494.

494. You obtain a peak velocity of 2.3 m/sec across the aortic valve from the apical five-chamber view for the patient seen in this video clip. The spectral Doppler signal is clear and parallel to the blood flow. If this patient also has a large ventricular septal defect, what do you think of the measurement of the aortic valve peak velocity?
   A. It is accurate.
   B. It is underestimated.
   C. It is overestimated.
   D. A mean gradient is more accurate.

495. You are asked to perform an echocardiogram on a newborn baby. From the suprasternal view, you see a good-sized aortic arch with a posterior "shelf" at the level of the aortic isthmus and a moderately sized patent ductus arteriosus (PDA). The peak velocity across the aortic isthmus is 2.0 m/sec. What is your diagnosis?
   A. Normal arch
   B. Aortic arch obstruction
   C. Potential coarctation of the aorta
   D. Hypoplastic aortic arch

496. Which echocardiographic view is the best to detect and evaluate an anterior muscular ventricular septal defect by color Doppler?
   A. Suprasternal coronal view
   B. Parasternal short-axis view
   C. Apical four-chamber view
   D. Subcostal coronal view

497. A patient has a perimembranous ventricular septal defect, and spectral Doppler shows a peak velocity across the defect of 4 m/sec. What is the peak gradient through the defect?
   A. 8 mmHg
   B. 16 mmHg
   C. 32 mmHg
   D. 64 mmHg

498. The same patient (see question 497) has a blood pressure of 120/70 mmHg. What is the estimated right ventricular systolic pressure?

A. 112 mmHg

B. 104 mmHg

C. 64 mmHg

D. 56 mmHg

499. While using a parasternal long-axis view, you sweep toward the tricuspid valve and suspect a ventricular septal defect (VSD) because you see red color flow that might be crossing the ventricular septum. What will you do to further investigate the red color flow profile?

A. Use continuous-wave spectral Doppler. If it is high velocity, a VSD is confirmed.

B. Use continuous-wave spectral Doppler. If the flow is systolic, a VSD is possible.

C. Lower the Nyquist limit.

D. Increase the color Doppler gain.

500. A 5-year-old patient with mitral stenosis due to a single papillary muscle (i.e., a parachute mitral valve) and no other form of congenital heart disease is being seen by a cardiologist. The mean pressure gradient for this mitral valve was recorded as 8 mmHg by echocardiography. The mean gradient tells you that the degree of mitral valve stenosis is:

A. Normal

B. Mild

C. Moderate

D. Severe

501. In which of the following conditions should the mean gradient across the atrial septum be measured because it could be important for acute clinical management?

A. Atrial septal defect

B. Transposition of the great arteries (d-TGA) with intact ventricular septum

C. Congenitally corrected transposition of the great arteries (ccTGA)

D. Double-inlet left ventricle

502. Spectral Doppler demonstrates a peak velocity of 1 m/sec across an atrial septal defect. Which of the following statements is correct?
   A. Left atrial pressure is low.
   B. Right atrial pressure is low.
   C. Right atrial pressure is high.
   D. The peak pressure gradient between the left and right atrium is 4 mmHg.

503. The mean gradient across your patient's aortic valve is 45 mmHg, and there is preserved left ventricular systolic function. What is the most likely diagnosis?
   A. Mild aortic valve stenosis
   B. Moderate aortic valve stenosis
   C. Severe aortic valve stenosis
   D. More information is required.

504. Your patient has normal left ventricular systolic function. Continuous-wave Doppler measurement of the peak velocity across the aortic valve is 3.5 m/sec. Based on this measurement, what is the severity of aortic valve stenosis?
   A. Mild
   B. Moderate
   C. Severe
   D. 2D images are needed to make a determination.

505. You have calculated the aortic valve area in your young adult patient to be 0.9 cm^2. Which of the following best describes the condition of this patient's aortic valve?
   A. Mildly stenotic
   B. Moderately stenotic
   C. Severely stenotic
   D. Normal

506. A patient had aortic valve regurgitation noted on the last office visit. Today the echocardiogram reveals that the left ventricle is more dilated compared to the last study. You measure the aortic valve regurgitation by spectral Doppler. Which of the following statements is correct?
   A. Aortic pressure half-time (PHT) became shorter.
   B. Aortic PHT became longer.

C. Aortic PHT remained the same.

D. Aortic PHT is not a parameter used to evaluate aortic valve regurgitation.

507. Your patient is a young adult who is noted on physical exam to have an Austin Flint murmur. An echocardiogram is obtained with the spectral Doppler characteristics seen in this image. What does this image demonstrate?

See Color Plate 25 on page xxxi.

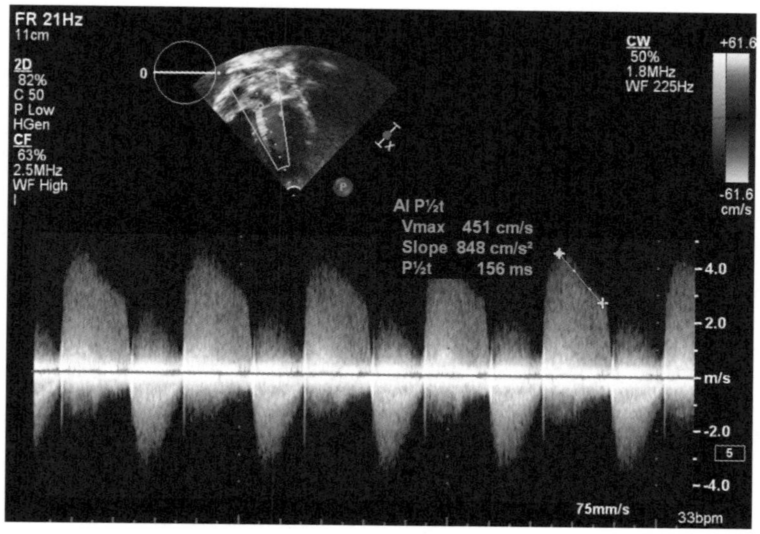

A. Severe aortic valve regurgitation

B. Mild pulmonary valve regurgitation

C. Moderate mitral valve stenosis

D. Moderate tricuspid valve stenosis

508. This image from a spectral Doppler tracing of the descending abdominal aorta most likely demonstrates which of the following?

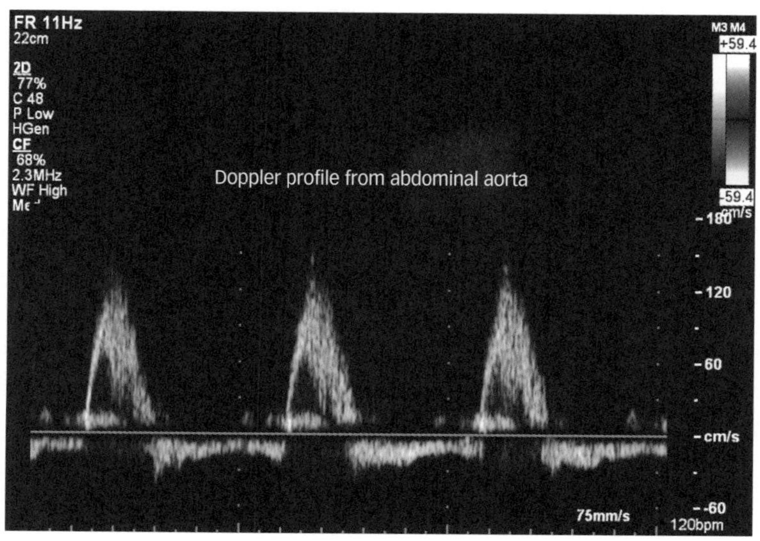

A. Normal Doppler profile
B. Coarctation of the aorta
C. Aortic valve regurgitation
D. Aortitis

509. Aside from 2D imaging and color flow Doppler of the aortic valve, what other echocardiographic parameters can be used to evaluate acute, moderate to severe aortic valve regurgitation?
A. Left ventricle tissue Doppler
B. Left ventricle dimension
C. Left ventricular ejection fraction
D. Reversal of flow in the descending aorta

Refer to video PER-Q510.

510. A color flow Doppler is obtained from the distal aortic arch and descending aorta, as seen in this video clip. The feature demonstrated in the video is NOT usually seen in the presence of:
A. A small patent ductus arteriosus
B. An aortopulmonary window
C. A large cerebral arteriovenous malformation
D. A Blalock-Taussig shunt

AIT—Hotspot

511. In a parasternal short-axis view, color flow Doppler demonstrates reversal of flow in both pulmonary arteries. Which diagnosis is most likely?
A. Moderate-sized patent ductus arteriosus
B. Aortopulmonary window
C. Branch pulmonary artery stenosis
D. Moderate to severe pulmonary valve regurgitation

512. Which of the following values is NOT needed for the echocardiographic calculation of cardiac output?
A. Aortic valve annulus diameter
B. Peak velocity across the aortic valve
C. Heart rate
D. Time velocity integral across the aortic valve

513. Shortening fraction (SF) is affected by several parameters. Assuming that left ventricular contractility is normal, what happens to SF when left ventricular volume acutely increases?

A. SF stays the same.

B. SF increases.

C. SF decreases.

D. SF may or may not be affected; more information is needed.

514. What is normal range for the resting left ventricular shortening fraction?

A. 15%–20%

B. 20%–25%

C. 28%–38%

D. Greater than 40%

515. Which of the following situations will NOT affect the reliability of the left ventricular shortening fraction (SF) calculation, as measured by M-mode echocardiography?

A. Ventricular septal dyskinesis

B. Paradoxical ventricular septum systolic motion

C. Reduced global ventricular wall motion

D. Abnormal ECG with bigeminy

516. Z-scores are often used to compare certain important cardiovascular structure measurements in the pediatric population. What is a Z-score for a specific cardiac structure?

A. A value based on the standard deviation around a mean value for that particular cardiac structure which varies by body surface area

B. A value based on the standard deviation around a mean value for that particular cardiac structure which varies by body weight

C. A fixed value (constant) for that particular cardiac structure for the entire pediatric population, irrespective of age, weight, or height

D. A value for that particular cardiac structure based on the comparable adult measurement, which has been modified for the pediatric population

517. Which of the following parameters is NOT applied in the calculation of left ventricular mass using M-mode measurements?
   A. Left ventricular end-diastolic dimension
   B. Posterior left ventricular wall thickness in end diastole
   C. Heart rate
   D. Interventricular septum wall thickness in end diastole

518. What does dP/dt measure?
   A. Ventricular contractility
   B. Ventricular diastolic function
   C. Ventricular elasticity
   D. The ratio between diastolic pressure and diastolic duration

519. What can you do to reduce measurement error when performing an assessment of dP/dt?
   A. Use a Doppler sweep speed of 150 cm/sec
   B. Use a Doppler sweep speed of 50 cm/sec
   C. Use a higher Nyquist limit to better demonstrate the peak Doppler velocity
   D. Use pulsed-wave Doppler

520. On an echocardiogram, you suspect a patient might have a left superior vena cava (SVC) draining directly into the left atrium. What will you do next to confirm this?
   A. Use a suprasternal coronal view.
   B. Use a subcostal view.
   C. Inject agitated saline into a vein in the right arm.
   D. Inject agitated saline into a vein in the left arm.

521. The use of agitated saline during echocardiography is NOT helpful for diagnosing:
   A. An unroofed coronary sinus
   B. Atrial septal defects
   C. Pulmonary arteriovenous fistulae
   D. Aortopulmonary collaterals

522. Your patient underwent a Fontan procedure, and his systemic arterial oxygen saturation is now in the lower 90s. Which simple method can help diagnose suspected hepatopulmonary syndrome (pulmonary arteriovenous malformations)?

A. Echocardiogram with color Doppler
B. Echocardiogram with contrast (bubble study)
C. Cardiac catheterization
D. Magnetic resonance imaging

523. In which scenario is contrast echocardiography using agitated saline NOT useful?

A. A young patient with a thromboembolic stroke
B. Unexplained hypoxemia
C. Possible intra-atrial baffle leak following an atrial switch procedure
D. Blalock-Taussig shunt patency

524. This spectral Doppler tracing was obtained from pulmonary venous Doppler inflow. Which number indicates pulmonary vein atrial flow reversal?

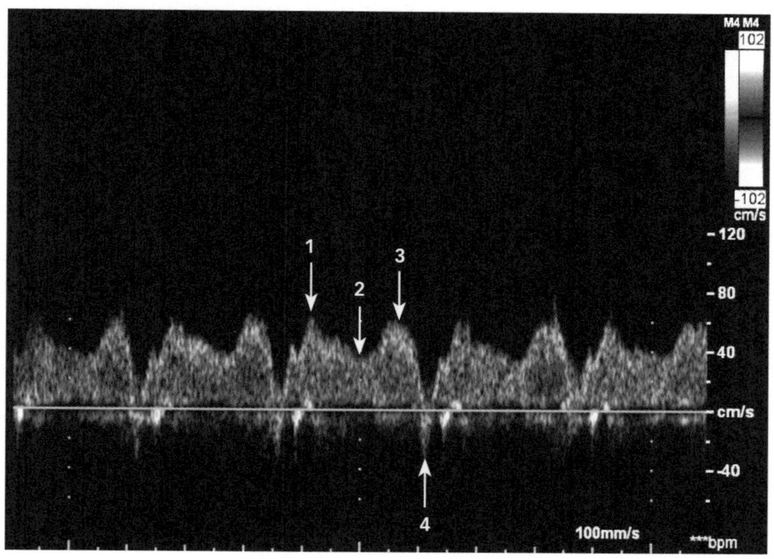

A. 1
B. 2
C. 3
D. 4

AIT—Hotspot

525. In the image in question 524, what is the arrow labeled 1 pointing to?

A. S wave

B. A wave

C. D wave

D. E wave

AIT—Hotspot

526. This image displays the spectral recording of a pulmonary vein Doppler tracing. Which number represents systole?

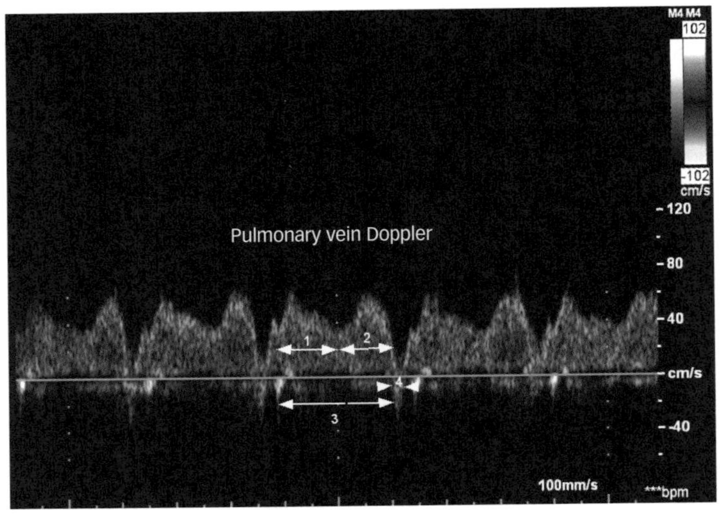

A. 1

B. 2

C. 3

D. 4

AIT—Hotspot

527. What maneuver can be performed to optimize the color flow Doppler evaluation of the pulmonary veins?

A. Reduce color Doppler sector

B. Increase Nyquist limit

C. Use color flow Doppler comparison

D. Increase Doppler gain as much as possible

528. Which of the following spectral Doppler features will NOT be found with pulmonary vein stenosis?

A. Deeper atrial reversal (Ar) wave

B. Increased peak velocity and mean gradient

C. Loss of phasic variation in the spectral Doppler signal

D. Turbulent flow by color Doppler

529. Which of the following coexisting cardiac defects can lead to underestimation of the severity of mitral valve stenosis?

A. Ventricular septal defect

B. Patent ductus arteriosus

C. Mitral valve regurgitation

D. Atrial septal defect

530. As mitral valve stenosis becomes worse, mitral valve pressure half-time:

A. Becomes longer

B. Becomes shorter

C. Does not change

D. Is indeterminate since more information is needed

531. Which of the following factors will NOT affect pressure half-time in the calculation of mitral valve area?

A. Left atrial pressure

B. Left ventricle diastolic pressure

C. Heart rate

D. Body surface area

532. Which of the following mean gradients is considered the threshold value for early or mild mitral valve stenosis?

A. >3 mmHg

B. >5 mmHg

C. >7 mmHg

D. >9 mmHg

533. Which of the following echocardiographic views of the left ventricle best demonstrates a cleft in the anterior leaflet of the mitral valve?

A. Parasternal long-axis view

B. Parasternal short-axis view

C. Apical four-chamber view

D. Subcostal long-axis view

534. What is the definition of mitral valve prolapse?
   A. Mitral valve displaced >1 mm in systole
   B. Mitral valve displaced >1.5 mm in diastole
   C. Mitral valve displaced >2 mm in systole
   D. Mitral valve displaced >2 mm in diastole

535. An infant boy has been diagnosed with a large ventricular septal defect (VSD). His vital signs include a blood pressure of 70/50 mmHg. The tricuspid valve regurgitation (TR) is trivial, with an incomplete spectral Doppler signal and a peak velocity measured at 2.5 m/sec. What is your estimation of right ventricular systolic pressure?
   A. 30 mmHg
   B. 70 mmHg
   C. Indeterminate; a complete TR spectral Doppler envelope is needed.
   D. Indeterminate; cardiac catheterization is needed to obtain the necessary data.

536. For a person reading an echocardiogram, which echocardiographic view best displays the spatial relationship between the great arteries?
   A. Parasternal long-axis view
   B. Parasternal short-axis view
   C. Apical four- or five-chamber view
   D. Subcostal long- or short-axis view

537. The Qp/Qs ratio represents the ratio of:
   A. Pulmonary artery diameter to aorta diameter
   B. Pulmonary blood flow to systemic blood flow
   C. Cardiac output to body surface area
   D. Systemic artery pressure to pulmonary artery pressure

538. What is the normal Qp/Qs value?
   A. <1
   B. >1
   C. 1
   D. Variable from one person to the next

539. A patient has an atrial septal defect with left-to-right shunting. Which of the following is most likely the Qp/Qs ratio for this patient?

A. 1.5:1

B. 1:1

C. 1:1.3

D. 0.7:1

540. A mean arterial blood pressure is needed to calculate left ventricular end-systolic wall stress in a heart transplant patient. The only information available is the measured blood pressure of 120/70 mmHg. What is the estimated mean blood pressure?

A. 80 mmHg

B. 87 mmHg

C. 95 mmHg

D. 100 mmHg

541. In pediatrics, how common is diastolic heart disease in the absence of congenital heart disease?

A. Frequent in neonates

B. Rare among all pediatric patients

C. Common in young athletes

D. Common in teenagers

542. How do spectral Doppler reference values for diastolic dysfunction differ in the pediatric population as compared with the values used for the adult population?

A. They are the same for both pediatric and adult patients.

B. They differ only for the neonatal population.

C. They do not exist for the neonatal population.

D. They vary by age.

543. The spectral Doppler inflow indices seen in this image are most likely:

See Color Plate 26 on page xxxi.

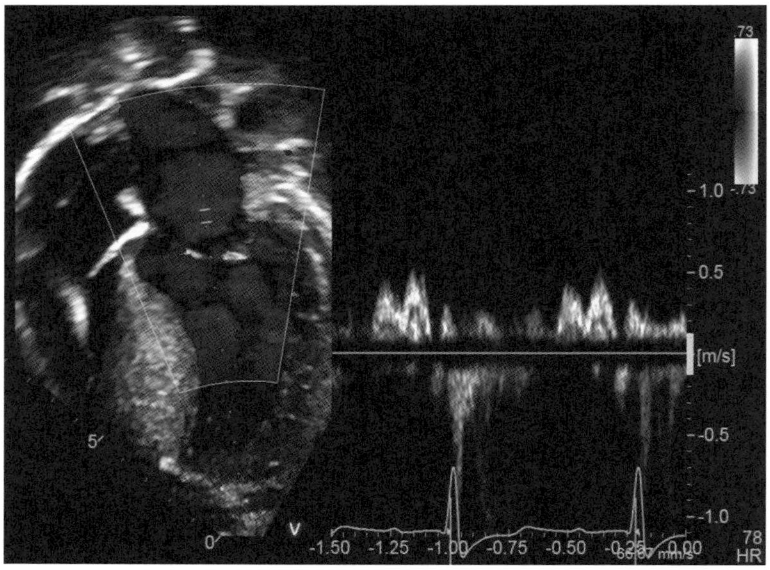

A. Normal filling velocities

B. Abnormal due to mitral valve morphology

C. Normal in the presence of the L wave

D. Abnormally decreased due to spectral gate position

544. In the continuous-wave spectral Doppler pattern seen in this image, what is being measured?

See Color Plate 27 on page xxxii.

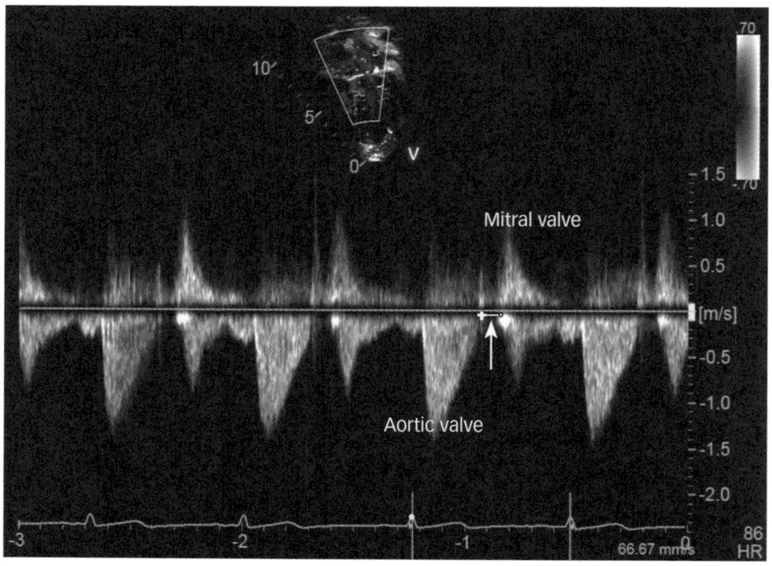

A. Exaggerated atrial A-wave reversal

B. Isovolumic relaxation time

C. Normal atrial A wave

D. Isovolumic contraction time

AIT—Hotspot

545. Isovolumic relaxation time is typically:

A. Increased in the presence of abnormal ventricular compliance and markedly elevated atrial pressure
B. Not affected by impaired relaxation
C. Increased with impaired left ventricular relaxation and normal left atrial pressure
D. Decreased with impaired left ventricular relaxation

546. Echocardiography was performed on a patient to evaluate for anthracycline cardiotoxicity. The previous echocardiogram showed normal left ventricular fractional shortening and a normal ejection fraction with normal sinus rhythm. On this visit the echocardiogram shows normal fractional shortening, a normal ejection fraction, and tachycardia. Which of the following is the most likely description of the mitral E wave on today's visit?

A. The E wave and A wave are not fused.
B. There is no change in E-wave deceleration time.
C. E-wave deceleration time is increased.
D. E-wave deceleration time is decreased.

547. You are about to perform an echocardiogram on a young adult with a parachute mitral valve and mitral stenosis. What will the mitral valve inflow pattern, recorded with pulsed-wave Doppler, tell you about diastolic function?

A. Left ventricular compliance can be assessed if used in conjunction with tissue Doppler imaging.
B. Impaired relaxation exists if there is a lower-velocity E wave as compared to a higher-velocity A wave.
C. A normal E/A-wave ratio indicates normal left ventricular diastolic function.
D. Findings are not reliable; diastolic function cannot be assessed in this setting.

548. Inspiration in a normal patient has the most effect on which of the following diastolic parameters?

A. Tricuspid annular a′ wave measured with tissue Doppler imaging
B. Tricuspid E wave, early right ventricular filling
C. Mitral valve a′ wave measured with tissue Doppler imaging
D. Mitral valve e′ wave measured with tissue Doppler imaging

549. In this image, which letter best represents early left ventricular filling?

See Color Plate 28 on page xxxii.

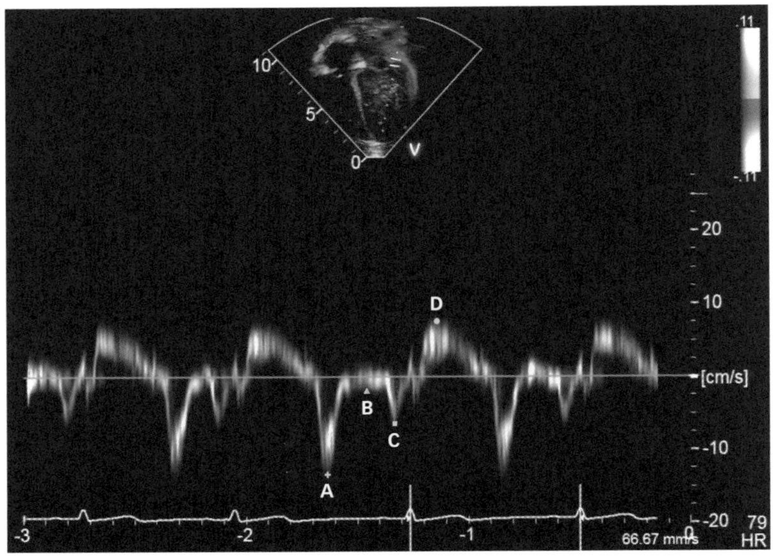

A. A

B. B

C. C

D. D

AIT—Hotspot

550. Increased left atrial volume is a marker of:

A. Acutely impaired left ventricular relaxation

B. Chronic left ventricular diastolic dysfunction

C. Normal left ventricular diastolic function

D. Improving left ventricular diastolic function

551. With echocardiography, left atrial volume is best determined by which of the following methods?

A. M-mode

B. Inclusion of the left atrial appendage

C. Simpson's method

D. Inclusion of the proximal pulmonary veins

552. In the normal neonatal heart what is the most common mitral Doppler inflow pattern?

A. Increased E-wave deceleration compared with that of a teenager

B. Increased isovolumic relaxation time compared with that of a teenager

C. Decreased E-wave/A-wave ratio as compared to that of older children

D. Increased E-wave velocity and very low A-wave velocity

553. A mitral valve E wave that is decreased in comparison to the A wave most likely represents which of the following?

A. Abnormal left ventricular relaxation with normal left atrial pressure

B. Restrictive cardiomyopathy

C. Normal finding in the young adult

D. Noncompliant left ventricle

554. An L wave is most often seen in which of the following settings?

A. Abnormal relaxation and slower heart rates

B. Abnormal relaxation and fast heart rates

C. Abnormal relaxation, elevated left atrial pressure, and fast heart rates

D. Abnormal left ventricular compliance

555. An increase in duration of the pulmonary vein Ar wave (atrial reversal with atrial contraction), as compared to the duration of the mitral valve inflow A wave (late left ventricular filling), is a sign of:

A. Decreased left ventricular filling pressure

B. Normal left ventricular filling pressure

C. Increased left ventricular filling pressure

D. Normal left atrial pressure

556. Which of these E/e′ ratios best correlates with an increased left ventricular end-diastolic pressure (LVEDP) by echocardiography?

A. E/e′ ratio of 2

B. E/e′ ratio of 5

C. E/e′ ratio of 8

D. E/e′ ratio of 12

557. This spectral Doppler image was taken from a structurally normal heart, with an E/A ratio of 3. What does it demonstrate?

See Color Plate 29 on page xxxiii.

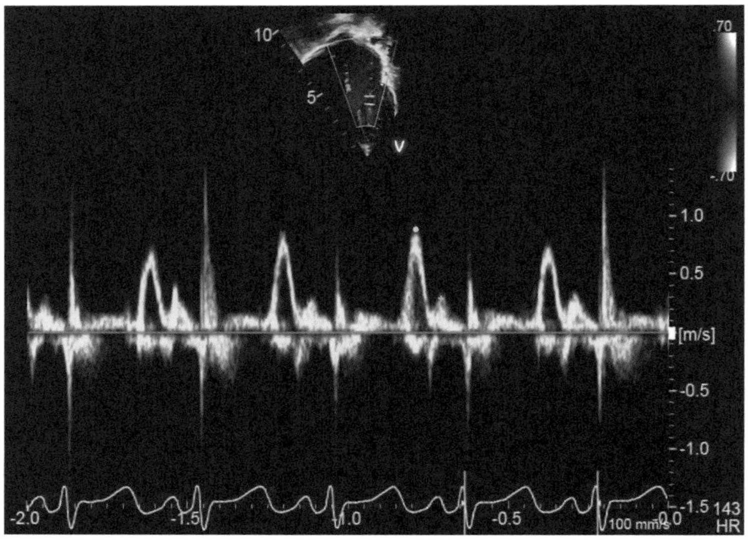

A. Normal left atrial pressure

B. Normal left ventricular filling pressure

C. Abnormal left ventricular diastolic compliance

D. Pseudonormal left ventricular filling pattern

558. A patient is scheduled for outpatient echocardiography and was referred to cardiology because of systemic hypertension. You find the patient to have left ventricular hypertrophy. Which option listed below most likely represents the chance that this patient has a diastolic filling abnormality?

A. 10%

B. 36%

C. 62%

D. 95%

559. Which of the following techniques is most important for accurately estimating left atrial volume?

A. Including the pulmonary vein ostia and excluding the left atrial appendage

B. Using the longest atrial length obtained from either the apical two-chamber or apical four-chamber view

C. Including both the pulmonary vein ostia and the left atrial appendage

D. Measuring atrial lengths in both the apical four-chamber and apical two-chamber views

560. This spectral Doppler image was obtained from the pulmonary vein of an infant. Which statement best describes the state of left ventricular diastolic function in this patient?

See Color Plate 30 on page xxxiii.

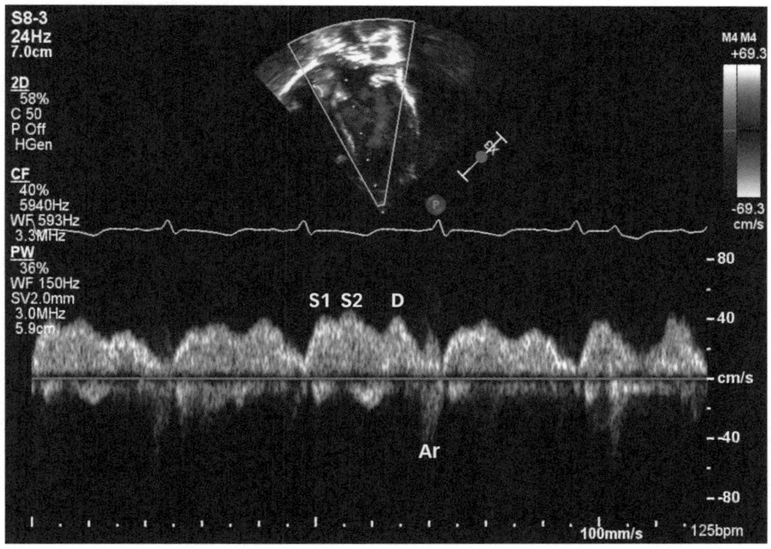

A. An Ar wave (atrial reversal with atrial contraction) suggests diastolic dysfunction.

B. Triphasic pulmonary venous inflow waves are not seen in this image, indicating diastolic disease.

C. Triphasic pulmonary venous inflow waves are seen during atrial filling and do not indicate diastolic disease.

D. This pulmonary vein tracing indicates diastolic dysfunction with abnormal relaxation.

561. You visualize an L wave in the spectral Doppler tracing from a patient with abnormal relaxation and a slow heart rate. Which option best describes the timing of the L wave?

A. Isovolumic relaxation

B. Late ventricular filling

C. Isovolumic contraction

D. Diastasis

562. In this image, identify the letter on the electrocardiogram that corresponds with late ventricular diastolic filling.

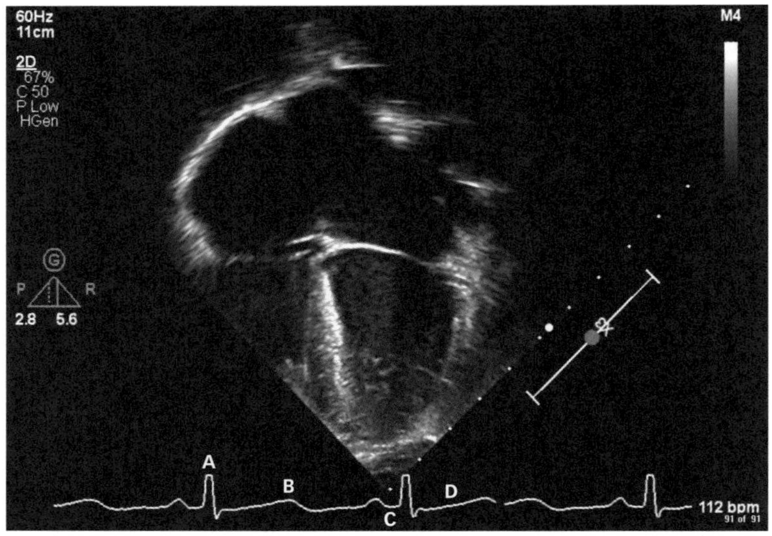

A. A
B. B
C. C
D. D

AIT—Hotspot

563. When would you see an E/A ratio of less than 1?
   A. With abnormal relaxation and normal left atrial pressure
   B. With restrictive cardiomyopathy
   C. In an athlete
   D. In a young adult

564. During echocardiography of a 13-year-old, you find an E/A ratio greater than 2.8, an E/e′ ratio greater than 15, biatrial enlargement, and a shortened deceleration time. These findings are most consistent with which of the following choices?
   A. Abnormal relaxation with normal left atrial pressure
   B. Normal compliance of the left ventricle
   C. Noncompliant, stiff left ventricle
   D. Normal relaxation with elevated left atrial pressure

565. What does a prolonged pulmonary vein Ar wave suggest in a pediatric patient?
   A. Atrial fibrillation
   B. Normal left ventricular relaxation with normal left atrial pressure
   C. Normal left ventricular filling pressure
   D. Diastolic dysfunction

566. Which of the following is the best technique for measuring the volume of a left atrium that appears enlarged?
   A. Measure in the parasternal short-axis plane by Simpson's method (summation of disks).
   B. Measure in the apical two-chamber plane by the area-length method.
   C. Using M-mode, measure in the parasternal long-axis plane from the posterior aortic wall to the posterior left atrial wall.
   D. Measure in both the apical two-chamber and apical four-chamber planes using biplane Simpson's method (summation of disks).

567. What is the appropriate point in the cardiac cycle to measure left atrial volume?
   A. At the onset of the P wave on the electrocardiogram (ECG)
   B. At end systole before mitral valve opening
   C. At end diastole during late ventricular filling with the mitral valve open
   D. At the onset of the QRS complex on the ECG

568. While scanning a patient with suspected mitral valve hypoplasia, you are asked: Is the mitral valve too small? Which of the following best describes what to do next?
   A. Go to a parasternal short-axis view and acquire the best en face view to perform 2D planimetry.
   B. Go to the apical four-chamber view and measure the mitral valve annulus from leading edge to leading edge.
   C. Go to a subcostal short-axis view and acquire the best en face view to perform 2D planimetry.
   D. Go to the apical four-chamber view and measure the mitral valve annulus from inner edge to inner edge.

569. In this image of the mitral valve annulus, how would you best characterize the placement of the calipers?

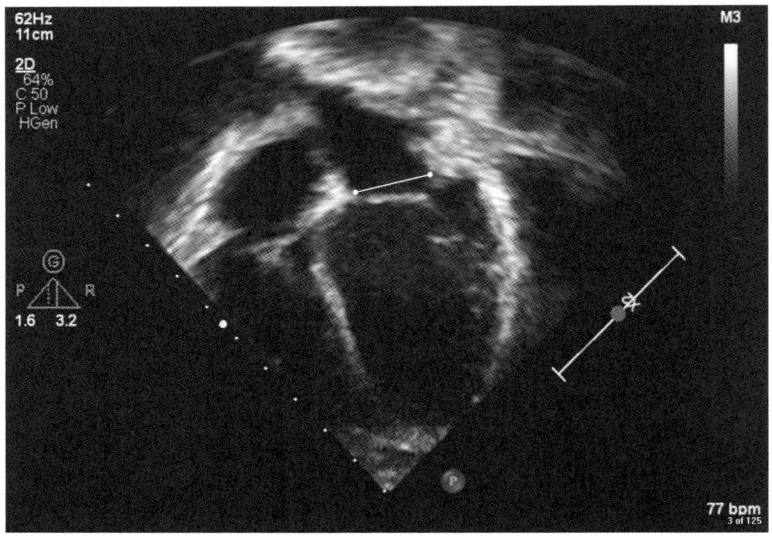

A. Incorrect for measurement of the annulus because the mitral valve is closed

B. Leading edge to leading edge and therefore acceptable for measuring the annulus

C. Inner edge to inner edge and therefore correct for measuring the annulus

D. Incorrect angulation of the calipers and therefore incorrect for measuring the annulus

570. Your 5-year-old patient has thickened, rolled leaflets and short chordae tendineae. Which measurement will you perform to evaluate for mitral valve stenosis?

A. Mean mitral valve gradient with pulsed-wave Doppler

B. Pressure half-time (PHT) to determine mitral valve area

C. Mean mitral valve gradient with continuous-wave Doppler

D. Mitral valve area using 2D planimetry in the parasternal short-axis plane

571. What does this image demonstrate about the mitral valve?

See Color Plate 31 on page xxxiv.

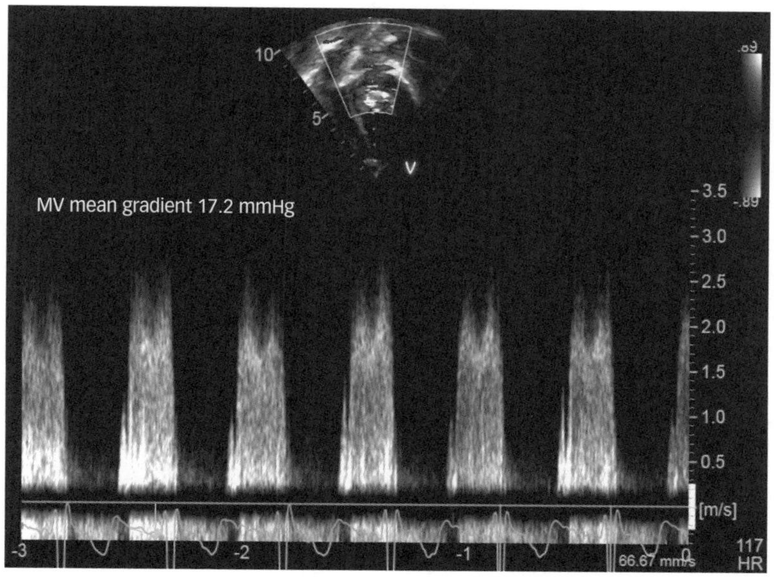

A. Normal mean mitral valve gradient

B. Mild mitral valve stenosis

C. Moderate mitral valve stenosis

D. Severe mitral valve stenosis

572. Which dimension of the tricuspid valve is being measured in this image?

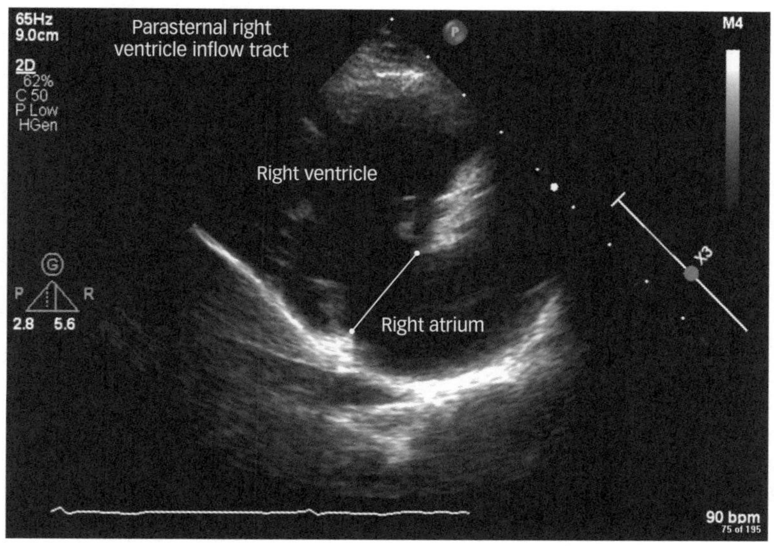

A. Septal–lateral diameter

B. Anterior–posterior diameter

C. Anterior–septal diameter

D. Posterior–septal diameter

Refer to video PER-Q573.

573. This video clip is from a patient with L-looped ventricles. For this patient, what should you measure to determine tricuspid valve diameter?

   A. Left-sided atrioventricular valve (AV valve) at the widest diameter in early diastole

   B. Left-sided AV valve at the widest diameter in late systole

   C. Right-sided AV valve at the widest diameter in early diastole

   D. Right-sided AV valve at the widest diameter in early systole

574. This spectral Doppler image is taken from a patient who has an atrial septal defect (ASD) with a large left-to-right shunt and no mitral valve regurgitation. There is a question as to whether this patient has mitral valve stenosis. Which of the following options will help the cardiologist make this determination?

See Color Plate 32 on page xxxiv.

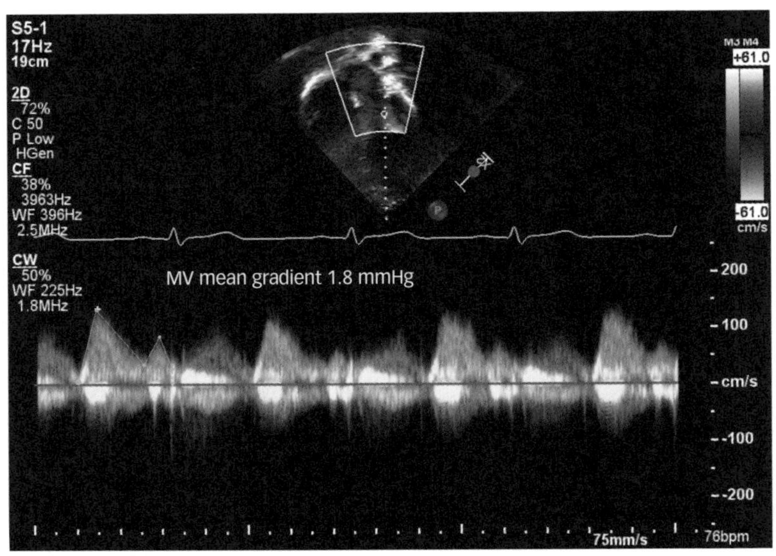

   A. The mean mitral pressure gradient is within normal range; no mitral valve stenosis.

   B. The mean mitral valve pressure gradient is increased.

   C. The mean mitral pressure gradient is underestimated due to the presence of an ASD.

   D. The mean mitral gradient should have been traced over three consecutive beats, so the measurement is incomplete and therefore not useful.

Refer to video PER-Q575.

575. What value would be most useful in diagnosing the anomaly demonstrated in this video clip?
   A. 2D planimetry of tricuspid valve orifice area
   B. Celermajer index
   C. Displacement index
   D. Tricuspid valve annulus size in early diastole

576. In the presence of Ebstein anomaly, a Celermajer index greater than 1 indicates:
   A. Normal cardiac function in the setting of tricuspid valve regurgitation
   B. Poor prognosis in the setting of Ebstein anomaly of the mitral valve
   C. Good prognosis in the setting of borderline pulmonary pressures
   D. Poor prognosis in the setting of Ebstein anomaly of the tricuspid valve

577. Tricuspid valve stenosis is LEAST associated with:
   A. Hepatomegaly
   B. Right atrial hypertrophy
   C. Right ventricular outflow tract obstruction
   D. Obligatory left-to-right atrial shunting

578. The right ventricular free wall thickness should be measured:
   A. Just below the pulmonary valve
   B. At end diastole
   C. With heavy trabeculations included
   D. Just past the QRS complex on the electrocardiogram tracing

579. In hypoplastic left heart syndrome, the anatomic variant with mitral stenosis and aortic atresia is most likely to be associated with:
   A. Endocardial fibroelastosis
   B. Absence of the left or right sixth aortic arch
   C. Unguarded mitral valve orifice
   D. Giant left atrium

580. This image is an apical four-chamber view in the setting of L-looped ventricles. What is being measured?

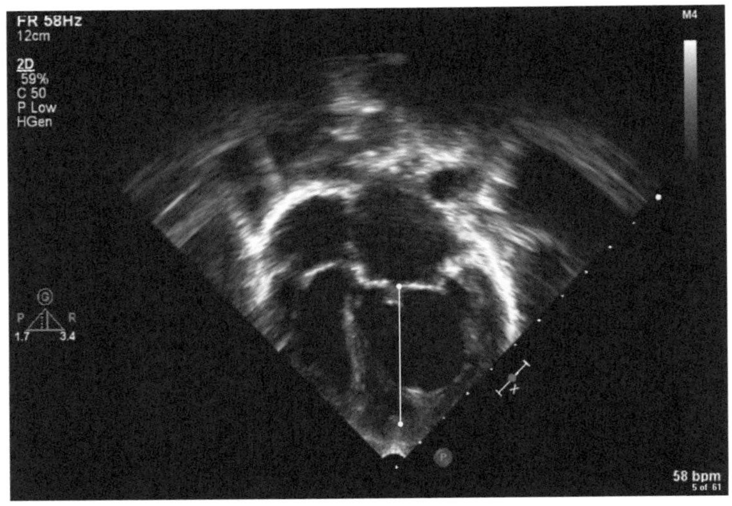

A. Left ventricular length

B. Right ventricular length

C. Fractional area change

D. Tricuspid annular plane systolic excursion

581. This image is an apical four-chamber view taken from a patient with a normal heart. The diastolic area for right ventricular fractional area change is being measured (see tracing in this image). Which of these statements best describes what is occurring?

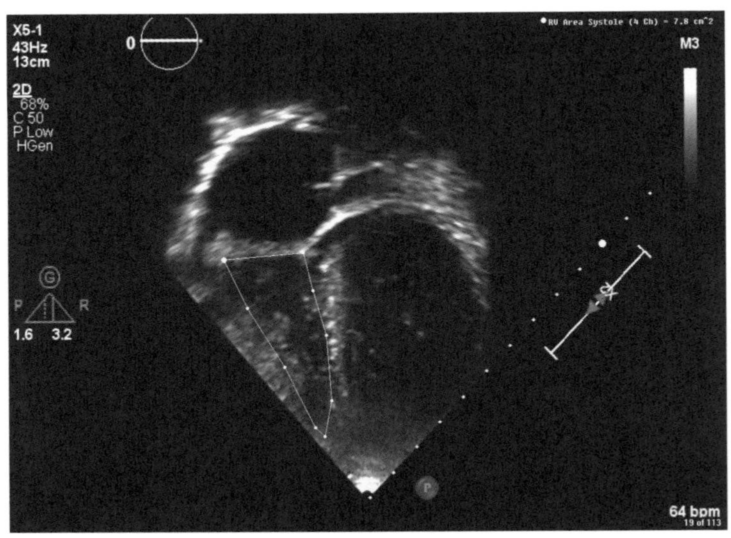

A. This is a standard apical four-chamber view.

B. The image is well centered in the right ventricle.

C. The image is not well centered in the right ventricle.

D. The right ventricular area is being incorrectly measured with the tricuspid valve open.

582. What is the normal value for right ventricular fractional area change (RVFAC)?

A. <20%

B. 20%–30%

C. 30%–35%

D. >35%

583. Which equation is used to calculate right ventricular fractional area change (RVFAC)? (RVEDA = right ventricular end-diastolic area and RVESA = right ventricular end-systolic area.)

A. RVFAC (%) = [(RVEDA − RVESA)/RVEDA] × 100

B. RVFAC (%) = [RVEDA/RVESA + RVEDA] × 100

C. RVFAC (%) = [(RVEDA + RVESA)/RVEDA] × 100

D. RVFAC (%) = [(RVEDA + RVESA) × RVEDA] × 100

Refer to video PER-Q584.

584. This video clip is of superoinferior ventricles (upstairs-downstairs heart). Which of the following is the most likely diagnosis?

A. Normal right ventricular dimensions

B. Hypoplasia of the left ventricle

C. Hypoplasia of the right ventricle

D. Atrial and ventricular septa that are aligned with each other

585. You have finished an echocardiogram on a patient in the cardiac intensive care unit who just underwent an arterial switch operation and is now found to have a hypokinetic left ventricular apex. Which of the following is the best option for assessing left ventricular function in this setting?

A. Fractional shortening derived by M-mode

B. Fractional shortening derived by 2D echocardiography

C. Ejection fraction derived by biplane Simpson's method

D. Ejection fraction derived by M-mode

586. What value, expressed as a percentage, is calculated by this formula:

$$(LVEDV - LVESV)/LVEDV \times 100$$

where LVEDV = left ventricular end-diastolic volume and LVESV = left ventricular end-systolic volume?

A. Left ventricular mass

B. Ejection fraction by biplane Simpson's method

C. Fractional shortening using M-mode

D. Fractional shortening using 2D technique

587. You are using the area-length method to calculate left ventricular ejection fraction. Which of the following views will you choose to obtain the left ventricular area?

A. Parasternal long-axis

B. Apical two-chamber

C. Subcostal short-axis

D. Subcostal long-axis

588. You are calculating left ventricular ejection fraction with the area-length method. Which of these views will you use to obtain the left ventricular length?

A. Subcostal short-axis

B. Subcostal long-axis

C. Parasternal short-axis

D. Parasternal long-axis

589. What is the formula for calculating left ventricular (LV) volume when you are using the area-length method?

A. $5/6 \times$ short-axis basal area $\times$ LV length

B. $.5/6 \times$ short-axis basal area $\times$ (LV length)^2

C. $5/6 \times$ (short-axis area)$^2 \times$ LV length

D. $5/6 +$ short-axis area/LV length

590. What does an ascending aortic Z-score of +3.2 signify in a patient with Marfan syndrome?

A. Normal value

B. Severely dilated ascending aorta

C. Mildly dilated ascending aorta

D. Nothing of significance; Z-scores are not considered useful in echocardiography.

591. This image was obtained from a patient with a normal heart. Which letter indicates the site of aortic enlargement generally seen early in Marfan syndrome?

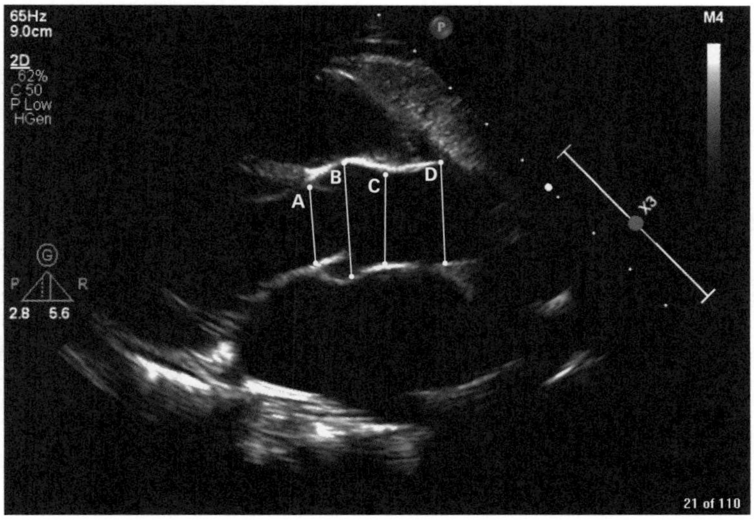

A. A

B. B

C. C

D. D

Refer to video PER-Q592.

592. This video clip displays an aortic arch. Which of these statements about the proximal transverse arch seen in this clip is correct?

A. It is measured between the innominate (brachiocephalic) artery and the left subclavian artery.

B. It is measured between the innominate artery and the left common carotid artery.

C. It is measured between the left common carotid artery and left subclavian artery.

D. It is generally described as the area closest to the ductus arteriosus.

593. Under normal circumstances a patent ductus arteriosus (PDA) is generally seen closest to which segment of the aortic arch?

A. Aortic isthmus

B. Ascending aorta

C. Proximal transverse aortic arch

D. Distal transverse aortic arch

594. In this image which letter marks the distal transverse aortic arch?

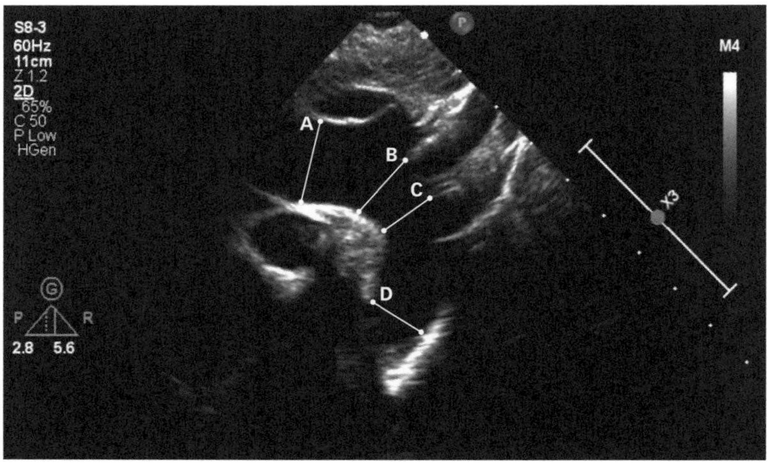

A. A

B. B

C. C

D. D

595. This image was described by the attending cardiologist as demonstrating tubular hypoplasia of the aortic arch. Which of the following options best defines tubular hypoplasia of the aortic arch?

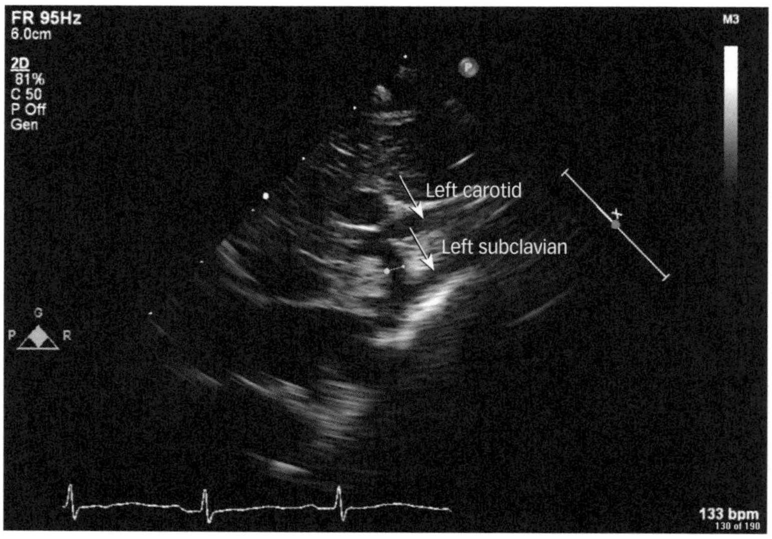

A. Small aortic isthmus only

B. Hypoplastic distal transverse arch, elongation of the area between the left common carotid artery and left subclavian artery, and a narrowed aortic isthmus

C. Discrete juxtaductal coarctation

D. Hypoplastic proximal and distal transverse arch with a normal-sized aortic isthmus

596. This is an M-mode image of the left ventricle in the parasternal short-axis view, just below the mitral valve leaflet tips. The Z-score for the measurements of the interventricular septum is +6.0. What does this Z-score suggest?

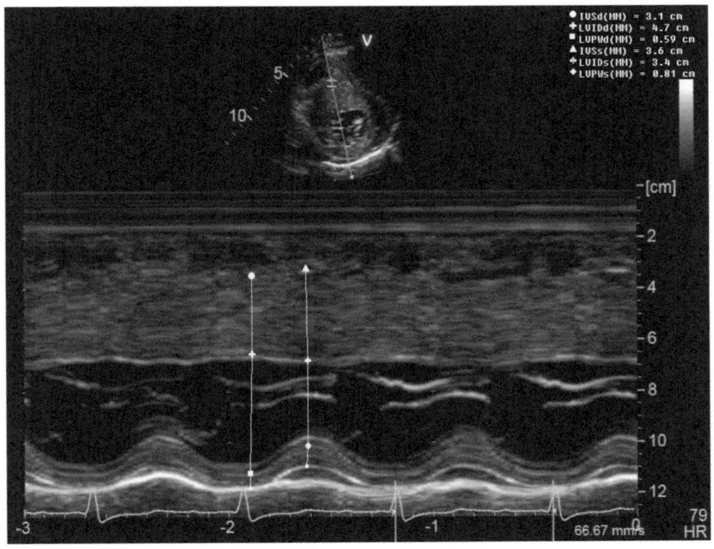

A. Interventricular septal hypertrophy
B. Upper limit of normal
C. Not predictive of hypertrophic cardiomyopathy
D. Systolic anterior motion of the mitral valve anterior leaflet

597. In the following equation SF stands for shortening fraction, ET for ejection time, and RR for the R wave to R wave interval. What value does this calculation provide?

$$[(SF) \times (RR)^{0.5}] / (ET)$$

A. Corrected geometrical assumptions about the left ventricle in biplane Simpson's method used for ejection fraction
B. Speed of left ventricular shortening, known as velocity of circumferential fiber shortening
C. Fractional shortening
D. Ejection fraction using M-mode echocardiography

598. Global left ventricular longitudinal strain:

A. Measures thickening of the left ventricular myocardium
B. Is positive when normal
C. Is negative when normal
D. Measures diastolic left ventricular volume

Refer to video PER-Q599.

599. What type of ventricular septal defect (VSD) is seen in this video clip, and when does shunting occur?
   A. Subpulmonary VSD with shunting seen in systole
   B. Perimembranous VSD with shunting seen in diastole
   C. Inlet VSD with shunting seen in diastole
   D. Muscular VSD with shunting seen in systole

600. While undergoing chemotherapy two years ago, the patient you are about to image had a reduced left ventricular ejection fraction of 40% and a global longitudinal strain (GLS) of −12%. Your echocardiogram now shows a normal left ventricular ejection fraction and a normal GLS. Which value below represents a normal GLS?
   A. +12%
   B. −2%
   C. −10%
   D. −20%

Refer to video PER-Q601.

601. This video clip is of a patient with a cleft mitral valve. When is the mitral regurgitation occurring?
   A. During diastasis, just before the P wave on the electrocardiogram
   B. At ventricular systole, closest to the QRS complex
   C. During late ventricular filling, just after the P wave on the electrocardiogram
   D. During early left ventricular filling

602. This image was obtained using tissue Doppler imaging. Which letter on the spectral tracing corresponds with isovolumic contraction time?

See Color Plate 33 on page xxxv.

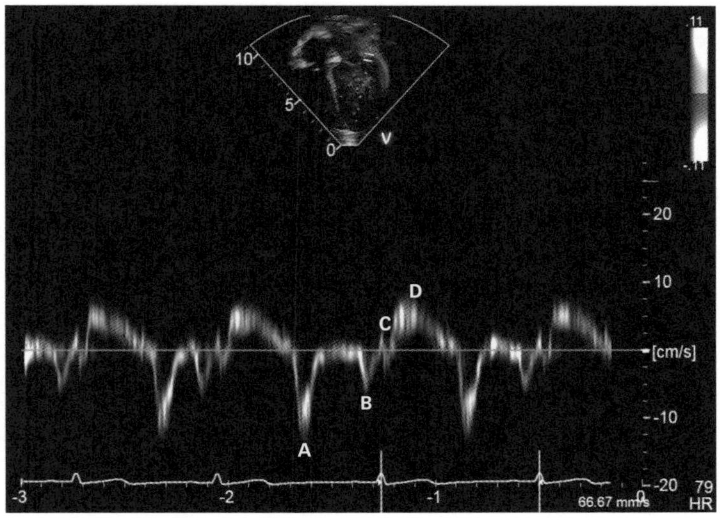

A. A

B. B

C. C

D. D

AIT—Hotspot

603. Which of these measurements is NOT needed when you are calculating the myocardial performance index for a left ventricle?

A. R wave to R wave interval

B. Isovolumic contraction time

C. Isovolumic relaxation time

D. Left ventricular ejection time

PART 7

Answers, Explanations, and References

Anatomy and physiology

Pathology and pathophysiology

Congenital anomalies

Postoperative anatomy

Clinical standards and guidelines

Measurement techniques and quantification

PART 1

Anatomy and Physiology

1. C. Eighth week.

By the eighth week of embryonic development (tenth week LMP), ventricular looping, arch formation, venous development, and septation of the atria, atrioventricular canal, ventricles, and outflow tracts are complete. In this question embryonic development is synonymous with conceptual age. Strictly speaking, menstrual age (time elapsed since the beginning of the last menstrual period, or LMP) is not the same as conceptual age (time elapsed since conception). "Gestational age" may refer to both, and often obstetric clinicians use LMP or menstrual age to refer to gestational age. Menstrual age is thus two weeks greater than conceptual age—so in terms of LMP, cardiac development is complete around week 10.

▶ Rychik J, Tian Z: *Fetal Cardiovascular Imaging: A Disease-Based Approach*. Philadelphia, Saunders, 2012, pp 1–15.

2. C. The left fourth aortic arch and left dorsal aorta.

There are six pairs of aortic arches in a developing embryo. In a normal left aortic arch, involution of the right dorsal aorta and right sixth arch occur. The definitive (normal) left arch then comprises the left fourth arch and left dorsal aorta.

▶ Allen HD, Driscoll DJ, Shaddy RE, et al: *Moss and Adams' Heart Disease in Infants, Children, and Adolescents: Including the Fetus and Young Adult*, 8th edition. Philadelphia, Lippincott Williams & Wilkins, 2013, pp 758–760.

3. C. The side where the aortic arch passes over the mainstem bronchus.

If the aortic arch is seen to the left of the trachea crossing over the left mainstem bronchus, the aortic arch is left-sided. If the aortic arch is seen to the right of the trachea crossing over the right mainstem bronchus, the aortic arch is right-sided. This is documented in a suprasternal long-axis view (suprasternal sagittal view), while visualizing the trachea and annotating the sweep to the left or right of the trachea. Alternatively, it can be documented in a suprasternal short-axis sweep (suprasternal coronal view) of the arch.

▶ Allen HD, Driscoll DJ, Shaddy RE, et al: *Moss and Adams' Heart Disease in Infants, Children, and Adolescents: Including the Fetus and Young Adult*, 8th edition. Philadelphia, Lippincott Williams & Wilkins, 2013, p 758.

4. D. Right and/or left sixth aortic arch.

In the fetus, the patent ductus arteriosus (PDA) connects the main pulmonary artery to the proximal descending aorta. It is one of the two main shunts (the other being the foramen ovale) that allow blood flow to bypass the developing fetal lungs and deliver oxygenated blood supply directly into the systemic circulation. Typically with a left aortic arch, the PDA is left-sided and derives from the left sixth aortic arch. The right sixth aortic arch usually disappears, but it can persist in unusual circumstances. For example, with discontinuous pulmonary arteries there can be persistent bilateral ducti. Normally the ductus arteriosus closes soon after birth, forming the ligamentum arteriosum. The right and left intersegmental arteries become the subclavian arteries, and the left and right third aortic arches form the left and right common carotid arteries. The right subclavian artery is derived from a portion of the right fourth arch.

- Allen HD, Driscoll DJ, Shaddy RE, et al: *Moss and Adams' Heart Disease in Infants, Children, and Adolescents: Including the Fetus and Young Adult*, 8th edition. Philadelphia, Lippincott Williams & Wilkins, 2013, pp 760–761, 768.
- Lai WW, Mertens LL, Cohen MS, et al (eds): *Echocardiography in Pediatric and Congenital Heart Disease: From Fetus to Adult*, 2nd edition. Chichester, UK, Wiley-Blackwell, 2016, p 327.

5. A. Innominate artery.

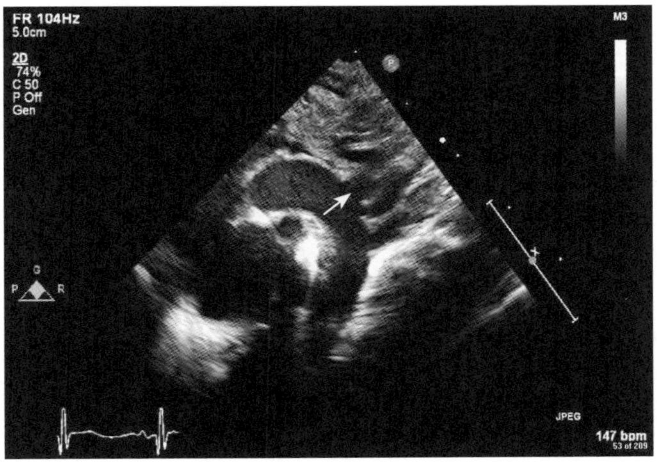

The arrow in this image is pointing to the innominate artery, also known as the brachiocephalic artery.

- Lai WW, Mertens LL, Cohen MS, et al (eds): *Echocardiography in Pediatric and Congenital Heart Disease: From Fetus to Adult*, 2nd edition. Chichester, UK, Wiley-Blackwell, 2016, p 54.

6. B. Coronary arteries and head and neck arteries.

Even in the presence of an anomaly such as anomalous left coronary artery from the pulmonary artery (ALCAPA), anomalous right coronary artery from the pulmonary artery (ARCAPA), or an isolated subclavian artery from the pulmonary artery, the coronary arteries and the head and neck vessels remain the anatomic landmarks used to identify the aorta.

▸ Allen HD, Driscoll DJ, Shaddy RE, et al: *Moss and Adams' Heart Disease in Infants, Children, and Adolescents: Including the Fetus and Young Adult*, 8th edition. Philadelphia, Lippincott Williams & Wilkins, 2013, pp 19–20.

▸ Anderson RH, Baker EJ, Penny D, et al: *Paediatric Cardiology*, 3rd edition. Philadelphia, Churchill Livingstone/Elsevier, 2010, p 27.

7. D. Bifurcation of the great artery.

Even when a pulmonary artery branch can be found arising from the ascending aorta, as in certain forms of congenital heart disease, the branch pulmonary arteries are anatomic landmarks used to identify the pulmonary artery. A trileaflet semilunar valve is nonspecific, also fitting the description of both the aortic and pulmonary valves. The ductus arteriosus connects the aorta to the pulmonary artery and therefore cannot be used to distinguish one from the other. The carina refers to the trachea, not branch pulmonary arteries.

▸ Anderson RH, Baker EJ, Penny D, et al: *Paediatric Cardiology*, 3rd edition. Philadelphia, Churchill Livingstone/Elsevier, 2010, p 27.

▸ Lai WW, Mertens LL, Cohen MS, et al (eds): *Echocardiography in Pediatric and Congenital Heart Disease: From Fetus to Adult*, 2nd edition. Chichester, UK, Wiley-Blackwell, 2016, p 327.

8. B. Left ventricle.

The left ventricle is identified by fine ventricular trabeculations and a mostly (two-thirds) smooth septal surface, as seen from an apical four-chamber view. The conus arteriosus (infundibulum) is normally associated with the right ventricle. Other landmarks of the left ventricle, under normal circumstances, are two well-formed papillary muscles and a mitral valve with attachments only to the free wall.

▸ Lai WW, Mertens LL, Cohen MS, et al (eds): *Echocardiography in Pediatric and Congenital Heart Disease: From Fetus to Adult*, 2nd edition. Chichester, UK, Wiley-Blackwell, 2016, p 38.

9. D. Right ventricle.

Coarse ventricular trabeculations, tricuspid valve attachments to the septal surface of the interventricular septum, a moderator band, and a conus arteriosus (infundibulum) are the morphologic characteristics of the normal right ventricle—known as a morphologic right ventricle. It is important to note that the normality of a cardiac structure is defined by its morphology, not by its position in space. A morphologic right ventricle can be either right-sided or left-sided.

▶ Lai WW, Mertens LL, Cohen MS, et al (eds): *Echocardiography in Pediatric and Congenital Heart Disease: From Fetus to Adult*, 2nd edition. Chichester, UK, Wiley-Blackwell, 2016, pp 37, 39.

*Refer to video PER-Q10.**

10. C. Increased right ventricular volume and pressure.

Video PER-Q10 demonstrates a dilated right ventricle and flattened ventricular septal contour in both systole and diastole. The flattened systolic ventricular septal contour indicates elevated right ventricular systolic pressure (which might be seen in the presence of pulmonary hypertension or significant pulmonary valve stenosis), and the flattened diastolic ventricular septal contour generally indicates increased right ventricular volume (which might be expected with conditions such as a large atrial septal defect or total anomalous pulmonary venous connection). A small restrictive PDA is usually not seen with elevated pulmonary pressure.

▶ Lai WW, Mertens LL, Cohen MS, et al (eds): *Echocardiography in Pediatric and Congenital Heart Disease: From Fetus to Adult*, 2nd edition. Chichester, UK, Wiley-Blackwell, 2016, pp 168, 281–282.

▶ Park MK: *Park's Pediatric Cardiology for Practitioners*, 6th edition. Philadelphia, Saunders, 2014, pp 157, 489.

11. C. The load at the end of diastole and before contraction.

A practical approach to understanding preload is to think of it as the end-diastolic volume just prior to the onset of ventricular systole, as described by the Frank-Starling mechanism.

▶ Park MK: *Park's Pediatric Cardiology for Practitioners*, 6th edition. Philadelphia, Saunders, 2014, p 453.

*To access the video clips that go with this mock exam, register your book with Davies Publishing by visiting DaviesPublishing.com/book-registration, or phone us at 1-877-792-0005 (toll-free in the U.S.) or 1-636-792-3046.

ANSWERS

12. A. Aortic stenosis.

According to Myung K. Park (2014), afterload *is best defined as the force that resists myofibrillar shortening during systole. Aortic valve stenosis is considered a cause of increased left ventricular afterload.*

- Lai WW, Mertens LL, Cohen MS, et al (eds): *Echocardiography in Pediatric and Congenital Heart Disease: From Fetus to Adult*, 2nd edition. Chichester, UK, Wiley-Blackwell, 2016, p 340.
- Park MK: *Park's Pediatric Cardiology for Practitioners*, 6th edition. Philadelphia, Saunders, 2014, p 454.

13. B. Dissolution of the left dorsal aorta distal to the origin of the seventh intersegmental artery, persistence of the right fourth aortic arch, and persistence of the right dorsal aorta.

In the right aortic arch with mirror-image branching, the left dorsal aorta "regresses" and the right dorsal aorta and right fourth aortic arch persist, becoming the right aortic arch. Please also note that the left seventh intersegmental artery and left third and left fourth aortic arches become the left innominate (brachiocephalic) artery.

- Allen HD, Driscoll DJ, Shaddy RE, et al: *Moss and Adams' Heart Disease in Infants, Children, and Adolescents: Including the Fetus and Young Adult*, 8th edition. Philadelphia, Lippincott Williams & Wilkins, 2013, pp 759, 767.

14. A. Right atrial appendage.

The right atrial appendage appears on echocardiography as broad-based, triangular in shape, and incorporated into the right atrium.

- Anderson RH, Baker EJ, Penny D, et al: *Paediatric Cardiology*, 3rd edition. Philadelphia, Churchill Livingstone/Elsevier, 2010, p 19.
- Lai WW, Mertens LL, Cohen MS, et al (eds): *Echocardiography in Pediatric and Congenital Heart Disease: From Fetus to Adult*, 2nd edition. Chichester, UK, Wiley-Blackwell, 2016, pp 36–37, 51.

15. B. Right atrium.

When ambiguity of the viscera is excluded, the right atrium can be described as the atrium that has a broad-based appendage and receives the inferior vena cava and the coronary sinus.

- Anderson RH, Baker EJ, Penny D, et al: *Paediatric Cardiology*, 3rd edition. Philadelphia, Churchill Livingstone/Elsevier, 2010, p 19.
- Lai WW, Mertens LL, Cohen MS, et al (eds): *Echocardiography in Pediatric and Congenital Heart Disease: From Fetus to Adult*. Chichester, UK, Wiley-Blackwell, 2009, pp 34–37.

16. C. An increase in arterial oxygen.

After the newborn takes a first breath, the neonatal lungs expand and pulmonary vascular resistance falls. There is increased return of pulmonary venous blood to the left atrium. However, none of these factors produces spontaneous closure of the patent ductus arteriosus (PDA). Rather, it is the increased oxygen level in the blood that stimulates the closure of the PDA. Note that in some clinical situations, PGE1 is used to keep the PDA open, and in other clinical situations indomethacin (a drug that antagonizes the effect of PGE1) is used to close the PDA.

▶ Park MK: *Park's Pediatric Cardiology for Practitioners*, 6th edition. Philadelphia, Saunders, 2014, p 121.

▶ Rudolph AM: *Congenital Diseases of the Heart: Clinical-Physiological Considerations*, 3rd edition. Chichester, UK, Wiley Blackwell, 2009, pp 118, 120.

17. C. Right to left.

In the normal fetal circulation, oxygenated placental blood flow is directed through the umbilical vein, ductus venosus, inferior vena cava, and then to the right atrium. Once in the right atrium, blood flow crosses through the foramen ovale and into the left atrium. In a fetus with hypoplastic left heart syndrome (HLHS), left-to-right atrial shunting can be seen. Bidirectional flow at the patent foramen ovale can be seen in cases of left ventricular outflow tract (LVOT) obstruction.

▶ Rychik J, Tian Z: *Fetal Cardiovascular Imaging: A Disease-Based Approach*. Philadelphia, Saunders, 2012, pp 144–146, 232–240.

18. D. Increase in left atrial pressure.

After birth the umbilical cord is cut so oxygenated placental blood no longer flows through the patent foramen ovale into the left atrium. Instead, blood flow through the expanded lungs increases, returning back through the pulmonary veins into the left atrium, which in turn increases left atrial volume and pressure. The atrial septum primum, instead of opening toward the left atrium, now moves rightward and buttresses up against the septum secundum, thereby closing the foramen ovale.

▶ Children's Hospital of Philadelphia: How does the fetal circulatory system work? Available at https://www.chop.edu/conditions-diseases/blood-circulation-fetus-and-newborn.

▶ Park MK: *Park's Pediatric Cardiology for Practitioners*, 6th edition. Philadelphia, Saunders, 2014, p 121.

19. C. Morphologic left atrium.

Visualization of the flap of the foramen ovale (atrial septum primum) in the left atrium is a marker of left atrial morphology. The septum secundum is a defining feature of a morphologic right atrium. In the scenario posed by this question, the morphologic left atrium is right-sided. Therefore, with situs inversus totalis, the septum primum flopping into the right-sided atrium indicates a morphologic left atrium.

▶ Lai WW, Mertens LL, Cohen MS, et al (eds): *Echocardiography in Pediatric and Congenital Heart Disease: From Fetus to Adult*, 2nd edition. Chichester, UK, Wiley-Blackwell, 2016, pp 35–37.

20. B. Tricuspid valve.

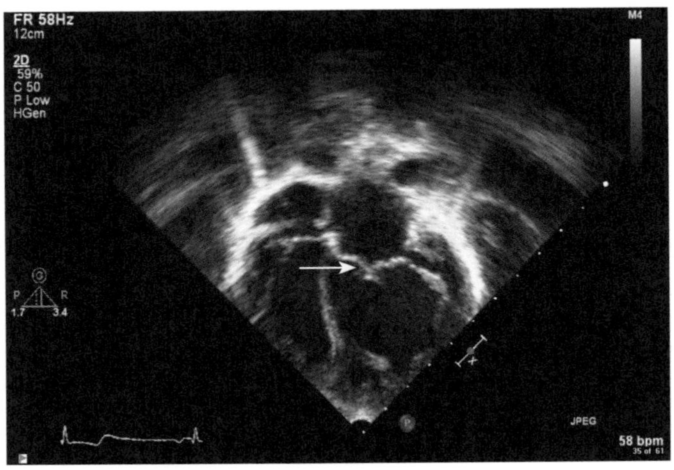

The two atrioventricular valves of the heart are the mitral and tricuspid (arrow) valves; there are also two semilunar valves, the pulmonary and the aortic valves. The mitral valve is associated with a morphologic left ventricle and the tricuspid valve with a morphologic right ventricle. This image demonstrates a left-sided tricuspid valve in the presence of L-looped ventricles. In this image the apical displacement of the left-sided atrioventricular valve as well as morphologic markers of the right ventricle are clearly seen. Excessive displacement of the left-sided tricuspid valve in the setting of L-looped ventricles can indicate Ebstein malformation and is typically associated with valve regurgitation. It is important to find morphologic markers like the moderator band, heavy trabeculations, and apical displacement of the tricuspid valve in order to identify the morphology of the right ventricle.

▶ Lai WW, Mertens LL, Cohen MS, et al (eds): *Echocardiography in Pediatric and Congenital Heart Disease: From Fetus to Adult*, 2nd edition. Chichester, UK, Wiley-Blackwell, 2016, pp 37–39, 231–240.

21. A. 1–2 weeks.

Pulmonary vascular resistance (PVR) in normal children and in children with small restrictive ventricular septal defects (VSDs) should drop to near normal levels within the first week after birth. If there is a larger VSD, PVR falls quickly after birth and then continues to drop until it reaches normal levels at 6–8 weeks after birth. If PVR were to be significantly high in this scenario, the same small muscular VSD would be expected to have a peak pressure gradient (PPG) much less than 88 mmHg. It is important to note that increased right-sided pressures can lead to small restrictive VSDs like the one described above having different physiologic characteristics from those of VSDs under normal right-sided pressures.

▶ Park MK: *Park's Pediatric Cardiology for Practitioners*, 6th edition. Philadelphia, Saunders, 2014, pp 121, 126–127.

22. A. L-looped.

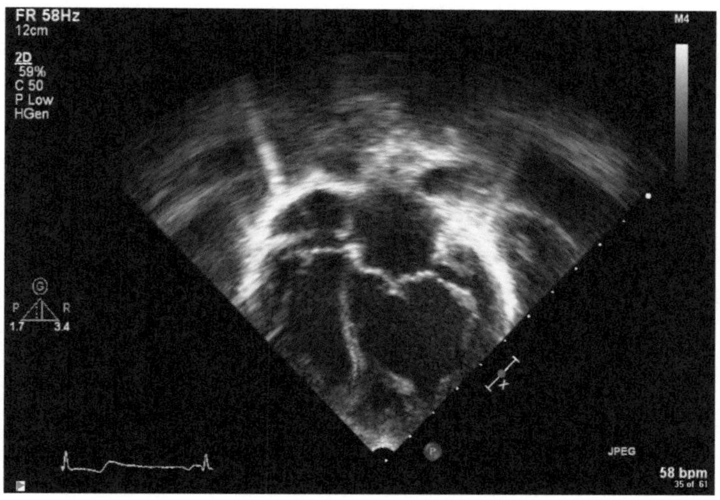

The image shows L-looped ventricles. In this case the patient has congenitally corrected transposition of the great arteries (ccTGA). The looping pattern of the ventricles can be determined by chirality (or handedness), which is the principle that a particular type of looping—D for "dextro" (right) and L for "levo" (left)—gives the morphologic right and left ventricles an identifiable 3D spatial arrangement.

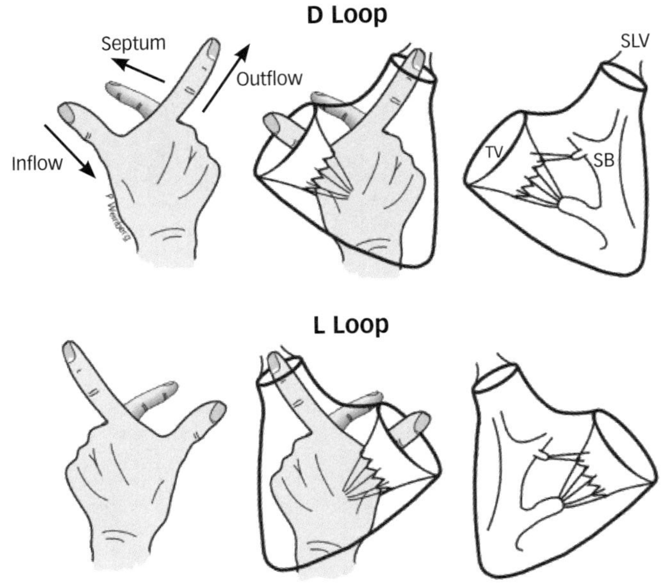

Source: Weinberg PM: Anatomy and classification of congenital heart disease. Courtesy of Thoracic Key, https://thoracickey.com/anatomy-and-classification-of-congenital-heart-disease/. TV = tricuspid valve, SB = septal band, SLV = semilunar valve. Reprinted with permission.

In general, the morphologic right ventricle is used to determine the looping pattern. In the case of D-looped ventricles, the right ventricle "fits" an imaginary right hand placed into the ventricle: The right thumb inserts into the inflow, the index finger into the outflow, and the middle finger into the septum (septal band, SB), with the palm resting upon the ventricular septum. Conversely, if the left hand could fit into the morphologic right ventricle (using the same corresponding ventricular/hand features as described previously), the ventricles are L-looped. If the looping pattern cannot be determined, then the looping is designated "X" or "indeterminate." There is no such thing as an "A" looping pattern.

▸ Lai WW, Mertens LL, Cohen MS, et al (eds): *Echocardiography in Pediatric and Congenital Heart Disease: From Fetus to Adult*, 2nd edition. Chichester, UK, Wiley-Blackwell, 2016, pp 37–39.

▸ Van Praagh R, Ongley PA, Swan HJ: Anatomic types of single or common ventricle in man: morphologic and geometric aspects of 60 necropsied cases. Am J Cardiol 13:367–386, 1964.

23. A. 24 hours after birth.

Closure of the ductus arteriosus typically occurs within the first day after birth. When echocardiography is performed within the first 24 hours after birth, it is not uncommon to see a small patent ductus arteriosus (PDA) shunting from left to right. Under circumstances when right-sided pressures are increased, the PDA can shunt from right to left, mimicking the visual characteristics of a branch pulmonary artery. Note that for echocardiography, both a suprasternal notch coronal view and a high left parasternal parasagittal view (ductal view) can be very helpful for PDA evaluation.

▶ Lai WW, Mertens LL, Cohen MS, et al (eds): *Echocardiography in Pediatric and Congenital Heart Disease: From Fetus to Adult*, 2nd edition. Chichester, UK, Wiley-Blackwell, 2016, pp 53–58.

▶ Park MK: *Park's Pediatric Cardiology for Practitioners*, 6th edition. Philadelphia, Saunders, 2014, p 122.

24. D. Prostaglandin E1 (PGE1).

Prostaglandin E1 (PGE1) is used to keep a duct open in cases of ductal-dependent congenital heart disease such as coarctation of the aorta (CoA), hypoplastic left heart syndrome (HLHS), severe pulmonary valve stenosis, and interrupted aortic arch. All the other agents cause ductal constriction.

▶ Le J, Gales MA, Gales BJ: Acetaminophen for patent ductus arteriosus. Ann Pharmacother 49:241–246, 2015.

▶ Park MK: *Park's Pediatric Cardiology for Practitioners*, 6th edition. Philadelphia, Saunders, 2014, pp 122–123, 171–172.

25. B. Right coronary artery.

See Color Plate 1 on page xix.

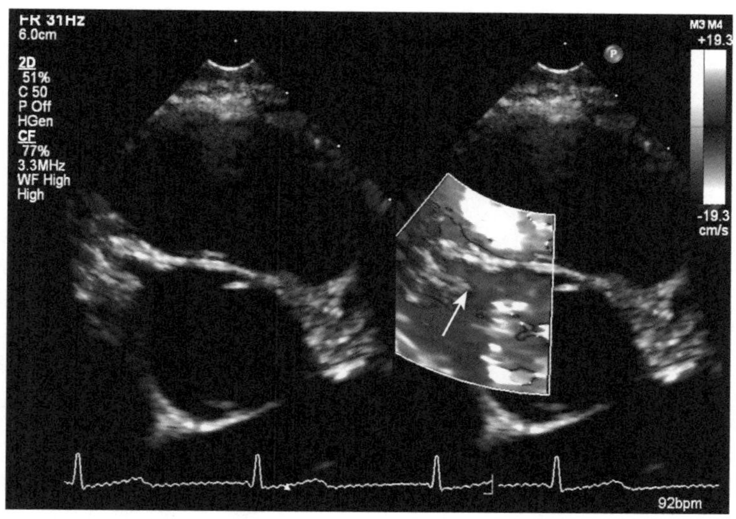

The arrow is pointing to the right coronary artery (RCA). In normal hearts the right coronary artery usually originates from the most anterior and rightward cusp.

▶ Anderson RH, Baker EJ, Penny D, et al: *Paediatric Cardiology*, 3rd edition. Philadelphia, Churchill Livingstone/Elsevier, 2010, p 933.

26. A. Left anterior descending coronary artery (LAD).

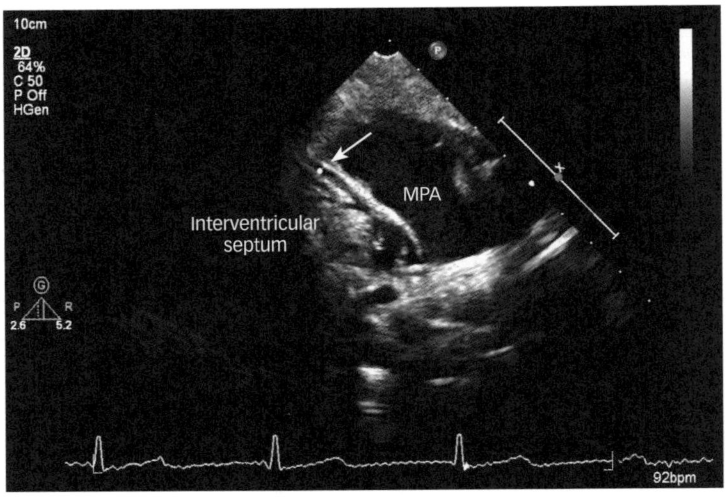

The structure indicated by the arrow is the left anterior descending coronary artery (LAD). This image is obtained from a parasternal long-axis view by sweeping superior and leftward toward the pulmonary valve. Note that the left main coronary artery (LMCA), LAD, interventricular septum, and posterior segment of the pulmonary artery are visualized in this view. This view can be useful when diagnosing anomalous left coronary artery from the pulmonary artery (ALCAPA). MPA = main pulmonary artery.

▶ Lai WW, Mertens LL, Cohen MS, et al (eds): *Echocardiography in Pediatric and Congenital Heart Disease: From Fetus to Adult*, 2nd edition. Chichester, UK, Wiley-Blackwell, 2016, pp 589, 591.

27. C. Left main coronary artery (LMCA).

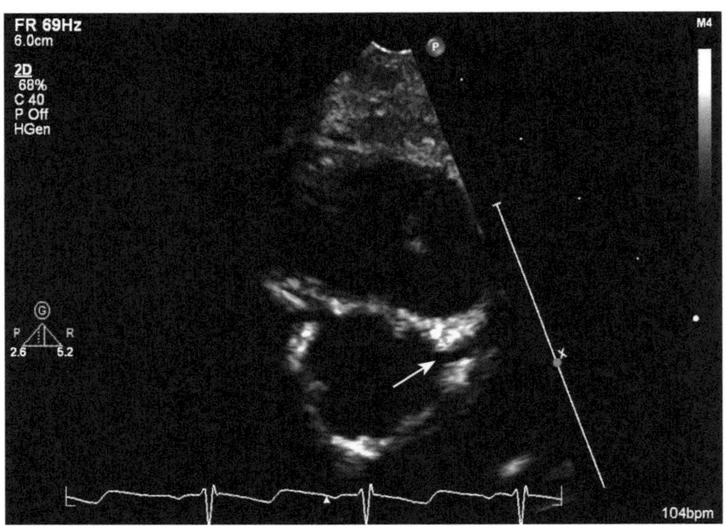

The left main coronary artery (LMCA, arrow) usually bifurcates into the left anterior descending (LAD) and circumflex (Cx) coronary arteries. The best views to confirm this normal

pattern are the subcostal long-axis, subcostal short-axis, parasternal short-axis, and parasternal long-axis to right ventricular outflow views.

▸ Lai WW, Mertens LL, Cohen MS, et al (eds): *Echocardiography in Pediatric and Congenital Heart Disease: From Fetus to Adult*, 2nd edition. Chichester, UK, Wiley-Blackwell, 2016, p 588.

Refer to video PER-Q28.

28. B. Circumflex from the right coronary artery.

The second most common coronary artery pattern in transposition of the great arteries (d-TGA) is the circumflex from the right coronary artery. The best echocardiographic sweeps to visualize this coronary artery pattern are the subcostal long-axis sweep and the apical four-chamber to five-chamber sweep, in which the circumflex coronary artery can be seen coursing posterior to the pulmonary artery and anterior to the mitral valve annulus, in the left atrioventricular groove.

▸ Lai WW, Mertens LL, Cohen MS, et al (eds): *Echocardiography in Pediatric and Congenital Heart Disease: From Fetus to Adult*, 2nd edition. Chichester, UK, Wiley-Blackwell, 2016, pp 450, 592.

29. D. Noncoronary cusp (NCC).

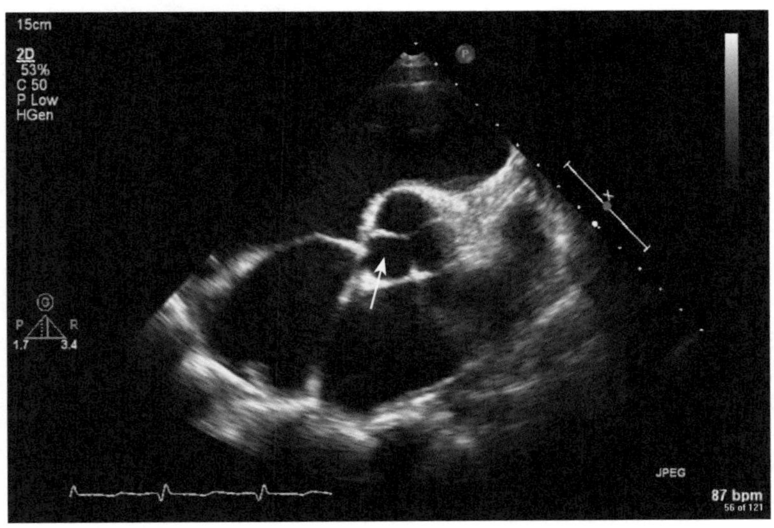

In the parasternal short-axis view the noncoronary cusp (NCC, arrow) is seen posterior to the right coronary cusp and rightward of the left coronary cusp.

▸ Anderson RH, Baker EJ, Penny D, et al: *Paediatric Cardiology*, 3rd edition. Philadelphia, Churchill Livingstone/Elsevier, 2010, p 934.

▸ Lai WW, Mertens LL, Cohen MS, et al (eds): *Echocardiography in Pediatric and Congenital Heart Disease: From Fetus to Adult*, 2nd edition. Chichester, UK, Wiley-Blackwell, 2016, p 588.

ANSWERS

30. C. Color flow Doppler.

Coronary artery imaging is one of the most challenging parts of echocardiographic evaluation, and one should use all the appropriate tools available. The use of 2D imaging and color flow Doppler imaging in combination is the best way to identify coronary artery origins.

▶ Lai WW, Mertens LL, Cohen MS, et al (eds): *Echocardiography in Pediatric and Congenital Heart Disease: From Fetus to Adult*, 2nd edition. Chichester, UK, Wiley-Blackwell, 2016, p 587.

31. A. Diastole.

Left main coronary artery filling occurs primarily during diastole.

▶ Lai WW, Mertens LL, Cohen MS, et al (eds): *Echocardiography in Pediatric and Congenital Heart Disease: From Fetus to Adult*, 2nd edition. Chichester, UK, Wiley-Blackwell, 2016, p 586.

32. D. Systole.

See Color Plate 1 on page xix.

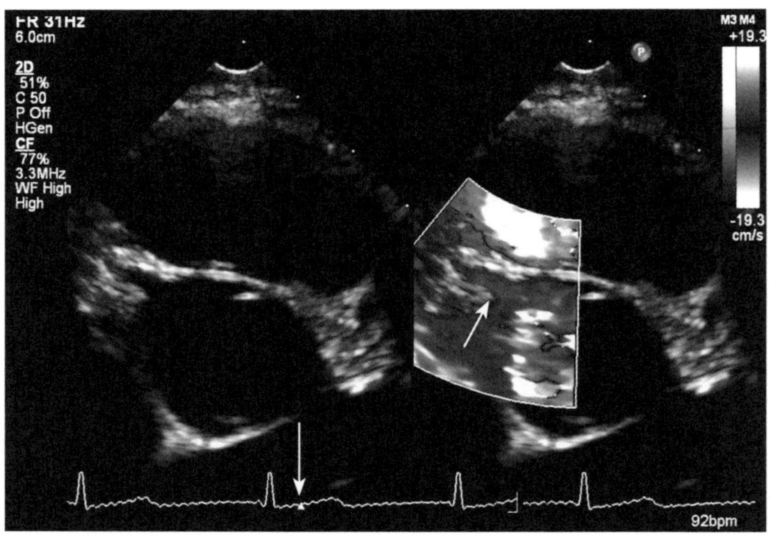

The image shows the right coronary artery (top arrow) filling during systole. The lower arrow marks the point on the electrocardiographic tracing when the image was frozen. According to Lai et al., compressive forces exerted by the right ventricle are ordinarily less than those of the left ventricle; therefore, coronary blood flow to the right ventricle is not interrupted during ventricular systole.

▶ Lai WW, Mertens LL, Cohen MS, et al (eds): *Echocardiography in Pediatric and Congenital Heart Disease: From Fetus to Adult*, 2nd edition. Chichester, UK, Wiley-Blackwell, 2016, p 586.

33. B. Coronary sinus.

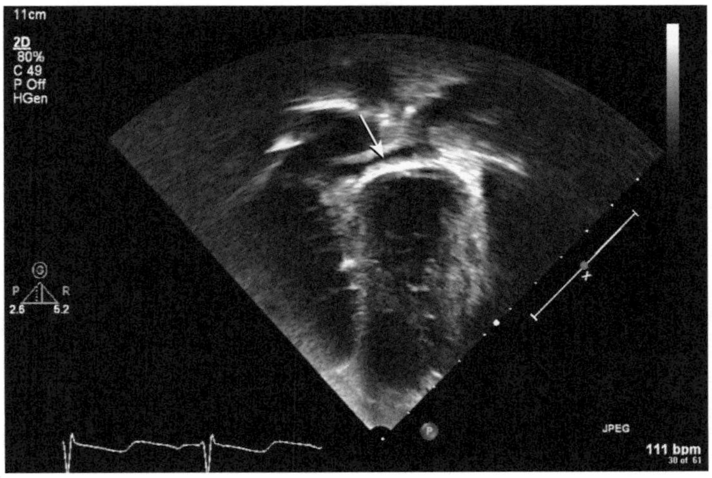

The coronary sinus (arrow) is a posterior structure that can be seen as it drains into the leftward and inferior portion of the right atrium. Additional views to evaluate the coronary sinus are the parasternal long-axis view, with a tilt toward the right hip to visualize the right ventricular inflow, and a subcostal long-axis (four-chamber) view, with posterior angulation.

▸ Lai WW, Mertens LL, Cohen MS, et al (eds): *Echocardiography in Pediatric and Congenital Heart Disease: From Fetus to Adult*, 2nd edition. Chichester, UK, Wiley-Blackwell, 2016, pp 47–51.

34. A. Left superior vena cava.

See Color Plate 2 on page xx.

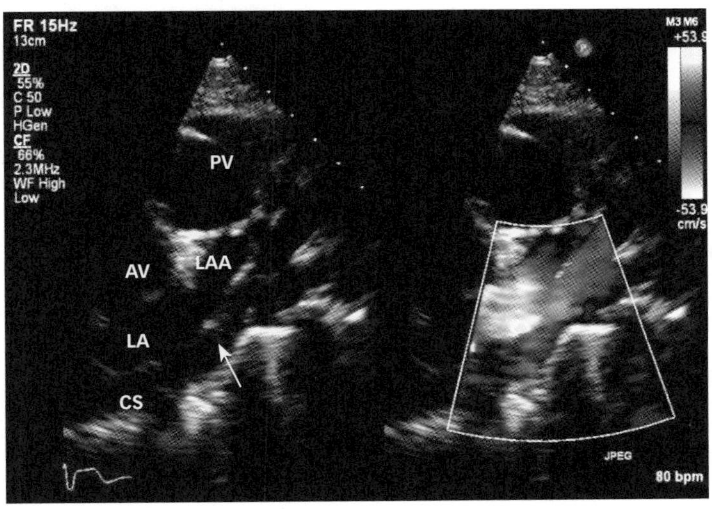

When a left superior vena cava (LSVC) is present, it usually connects to the coronary sinus (CS). In such cases, the CS will be dilated compared to its usual size when an LSVC is not present. Therefore, a clue to a persistent LSVC is a dilated CS. A bridging vein (innominate vein) is usually absent, but rarely it can remain present, connecting right and left SVCs.

ANSWERS

When a bridging vein is present, its caliber can vary in size but is usually small. When an LSVC is present, care should also be taken to rule out partial pulmonary venous drainage to an LSVC. Color flow imaging and a spectral Doppler profile aid in identifying anomalous pulmonary venous drainage to an LSVC. Other possible reasons for a dilated CS include hepatic veins draining into the CS, total anomalous pulmonary venous connection (TAPVC) to the CS, or CS ostial stenosis. Arrow = left superior vena cava, CS = coronary sinus, PV = pulmonary valve, AV = aortic valve, LAA = left atrial appendage, and LA = left atrium.

▶ Lai WW, Mertens LL, Cohen MS, et al (eds): *Echocardiography in Pediatric and Congenital Heart Disease: From Fetus to Adult*, 2nd edition. Chichester, UK, Wiley-Blackwell, 2016, pp 160–166, 182–186.

35. B. Innominate vein.

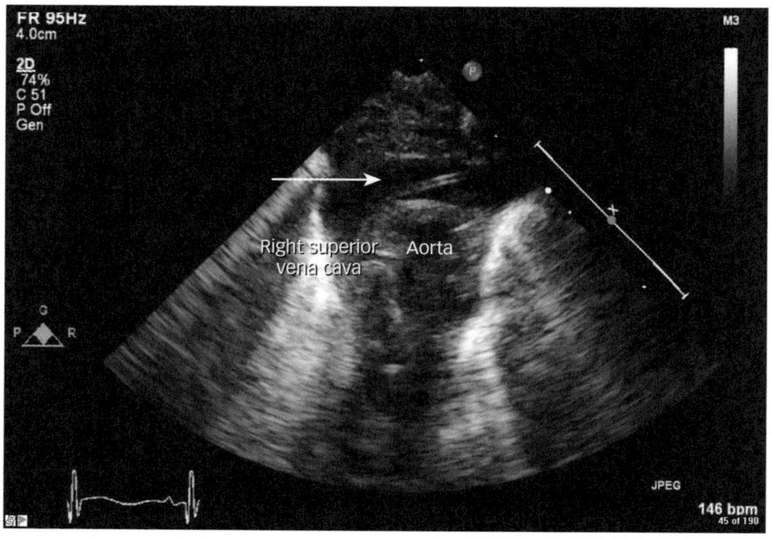

This image shows the innominate, or brachiocephalic, vein (arrow) in the suprasternal short-axis view. This view was obtained with the transducer in the suprasternal notch with the index marker positioned at 3 o'clock. An additional view to visualize the innominate vein can be acquired with the transducer in the suprasternal notch with the index marker positioned at 1–2 o'clock. In this view you will see the innominate vein superior to the aortic arch.

▶ Lai WW, Mertens LL, Cohen MS, et al (eds): *Echocardiography in Pediatric and Congenital Heart Disease: From Fetus to Adult*, 2nd edition. Chichester, UK, Wiley-Blackwell, 2016, pp 54, 56, 184.

36. D. Coronary sinus.

The coronary sinus (CS) is a posterior structure and can be visualized by a posterior angulation of the transducer in the apical four-chamber view. In this view, the CS can be seen perpendicular to the angle of insonation, returning to the right atrium.

- Lai WW, Mertens LL, Cohen MS, et al (eds): *Echocardiography in Pediatric and Congenital Heart Disease: From Fetus to Adult*, 2nd edition. Chichester, UK, Wiley-Blackwell, 2016, p 49.

37. B. Coronary sinus.

The left horn of the sinus venosus eventually develops into the coronary sinus. The Eustachian valve is a remnant of the right valve of the sinus venosus. The superior vena cava is derived from the right anterior cardinal vein. The levoatrial cardinal vein is not present in the normal four-chambered heart; when present, it is frequently seen in association with hypoplastic left heart syndrome and a restrictive atrial septum.

- Lai WW, Mertens LL, Cohen MS, et al (eds): *Echocardiography in Pediatric and Congenital Heart Disease: From Fetus to Adult*, 2nd edition. Chichester, UK, Wiley-Blackwell, 2016, p 185.
- Moore KL, Persaud TVN, Torchia MG: *The Developing Human: Clinically Oriented Embryology*, 9th edition. Philadelphia, Elsevier Saunders, 2013, pp 292, 305–306.

38. C. Right atrium.

In normal heart development the right horn of the sinus venosus eventually becomes the smooth-walled portion of the right atrium. The pulmonary veins are derived from a common pulmonary vein arising from the primitive lung buds, and this common pulmonary vein eventually forms a portion of the left atrium in conjunction with the embryonic left atrium of the primitive heart tube. The left atrial appendage also derives from the embryonic left atrium.

- Moore KL, Persaud TVN, Torchia MG: *The Developing Human: Clinically Oriented Embryology*, 9th edition. Philadelphia, Elsevier Saunders, 2013, pp 150, 204, 210, 305–306.

39. C. Eustachian valve.

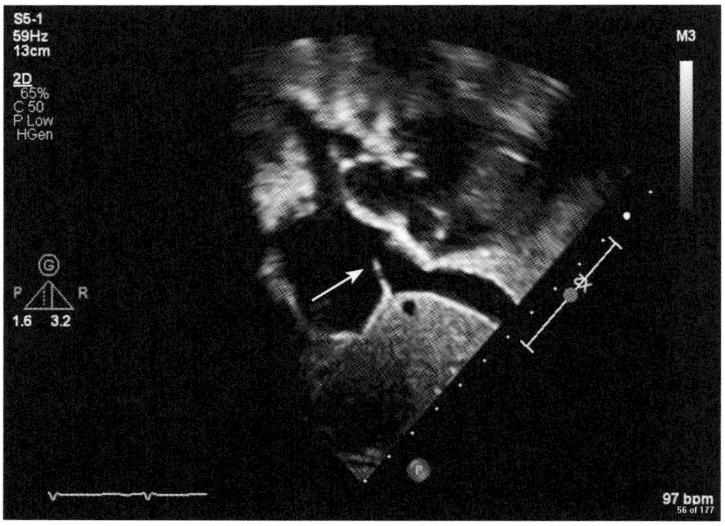

The valve of the inferior vena cava is the Eustachian valve (arrow). Care must be taken to clearly identify this structure because in the setting of an atrial septal defect (ASD) the Eustachian valve can wrongly be identified as an inferior rim of the defect. This is important in the setting of an ASD device closure as well as surgical closure of an ASD.

- Lai WW, Mertens LL, Cohen MS, et al (eds): *Echocardiography in Pediatric and Congenital Heart Disease: From Fetus to Adult*, 2nd edition. Chichester, UK, Wiley-Blackwell, 2016, pp 207–210, 240.

40. A. Interruption of the hepatic portion of the IVC.

Interruption of the hepatic portion of the inferior vena cava (IVC) does not mean that all components that form the IVC are missing; only the hepatic segment of the IVC is not present. Study of the embryologic venous system can enhance understanding of hepatic duplication of the inferior vena cava, interruption of the hepatic segment of the IVC, and other systemic venous malformations.

- Lai WW, Mertens LL, Cohen MS, et al (eds): *Echocardiography in Pediatric and Congenital Heart Disease: From Fetus to Adult*, 2nd edition. Chichester, UK, Wiley-Blackwell, 2016, p 181.
- Moore KL, Persaud TVN, Torchia MG: *The Developing Human: Clinically Oriented Embryology*, 9th edition. Philadelphia, Elsevier Saunders, 2013, pp 292, 295.

41. D. Patent ductus arteriosus (PDA).

A moderate to large sized patent ductus arteriosus (PDA) will generally be associated with prominent reversal of flow within the abdominal aorta. Other examples of cardiac pathology that can present with prominent diastolic flow reversal include significant aortic regurgitation, aortico–left ventricular tunnel (ALVT), and sinus of Valsalva rupture.

▶ Lai WW, Mertens LL, Cohen MS, et al (eds): *Echocardiography in Pediatric and Congenital Heart Disease: From Fetus to Adult*, 2nd edition. Chichester, UK, Wiley-Blackwell, 2016, pp 83, 320, 350.

42. C. A left-sided patent ductus arteriosus.

As a rule of thumb, the aortic arch, descending aorta, and ductus arteriosus should all be on the same side to exclude a vascular ring. Special care must be taken when imaging a right-sided aortic arch, an aberrant left subclavian artery, and a left-sided ductus arteriosus (originating from the left subclavian artery or a diverticulum of Kommerell), which can be a setup for a vascular ring. One exception to this statement would be a right-sided aortic arch and a left-sided patent ductus arteriosus originating from the left innominate (brachiocephalic) artery. In choice D, the patent ductus arteriosus is too far anterior to cause a vascular ring.

▶ Allen HD, Driscoll DJ, Shaddy RE, et al: *Moss and Adams' Heart Disease in Infants, Children, and Adolescents: Including the Fetus and Young Adult*, 8th edition. Philadelphia, Lippincott Williams & Wilkins, 2013, pp 758–788.

43. C. Finger-like appendage.

Hallmarks of left atrial morphology include a finger-like atrial appendage and the flap valve of the foramen ovale (atrial septum primum). The crista terminalis and septum secundum are characteristics of the morphologic right atrium; these structures cannot be readily visualized on transthoracic echocardiography. The site of pulmonary venous connection is not a reliable marker of left atrial morphology.

▶ Anderson RH, Baker EJ, Penny D, et al: *Paediatric Cardiology*, 3rd edition. Philadelphia, Churchill Livingstone/Elsevier, 2010, p 21.

▶ Lai WW, Mertens LL, Cohen MS, et al (eds): *Echocardiography in Pediatric and Congenital Heart Disease: From Fetus to Adult*, 2nd edition. Chichester, UK, Wiley-Blackwell, 2016, pp 35–37.

44. D. Situs solitus.

A right-sided liver, left-sided stomach, left-sided spleen, and right-sided cecum are all typical of normally positioned abdominal viscera, or situs solitus.

▶ Lai WW, Mertens LL, Cohen MS, et al (eds): *Echocardiography in Pediatric and Congenital Heart Disease: From Fetus to Adult*, 2nd edition. Chichester, UK, Wiley-Blackwell, 2016, pp 33–35.

ANSWERS

45. B. Situs solitus.

A right-sided morphologic right atrium and left-sided morphologic left atrium constitute the normal arrangement and morphology of the atria—situs solitus.

- Lai WW, Mertens LL, Cohen MS, et al (eds): *Echocardiography in Pediatric and Congenital Heart Disease: From Fetus to Adult*, 2nd edition. Chichester, UK, Wiley-Blackwell, 2016, pp 35–37.

46. C. L-looped ventricle.

The looping pattern of the ventricles is determined by the hand, left or right, that is used to identify the arrangement of the right ventricle. This is an imaginary exercise in which you place one or the other hand into the right ventricle from an anterior approach. If you could place only your right hand inside the right ventricle with the right thumb inserting into the inflow, the index finger inserting into the outflow, and the middle finger pointing to the septum, there is a dextro- *or* D-looping *pattern. D-looping is the normal pattern. Conversely, if you could fit only your left hand into the right ventricle in the same way, the looping pattern is leftward—i.e., the ventricle is* levo- *or* L-looped*.* X looping *refers to a looping pattern that cannot be determined. There is no such thing as an "A-looped" ventricular arrangement.*

- Lai WW, Mertens LL, Cohen MS, et al (eds): *Echocardiography in Pediatric and Congenital Heart Disease: From Fetus to Adult*, 2nd edition. Chichester, UK, Wiley-Blackwell, 2016, pp 37–39.
- Schallert EK, Danton GH, Kardon R, et al: Describing congenital heart disease using three-part segmental notation. RadioGraphics 33:E33–E47, 2013.
- Van Praagh R, Ongley PA, Swan HJ: Anatomic types of single or common ventricle in man: morphologic and geometric aspects of 60 necropsied cases. Am J Cardiol 13:367–386, 1964.

47. A. Tricuspid valve.

When the hand is used to determine a D-looped or L-looped right ventricle, the thumb represents inflow, the index finger represents the right ventricular outflow tract, the middle finger points to the ventricular septum, and the palm rests on the septum. Using this model, if the morphologic right ventricle being examined fits a right hand, it is a D-looped ventricle. If it fits a left hand, it is an L-looped ventricle. (See also the answers to questions 22 and 46.)

- Lai WW, Mertens LL, Cohen MS, et al (eds): *Echocardiography in Pediatric and Congenital Heart Disease: From Fetus to Adult*, 2nd edition. Chichester, UK, Wiley-Blackwell, 2016, p 39.

48. D. Normally related great arteries, situs inversus.

With inversus normally related great arteries, the aorta is posterior, leftward, and normally connected/assigned to the left ventricle with its ascending segment crossing over the left-sided pulmonary artery. This is seen in the patient with complete situs inversus and a segmental set of {I, L, I}, sometimes known as mirror-image dextrocardia. Note that this arrangement is the complete opposite (mirror image) of that seen in normal hearts {S, D, S}.

▶ Ezon DS, Goldberg JF, Kyle WB: *Atlas of Congenital Heart Disease Nomenclature: An Illustrated Guide to the Van Praagh and Anderson Approaches to Describing Congenital Cardiac Pathology*. Houston, Ezon Educational Services/CreateSpace, 2015, pp 22–23, 40–41.

▶ Lai WW, Mertens LL, Cohen MS, et al (eds): *Echocardiography in Pediatric and Congenital Heart Disease: From Fetus to Adult*, 2nd edition. Chichester, UK, Wiley-Blackwell, 2016, pp 44, 559–561.

49. B. Morphologic right ventricle in the setting of L-looped ventricles.

Irrespective of ventricular looping, an infundibulum is generally associated with a morphologic right ventricle. Other important morphologic right ventricular markers include a moderator band, coarse trabeculations, the tricuspid valve, and ventricular septal attachments of the tricuspid valve.

▶ Ezon DS, Goldberg JF, Kyle WB: *Atlas of Congenital Heart Disease Nomenclature: An Illustrated Guide to the Van Praagh and Anderson Approaches to Describing Congenital Cardiac Pathology*. Houston, Ezon Educational Services/CreateSpace, 2015, pp 10–11.

▶ Lai WW, Mertens LL, Cohen MS, et al (eds): *Echocardiography in Pediatric and Congenital Heart Disease: From Fetus to Adult*, 2nd edition. Chichester, UK, Wiley-Blackwell, 2016, pp 37–39.

50. D. Atrioventricular junction and ventriculoarterial junction.

The connecting segments are the atrioventricular junction and ventriculoarterial junction, as defined by Dr. Robert Anderson. Alternatively, Dr. Richard Van Praagh defines the connecting segments as the atrioventricular canal and the infundibulum (conus arteriosus). The atria, ventricles, and great arteries are the three main segments in the segmental approach, and both Dr. Anderson and Dr. Van Praagh define these three main segments using similar terminology.

▶ Anderson RH, Becker AE, Freedom RM, et al: Sequential segmental analysis of congenital heart disease. Pediatr Cardiol 5:281–288, 1984.

▶ Ezon DS, Goldberg JF, Kyle WB: *Atlas of Congenital Heart Disease Nomenclature: An Illustrated Guide to the Van Praagh and Anderson*

ANSWERS

ANSWERS

Approaches to Describing Congenital Cardiac Pathology. Houston, Ezon Educational Services/CreateSpace, 2015, pp 2–3, 40–41.

▸ Lai WW, Mertens LL, Cohen MS, et al (eds): *Echocardiography in Pediatric and Congenital Heart Disease: From Fetus to Adult*, 2nd edition. Chichester, UK, Wiley-Blackwell, 2016, pp 32–38.

51. C. Atria, ventricles, and great arteries.

The atria, ventricles (Dr. Van Praagh) or ventricular mass (Dr. Anderson), and great arteries are the three main segments in the segmental approach to congenital heart disease. The connecting segments are the atrioventricular junction and ventriculoarterial junction, as defined by Dr. Anderson. Alternatively, Dr. Van Praagh defines the connecting segments as the atrioventricular canal and the infundibulum.

▸ Anderson RH, Becker AE, Freedom RM, et al: Sequential segmental analysis of congenital heart disease. Pediatr Cardiol 5:281–288, 1984.

▸ Ezon DS, Goldberg JF, Kyle WB: *Atlas of Congenital Heart Disease Nomenclature: An Illustrated Guide to the Van Praagh and Anderson Approaches to Describing Congenital Cardiac Pathology*. Houston, Ezon Educational Services/CreateSpace, 2015, pp 2–3, 40–41.

▸ Lai WW, Mertens LL, Cohen MS, et al (eds): *Echocardiography in Pediatric and Congenital Heart Disease: From Fetus to Adult*, 2nd edition. Chichester, UK, Wiley-Blackwell, 2016, pp 32–38.

Refer to video PER-Q52.

52. A. Situs solitus.

Video PER-Q52 is a subxiphoid (subcostal) long-axis view with the index marker positioned at 3 o'clock. This video clip demonstrates normal arrangement of the abdominal visceral organs with a right-sided liver, right-sided inferior vena cava, left-sided aorta, and left-sided stomach.

▸ Lai WW, Mertens LL, Cohen MS, et al (eds): *Echocardiography in Pediatric and Congenital Heart Disease: From Fetus to Adult*, 2nd edition. Chichester, UK, Wiley-Blackwell, 2016, pp 32–33, 46, 573.

53. C. Left atrial appendage.

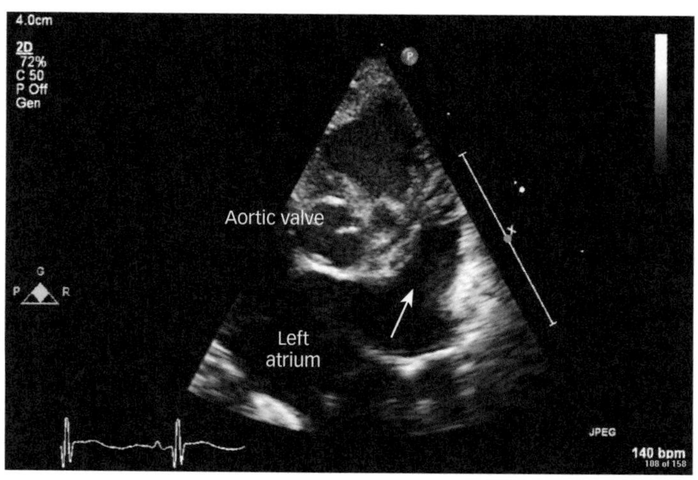

This is a parasternal short-axis view below the level of the aortic valve and just above the mitral valve. In this image the left atrium and left atrial appendage (arrow) are seen. The left atrial appendage can be differentiated from a left pulmonary vein by adding color Doppler over the area of interest. To-and-fro flow is seen with the left atrial appendage and a pulmonary venous spectral Doppler profile in the presence of a left pulmonary vein.

▸ Lai WW, Mertens LL, Cohen MS, et al (eds): *Echocardiography in Pediatric and Congenital Heart Disease: From Fetus to Adult*, 2nd edition. Chichester, UK, Wiley-Blackwell, 2016, pp 52–55, 134–135.

54. D. Superior vena cava.

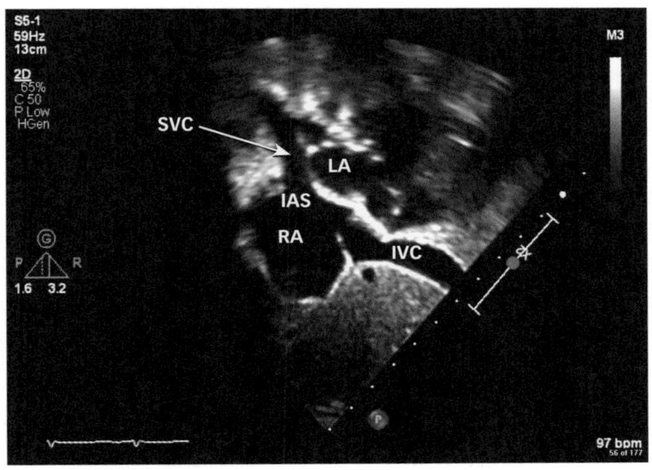

This is a subcostal short-axis (sagittal) view in a normal heart, with the arrow pointing to the superior vena cava (SVC). In this image the SVC, inferior vena cava (IVC), and interatrial septum (IAS) are visualized. RA = right atrium, LA = left atrium.

▸ Lai WW, Mertens LL, Cohen MS, et al (eds): *Echocardiography in Pediatric and Congenital Heart Disease: From Fetus to Adult*, 2nd edition. Chichester, UK, Wiley-Blackwell, 2016, pp 46–48.

Refer to video PER-Q55.

55. A. Levocardia.

Video PER-Q55 is a subcostal long-axis (frontal) sweep demonstrating levocardia. The sweep is obtained with an invert or up-down option selected on the ultrasound equipment in order to reflect structures like the liver and stomach inferior to the heart as the sweep progresses. The transducer's notch/dot is set to 3 o'clock. This video clip demonstrates the majority of the cardiac mass in the left thoracic cavity as well as the heart's apex pointing leftward.

In dextrocardia the majority of the cardiac mass, as well as the heart's apex (which is pointing to the right), is in the right thoracic cavity. In mesocardia the heart is mostly behind the sternum with the apex pointing inferiorly or anteriorly.

▸ Lai WW, Mertens LL, Cohen MS, et al (eds): *Echocardiography in Pediatric and Congenital Heart Disease: From Fetus to Adult*, 2nd edition. Chichester, UK, Wiley-Blackwell, 2016, pp 33–35, 46–48.

56. B. Thebesian valve.

The Thebesian valve is the valve of the coronary sinus.

▸ Lai WW, Mertens LL, Cohen MS, et al (eds): *Echocardiography in Pediatric and Congenital Heart Disease: From Fetus to Adult*, 2nd edition. Chichester, UK, Wiley-Blackwell, 2016, p 240.

57. B. Chiari network.

This structure represents a Chiari network. *The multiple fenestrations in this scenario prevent obstruction and distinguish a Chiari network from cor triatriatum dextrum.* Cor triatriatum dextrum *is present when a prominent membrane subdivides the right atrial appendage portion of the right atrium from the portion that receives the inferior vena cava, superior vena cava, and coronary sinus. The subdivision caused by the membrane in cor triatriatum dextrum can cause right-to-left shunting if the membrane is significantly obstructive.*

▸ Anderson RH, Baker EJ, Penny D, et al: *Paediatric Cardiology*, 3rd edition. Philadelphia, Churchill Livingstone/Elsevier, 2010, p 550.

▸ Lai WW, Mertens LL, Cohen MS, et al (eds): *Echocardiography in Pediatric and Congenital Heart Disease: From Fetus to Adult*, 2nd edition. Chichester, UK, Wiley-Blackwell, 2016, p 240.

58. A. Small patent ductus arteriosus.

See Color Plate 3 on page xx.

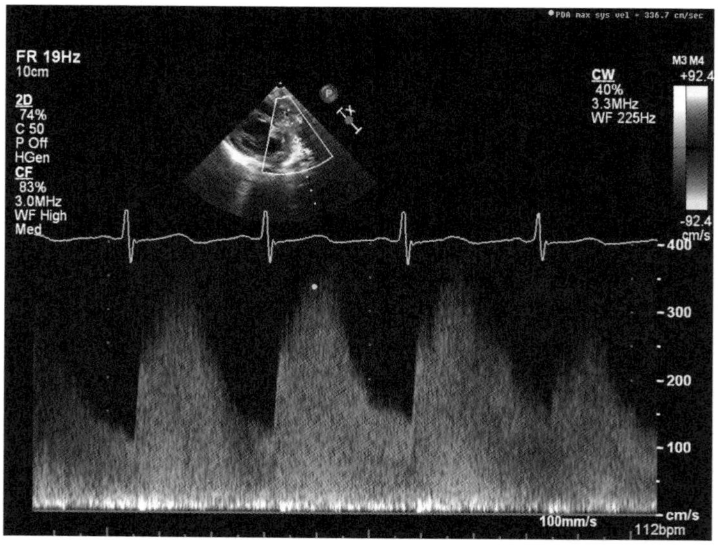

This spectral Doppler image is from an infant with a small restrictive patent ductus arteriosus (PDA), with continuous left-to-right shunting when pulmonary vascular resistance is less than systemic vascular resistance. Choices B (pulmonary vein) and C (superior vena cava) are incorrect, as these vessels generally have low-velocity phasic flow with return close to the baseline. Choice D (left pulmonary artery) is incorrect because left pulmonary artery flow would be seen moving in the opposite direction, away from the transducer.

▶ Lai WW, Mertens LL, Cohen MS, et al (eds): *Echocardiography in Pediatric and Congenital Heart Disease: From Fetus to Adult*, 2nd edition. Chichester, UK, Wiley-Blackwell, 2016, pp 135, 165, 389.

▶ Zwiebel WJ, Pellerito JS: *Introduction to Vascular Ultrasonography*, 5th edition. Philadelphia, Saunders, 2005, p 13.

59. D. Aortic valve.

See Color Plate 4 on page xxi.

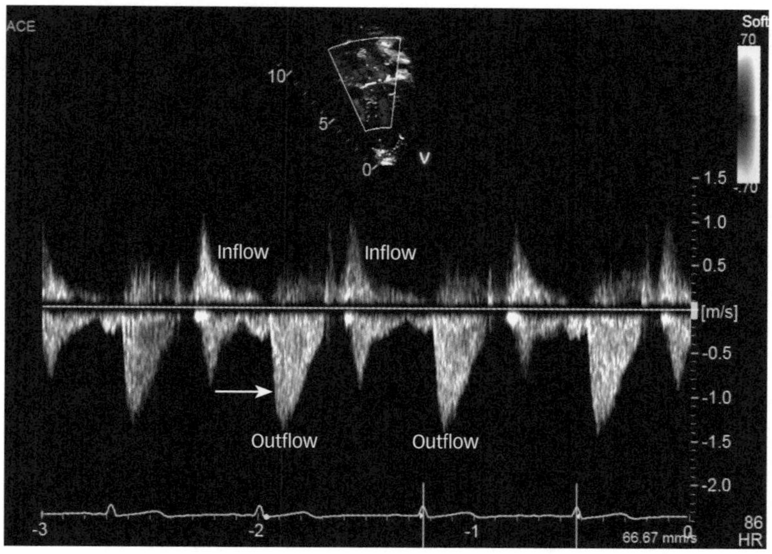

The arrow in this image represents aortic valve spectral Doppler. Both aortic and mitral valve spectral Doppler waveforms are seen. In the structurally normal heart, the Doppler waveforms of both the aortic valve and the mitral valve can be documented at the same time due to their proximity to each other (mitral to aortic fibrinous continuity). In contrast, the pulmonary valve and tricuspid valve spectral Doppler waveforms are generally not obtained simultaneously because of the separation created by the infundibulum (conus arteriosus).

▶ Lai WW, Mertens LL, Cohen MS, et al (eds): *Echocardiography in Pediatric and Congenital Heart Disease: From Fetus to Adult*, 2nd edition. Chichester, UK, Wiley-Blackwell, 2016, pp 38, 106–107, 135.

ANSWERS

PART 2

Pathology and Pathophysiology

60. A. Dilated cardiomyopathy.

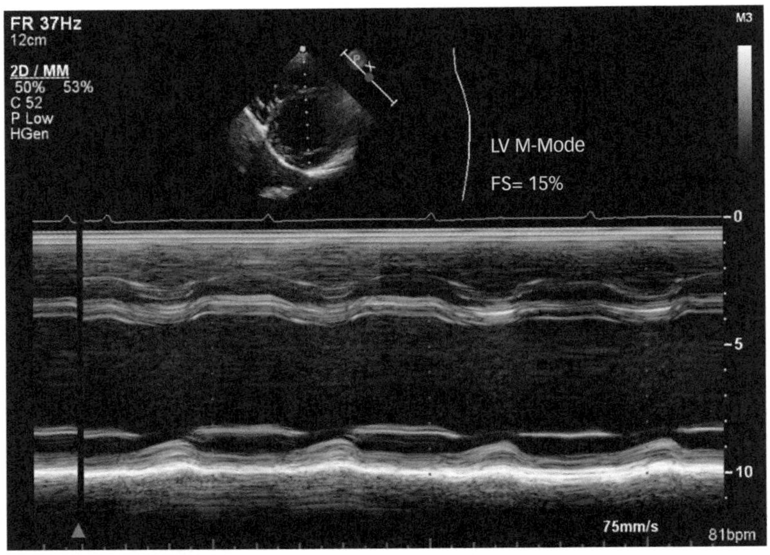

In this patient the left ventricle (LV) is larger than normal, with a Z-score of +5.5, indicating dilatation. Fractional shortening (FS) is only 15%; normal FS is greater than 27%. The LV free wall and septum appear thin, not thick, so the answer is not choice C. Pulmonary hypertension affects the right ventricle, which would be expected to be more dilated than the left ventricle, so choice D is also incorrect. (See also the answer to question 516.)

▸ Lai WW, Mertens LL, Cohen MS, et al (eds): *Echocardiography in Pediatric and Congenital Heart Disease: From Fetus to Adult*, 2nd edition. Chichester, UK, Wiley-Blackwell, 2016, p 653.

61. C. Anomalous left coronary artery from the pulmonary artery.

In patients with anomalous left coronary artery from the pulmonary artery (ALCAPA), the left main coronary artery (LMCA) originates from the main pulmonary artery instead of the aortic root, and antegrade perfusion into the LMCA depends on high pulmonary artery pressures (typically found in utero and at birth). When pulmonary vascular resistance and pulmonary artery pressure fall a few weeks after birth, there is reduced antegrade flow through the LMCA. Instead, LMCA flow reverses and proceeds in a retrograde manner from the coronary artery into the pulmonary artery, resulting in a "steal" of blood flow from the left ventricular (LV) myocardium. To compensate, right coronary artery blood flow increases and perfuses the left coronary artery through collateral arteries connecting the right and left coronary artery systems (often visible by echocardiography). Nonetheless, the steal often leads to the LV developing signs of ischemia, chamber dilatation, poor systolic function, and mitral valve regurgitation due to papillary muscle ischemia. With early diagnosis and surgical correction, LV function can recover. A small right coronary artery fistula usually will not cause significant hemodynamic change; there is no left or right ventricular dilatation. Bacterial myocarditis and juvenile rheumatoid arthritis are treated with medications; surgery is not necessary.

▸ Allen HD, Driscoll DJ, Shaddy RE, et al: *Moss and Adams' Heart Disease in Infants, Children, and Adolescents: Including the Fetus and Young Adult*, 8th edition. Philadelphia, Lippincott Williams & Wilkins, 2013, pp 749–751.

▸ Lai WW, Mertens LL, Cohen MS, et al (eds): *Echocardiography in Pediatric and Congenital Heart Disease: From Fetus to Adult*, 2nd edition. Chichester, UK, Wiley-Blackwell, 2016, pp 591–593.

62. C. Hypertrophic cardiomyopathy.

A ventricular septal defect (VSD), bicuspid aortic valve, or pericardial effusion will not cause death that is unexpected, abrupt, and related to a cardiovascular condition—known as sudden cardiac death (SCD). Hypertrophic cardiomyopathy is the most common cause of SCD in children and young adults. Most patients with hypertrophic cardiomyopathy are asymptomatic. Life-threatening arrhythmia, syncope, and sometimes sudden death may be the first clinical symptoms.

▸ Allen HD, Driscoll DJ, Shaddy RE, et al: *Moss and Adams' Heart Disease in Infants, Children, and Adolescents: Including the Fetus and Young Adult*, 8th edition. Philadelphia, Lippincott Williams & Wilkins, 2013, pp 1228–1231.

▸ Lai WW, Mertens LL, Cohen MS, et al (eds): *Echocardiography in Pediatric and Congenital Heart Disease: From Fetus to Adult*, 2nd edition. Chichester, UK, Wiley-Blackwell, 2016, pp 677–678.

63. A. Dilated right and left atria.

Restrictive cardiomyopathy impairs ventricular relaxation and subsequent ventricular filling, so the left ventricle would not be dilated. Systolic function and wall thickness may appear normal. Due to abnormal ventricular filling, the left and right atria are dilated. Doppler demonstrates little change in mitral valve and tricuspid valve inflow with inspiration and expiration.

These features distinguish restrictive cardiomyopathy from tamponade physiology and constrictive pericarditis, both of which are associated with pericardial effusion.

▶ Armstrong WF, Ryan T: *Feigenbaum's Echocardiography*, 7th edition. Philadelphia, Lippincott Williams & Wilkins, 2010, p 259.

▶ Lai WW, Mertens LL, Cohen MS, et al (eds): *Echocardiography in Pediatric and Congenital Heart Disease: From Fetus to Adult*, 2nd edition. Chichester, UK, Wiley-Blackwell, 2016, pp 694–703.

64. B. Avoiding mitral valve regurgitant flow.

See Color Plate 5 on page xxi.

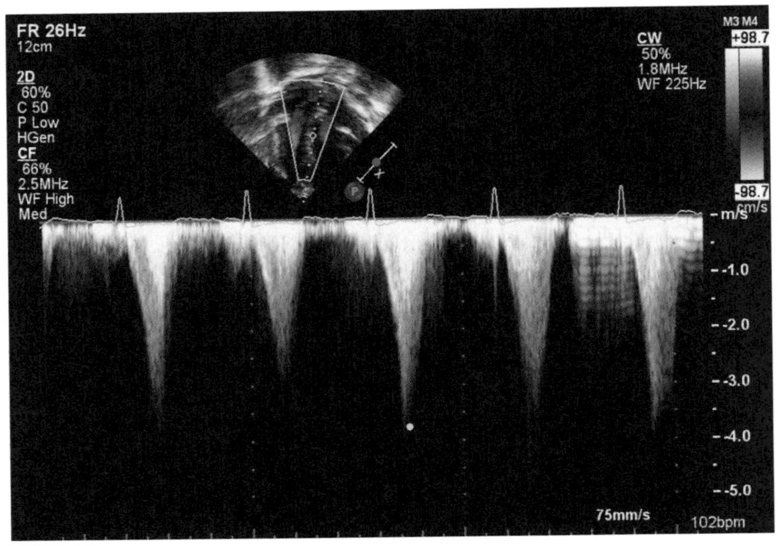

Evaluating left ventricular outflow tract (LVOT) obstruction for hypertrophic cardiomyopathy can be technically challenging. Color flow Doppler should be used to visualize the exact location of outflow obstruction. Pulsed-wave Doppler can be used sequentially across the outflow tract, but it might not be adequate to measure a high-velocity jet due to a lower Nyquist limit. Therefore it is necessary to use continuous-wave (CW) Doppler, but it is important to distinguish the true LVOT velocity from mitral valve regurgitation velocity. Typically, with CW Doppler evaluation of LVOT obstruction, the waveform displays a dagger-like shape that distinguishes it from a mitral valve regurgitation flow pattern. Using an apical five-chamber view and orienting the transducer parallel to the LVOT will help you avoid unintentionally imaging mitral valve regurgitant flow.

▶ Lai WW, Mertens LL, Cohen MS, et al (eds): *Echocardiography in Pediatric and Congenital Heart Disease: From Fetus to Adult*, 2nd edition. Chichester, UK, Wiley-Blackwell, 2016, pp 683–685.

65. D. Hypertrophic cardiomyopathy.

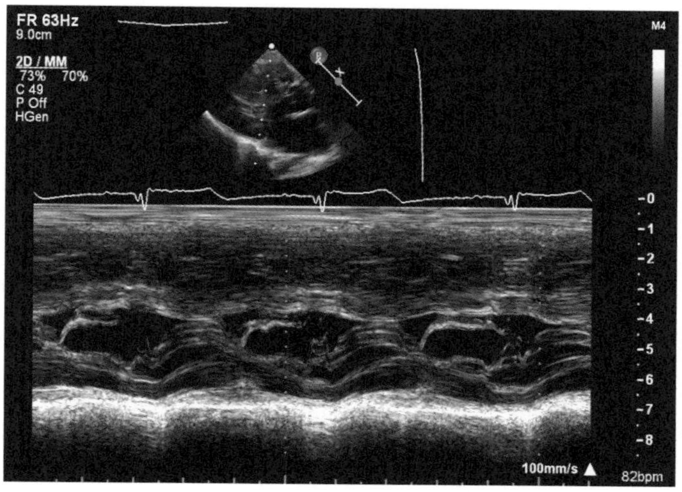

Systolic anterior motion (SAM) is seen in hypertrophic cardiomyopathy with left ventricular outflow tract (LVOT) obstruction, and of the choices offered hypertrophic cardiomyopathy is the only one in which SAM can be found. However, this type of mitral valve motion can also be found in the presence of other conditions, such as after mitral valve repair or with an anomalous papillary muscle.

- Armstrong WF, Ryan T: *Feigenbaum's Echocardiography*, 7th edition. Philadelphia, Lippincott Williams & Wilkins, 2010, p 540.
- Lai WW, Mertens LL, Cohen MS, et al (eds): *Echocardiography in Pediatric and Congenital Heart Disease: From Fetus to Adult*, 2nd edition. Chichester, UK, Wiley-Blackwell, 2016, pp 681–682.

66. C. Hypertrophic cardiomyopathy.

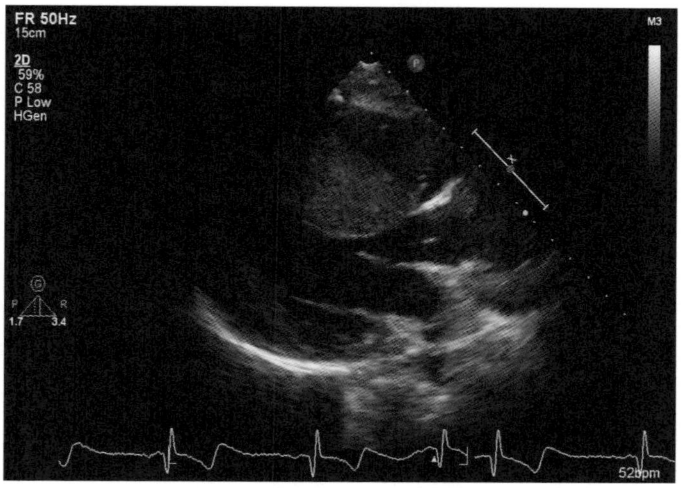

Significant left ventricular hypertrophy is seen in this image, so hypertrophic cardiomyopathy is the answer. In dilated cardiomyopathy (choice B), the left ventricle (LV)

ANSWERS

is often significantly dilated and thin-walled. The LV is not dilated in this image, so choice B is incorrect. Restrictive cardiomyopathy (choice D) is generally associated with a large left atrium, and in this image the left atrial size appears normal; therefore choice D is incorrect. Myocarditis (choice A) usually will not have the significant LV hypertrophy seen in this image, so choice A is also incorrect.

▶ Lai WW, Mertens LL, Cohen MS, et al (eds): *Echocardiography in Pediatric and Congenital Heart Disease: From Fetus to Adult*, 2nd edition. Chichester, UK, Wiley-Blackwell, 2016, pp 677–681.

67. B. Mitral valve inflow E-wave deceleration time less than 160 ms.

Restrictive cardiomyopathy is characterized by the following: a mitral valve inflow E/A ratio greater than 2.0; a mitral valve inflow E-wave deceleration time less than 160 ms; increased pulmonary vein A-wave reversal velocity and duration; an E/Ea ratio greater than 15; and no respiratory variation in isovolumetric relaxation time (IVRT) or left ventricular (LV) inflow. This last factor helps to distinguish restrictive cardiomyopathy from constrictive pericarditis.

▶ Armstrong WF, Ryan T: *Feigenbaum's Echocardiography*, 7th edition. Philadelphia, Lippincott Williams & Wilkins, 2010, p 556.

▶ Lai WW, Mertens LL, Cohen MS, et al (eds): *Echocardiography in Pediatric and Congenital Heart Disease: From Fetus to Adult*, 2nd edition. Chichester, UK, Wiley-Blackwell, 2016, p 695.

68. A. Increased cardiac output.

Sickle cell disease is a chronic red blood cell (RBC) disorder characterized by abnormal, sickle-shaped RBCs. Sickled RBCs typically survive only 10–20 days, compared to a lifespan of 90–120 days for normal RBCs. Because of the reduced lifespan of sickled RBCs, patients suffer from chronic anemia and inefficient oxygenation of the blood supply, resulting in an increase in cardiac output (accompanied by increased stroke volume and a minimally increased heart rate) to optimize oxygen delivery to the body. The increase in stroke volume results in left ventricular (LV) dilatation, not chamber size reduction.

▶ Gladwin MT, Sachdev V: Cardiovascular abnormalities in sickle cell disease. J Am Coll Cardiol 59:1123–1133, 2012.

69. D. Duchenne muscular dystrophy.

Mitochondrial disease, Noonan syndrome, and LEOPARD syndrome (an acronym for ***l****entigines,* ***e****lectrocardiographic conduction abnormalities,* ***o****cular hypertelorism,* ***p****ulmonary stenosis,* ***a****bnormal genitalia,* ***r****etarded growth, and* ***d****eafness) are all related to hypertrophic cardiomyopathy. Muscular dystrophy usually causes dilated (not hypertrophic) cardiomyopathy.*

▶ Lai WW, Mertens LL, Cohen MS, et al (eds): *Echocardiography in Pediatric and Congenital Heart Disease: From Fetus to Adult*, 2nd edition. Chichester, UK, Wiley-Blackwell, 2016, p 679.

70. D. Left atrial and left ventricular end-diastolic pressures are both elevated.

In restrictive cardiomyopathy, the left ventricular walls become stiff and noncompliant, and this causes impaired left ventricular diastolic filling, resulting in elevated left atrial and left ventricular end-diastolic pressures. Choice A is incorrect because left ventricular end-diastolic pressure will be higher than that in the right ventricle. Choice C is incorrect because left atrial and left ventricular end-diastolic pressures are equal.

▶ Lai WW, Mertens LL, Cohen MS, et al (eds): *Echocardiography in Pediatric and Congenital Heart Disease: From Fetus to Adult*, 2nd edition. Chichester, UK, Wiley-Blackwell, 2016, pp 694–695.

71. C. Fatty replacement of the right ventricular myocardium.

Arrhythmogenic right ventricular cardiomyopathy/dysplasia (ARVC/D) is a genetic disorder that mainly affects the right ventricle. With ARVC/D fibrofatty tissue replaces right ventricular muscle gradually, often leading to a potentially lethal arrhythmia. With parchment heart, also known as Uhl's cardiomyopathy, a parchment-thin right ventricular wall results in a dilated congestive cardiomyopathy, primarily involving the right ventricle. Endocardial fibroelastosis (EFE) is characterized by prominent thickening of the ventricular endocardium; a thick and bright endocardium will be seen with echocardiography. Metabolic cardiomyopathy is a nonspecific term referring to a broad range of metabolic disorders that can produce systolic and/or diastolic dysfunction of the ventricles, but they do not result in fibrofatty replacement of the muscle.

▶ Lai WW, Mertens LL, Cohen MS, et al (eds): *Echocardiography in Pediatric and Congenital Heart Disease: From Fetus to Adult*, 2nd edition. Chichester, UK, Wiley-Blackwell, 2016, p 727.

72. B. 64 mmHg + right atrial (RA) pressure.

Using the simplified Bernoulli equation, right ventricular pressure (RVP) = 4 × tricuspid regurgitant (TR) velocity² + right atrial pressure (RAP). Therefore the TR gradient = 4 × (4)² = 64 mmHg. Normal RAP = 5–10 mmHg, and normal RVP = 64 + (5 or 10 mmHg) = 69–74 mmHg.

▶ Lai WW, Mertens LL, Cohen MS, et al (eds): *Echocardiography in Pediatric and Congenital Heart Disease: From Fetus to Adult*, 2nd edition. Chichester, UK, Wiley-Blackwell, 2016, pp 79–80.

73. C. Pulmonary hypertension.

A

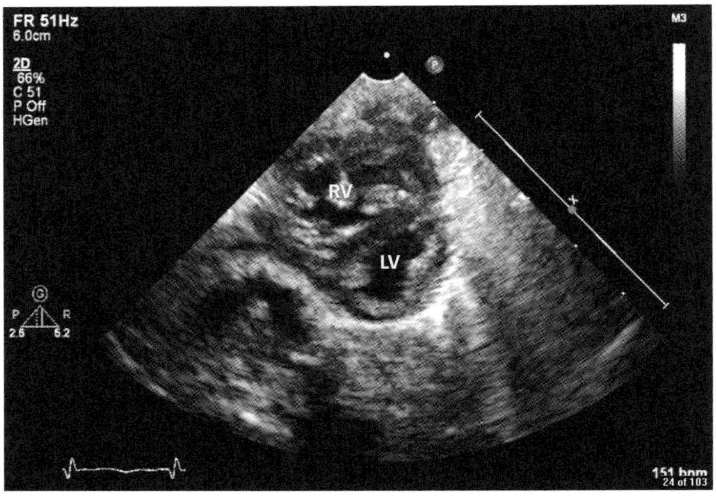

B

See Color Plate 6 on page xxii.

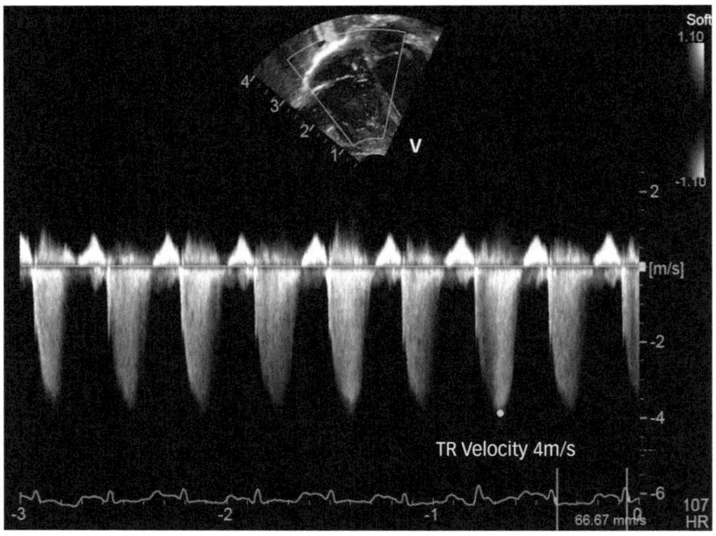

A congenital diaphragmatic hernia (CDH) can impair lung development and increase the risk of pulmonary hypertension. Postnatally, the infant may have significant respiratory distress; the echocardiogram often demonstrates dextroposition of the heart (when the CDH is left-sided) and a flattened ventricular

*septum due to increased right ventricular (RV) pressure. If the patient has tricuspid valve regurgitation, often the regurgitant jet velocity is high. In image **A** the ventricular septum is flat; in image **B** tricuspid regurgitant velocity is 4.0 m/sec. The estimated RV pressure will be 64 mmHg + RA pressure. An atrial septal defect generally does not cause pulmonary hypertension in a newborn. Pulmonary artery (PA) pressure can be elevated with a VSD, but this is not the most common etiology of high PA pressure in a patient with a known CDH.*

74. C. Pulmonary valve motion with an absent A-dip on M-mode.

With normal pulmonary artery pressure, M-mode of the pulmonary valve shows an A-dip. When there is pulmonary hypertension, this A-dip disappears. Mitral valve systolic anterior motion and aortic valve reopening are features typical of hypertrophic cardiomyopathy. Mitral valve vibration in diastole is caused by aortic valve regurgitation.

▸ Lai WW, Mertens LL, Cohen MS, et al (eds): *Echocardiography in Pediatric and Congenital Heart Disease: From Fetus to Adult*. Chichester, UK, Wiley-Blackwell, 2009, p 756.

75. A. VSD with normal pulmonary artery pressure.

See Color Plate 7 on page xxii.

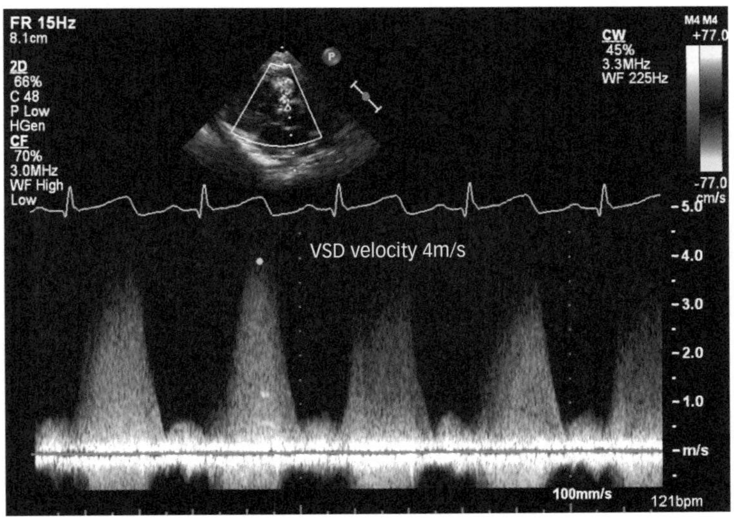

The velocity of blood flow through the ventricular septal defect (VSD) is 4 m/sec, using the simplified Bernoulli equation:

$$\begin{aligned} \Delta P_{max} &= \text{LV pressure} - \text{RV pressure} \\ &= 4V^2 \\ &= 4 \times 4 \times 4 \\ &= 64 \text{ mmHg} \end{aligned}$$

Since left ventricular (LV) systolic pressure should equal systolic arterial blood pressure of 90 mmHg, right ventricular (RV) systolic pressure can be estimated at 90 mmHg − 64 mmHg = 26 mmHg. In the absence of right ventricular outflow tract (RVOT) obstruction, pulmonary artery systolic pressure should be equivalent to RV systolic pressure; therefore pulmonary artery systolic pressure equals 26 mmHg, which is normal for this infant patient.

▶ Lai WW, Mertens LL, Cohen MS, et al (eds): *Echocardiography in Pediatric and Congenital Heart Disease: From Fetus to Adult*, 2nd edition. Chichester, UK, Wiley-Blackwell, 2016, p 878.

76. D. Changes in IVC size with respiration.

The pulmonary regurgitant velocity can also be used to calculate pulmonary artery pressures, as previous studies have demonstrated good correlation of the pulmonary regurgitant jet with both end-diastolic pressure and mean pulmonary artery pressures. Without calculating the velocity of tricuspid valve regurgitation or pulmonary valve regurgitation, we cannot <u>*directly*</u> *calculate pulmonary artery pressure. However, we can use changes in the size of the inferior vena cava (IVC) to estimate right ventricular pressure* <u>*indirectly*</u>*. With a normal right atrial (RA) pressure of 5–10 mmHg, IVC diameter will decrease 50% during inspiration. When RA pressure exceeds 10 mmHg, IVC size is often unchanged during inspiration. If RA pressure exceeds 20 mmHg, the IVC is dilated. With pulmonary hypertension, RA pressure can equal or exceed 10 mmHg. Therefore an IVC diameter that does not change with respiration can be an* <u>*indirect*</u> *indicator of pulmonary hypertension. See the answer to question 75, which illustrates the calculation of PA pressure in the setting of a systemic-to-pulmonary shunt, using the shunt velocity.*

▶ Lai WW, Mertens LL, Cohen MS, et al (eds): *Echocardiography in Pediatric and Congenital Heart Disease: From Fetus to Adult*, 2nd edition. Chichester, UK, Wiley-Blackwell, 2016, p 87.

77. B. Truncus arteriosus.

Congenital heart defects—including truncus arteriosus (TA), ventricular septal defect (VSD), atrial septal defect (ASD), aortopulmonary window, and patent ductus arteriosus (PDA)—are characterized by excessive blood flow entering the pulmonary artery. Without surgical correction, many patients with these anomalies will develop significant pulmonary vascular disease that can eventually be irreversible (Eisenmenger syndrome). When a VSD is associated with pulmonary stenosis, however, the pulmonary stenosis limits excessive blood flow into the lung and can actually protect the lungs from developing pulmonary vascular disease. Scimitar syndrome involves partial anomalous pulmonary venous connection, with a small amount of extra flow to the right side of the heart; the accompanying right lung hypoplasia (not unrestricted flow to the lungs) may cause pulmonary hypertension. Mitral valve stenosis causes pulmonary hypertension due to elevated left atrial and pulmonary venous pressure, and this elevated pressure then leads to elevated pulmonary artery pressure, similar to the mechanism of pulmonary hypertension found in patients with pulmonary venous obstruction. In this condition, there is no left-to-right shunting and therefore no excess blood flow to the lungs.

- Allen HD, Driscoll DJ, Shaddy RE, et al: *Moss and Adams' Heart Disease in Infants, Children, and Adolescents: Including the Fetus and Young Adult*, 8th edition. Philadelphia, Lippincott Williams & Wilkins, 2013, p 1401.
- Lai WW, Mertens LL, Cohen MS, et al (eds): *Echocardiography in Pediatric and Congenital Heart Disease: From Fetus to Adult*, 2nd edition. Chichester, UK, Wiley-Blackwell, 2016, p 872.

78. D. Aortopulmonary (AP) window.

Before idiopathic pulmonary hypertension can be diagnosed, one must exclude cardiac defects that can cause pulmonary hypertension, such as a large ventricular septal defect (VSD) or a patent ductus arteriosus (PDA). These defects are difficult to overlook with a standard echocardiographic evaluation. Shunting across the atrial septum is also readily seen on echocardiography even in a setting of pulmonary hypertension. An aortopulmonary (AP) window, however, is easy to miss because on echocardiography it is characterized by an echo "dropout" due to absence of the wall between the aorta and the pulmonary artery. This finding, however, also occurs with normal patients: There is often an echo dropout in the wall between the aorta and the pulmonary artery as seen from the parasternal short-axis window. Therefore, it can be difficult to determine whether this echo dropout is normal or represents a defect. To complicate matters, color flow Doppler of this area can be deceiving: Even when the AP window is large (although this is usually the case), pulmonary artery pressure will be elevated, and only a subtle left-to-right shunt can be seen. The pitfall would be to assume normality when the possibility of an AP window exists. Hence it is important to investigate this area carefully to avoid missing a possible AP window.

- Lai WW, Mertens LL, Cohen MS, et al (eds): *Echocardiography in Pediatric and Congenital Heart Disease: From Fetus to Adult*, 2nd edition. Chichester, UK, Wiley-Blackwell, 2016, p 873.

79. A. Kawasaki disease.

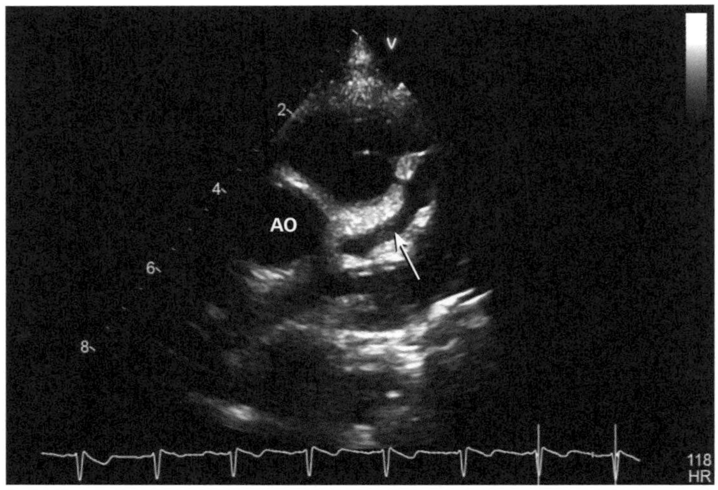

The findings for this patient are highly suggestive of Kawasaki disease. Typical symptoms include a high fever lasting more than 5 days, changes in the skin of the extremities (palmar erythema/desquamation), cracked lips, conjunctivitis, and a red, swollen tongue known as a "strawberry" tongue. Some patients will also develop involvement of the coronary arteries, which can include dilatation, ectasia, and aneurysm(s). Coronary involvement can affect one area or can be diffuse, affecting both right and left coronary arteries. In this image note dilatation and a saccular aneurysm in the proximal left anterior descending artery (LAD, arrow). None of the other possibilities mentioned exhibits the same typical clinical findings or coronary artery findings seen on the echocardiogram. AO = aorta.

- Lai WW, Mertens LL, Cohen MS, et al (eds): *Echocardiography in Pediatric and Congenital Heart Disease: From Fetus to Adult*, 2nd edition. Chichester, UK, Wiley-Blackwell, 2016, p 739.

80. B. Left circumflex coronary artery.

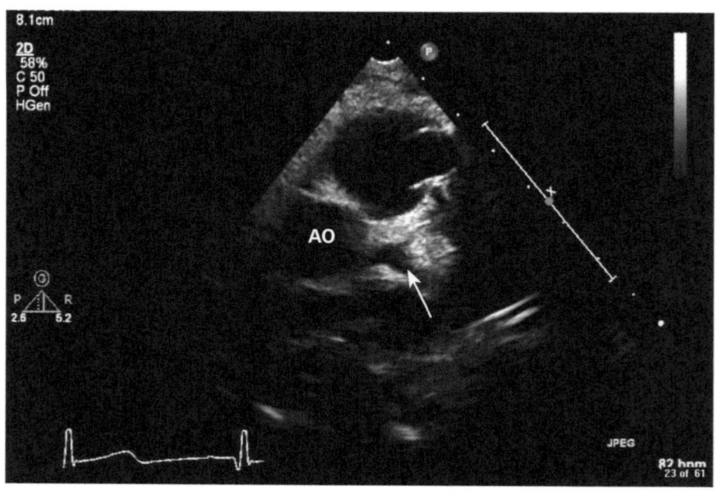

In a parasternal short-axis image, the location indicated by the arrow is typical for visualization of the left circumflex coronary artery. AO = aorta.

▶ Lai WW, Mertens LL, Cohen MS, et al (eds): *Echocardiography in Pediatric and Congenital Heart Disease: From Fetus to Adult*, 2nd edition. Chichester, UK, Wiley-Blackwell, 2016, p 741.

81. A. Right atrial wall collapse in diastole.

A pericardial effusion that produces an increase in intrapericardial pressure can result in tamponade physiology. This occurs when the intrapericardial pressure exceeds right ventricular (RV) pressure in diastole, leading to diastolic collapse of the RV free wall as well as the right atrial (RA) wall. However, the development of tamponade physiology depends not so much on the size of the effusion as on the rapidity of accumulation and the relative compliance (stiffness) of the pericardium. A large pericardial effusion might not produce signs of tamponade if it has accumulated chronically over a long period of time and thus if pericardial compliance and ventricular compliance have slowly increased such that the intrapericardial pressure remains low. Intrathoracic pressure changes during expiration and inspiration, along with some variation in mitral valve inflow, are to be expected with respiratory changes. However, when a patient has tamponade physiology, intrathoracic pressure will produce a much more pronounced respiratory variation in mitral valve inflow compared with a normal heart or a non-tamponade situation. In general this variation in mitral valve inflow between inspiration and expiration is greater than 30%.

▶ Armstrong WF, Ryan T: *Feigenbaum's Echocardiography*, 7th edition. Philadelphia, Lippincott Williams & Wilkins, 2010, pp 249–251.

▶ Lai WW, Mertens LL, Cohen MS, et al (eds): *Echocardiography in Pediatric and Congenital Heart Disease: From Fetus to Adult*, 2nd edition. Chichester, UK, Wiley-Blackwell, 2016, pp 709–713.

82. B. Pericardial effusion.

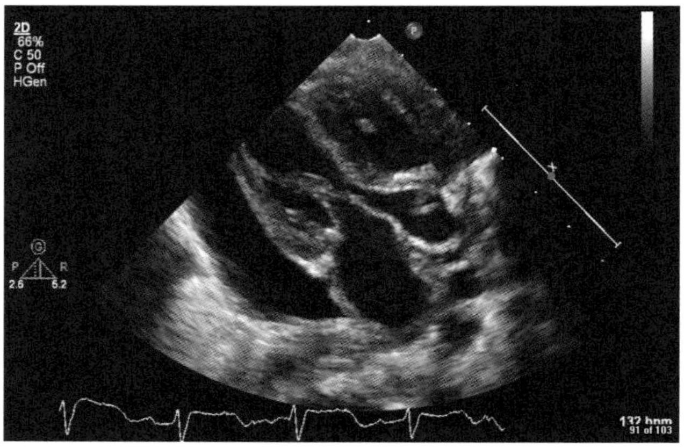

This image shows a posterior wall "echo-free" space, which is typical of a pericardial effusion. Pleural effusion can be confused for pericardial effusion. Pleural effusions are located in the chest, posterior to the descending thoracic aorta. Peritoneal fluid may have a similar sonographic appearance but is not well seen with this view. Pericardial effusion is located anterior to the descending thoracic aorta.

- Armstrong WF, Ryan T: *Feigenbaum's Echocardiography*, 7th edition. Philadelphia, Lippincott Williams & Wilkins, 2010, p 248.
- Lai WW, Mertens LL, Cohen MS, et al (eds): *Echocardiography in Pediatric and Congenital Heart Disease: From Fetus to Adult*, 2nd edition. Chichester, UK, Wiley-Blackwell, 2016, pp 709–713.

83. C. Posterior and inferior wall.

Small pericardial effusions are often first seen along the posterior and inferior walls. As the effusion grows, it can expand to areas next to the right atrium, apex, and finally along the right ventricular anterior wall. The exception is a loculated effusion, in which the fluid collections are separated by tissue.

- Armstrong WF, Ryan T: *Feigenbaum's Echocardiography*, 7th edition. Philadelphia, Lippincott Williams & Wilkins, 2010, p 242.
- Lai WW, Mertens LL, Cohen MS, et al (eds): *Echocardiography in Pediatric and Congenital Heart Disease: From Fetus to Adult*, 2nd edition. Chichester, UK, Wiley-Blackwell, 2016, p 710.

84. D. The rapidity of the effusion's development.

Tamponade physiology occurs when a pericardial effusion is significant enough to lead to reduced ventricular filling, which can in turn lead to hemodynamic compromise. Usually, tamponade physiology arises when the effusion accumulates rapidly over a short period of time. The size of the effusion does not necessarily correspond with hemodynamic significance: A patient could have a large effusion that has developed over a long period of time and does not produce tamponade physiology because the effusion has accumulated slowly. In these cases, the pericardial and ventricular compliance has had time to increase slowly to accommodate the effusion, and intrapericardial pressure remains low; thus there is no cardiac compromise. However, if the effusion continues to increase, at some point the pericardium can no longer expand, leading to a significant rise in intrapericardial pressure (exceeding right atrial and right ventricular diastolic pressures), at which point tamponade physiology ensues.

▶ Armstrong WF, Ryan T: *Feigenbaum's Echocardiography*, 7th edition. Philadelphia, Lippincott Williams & Wilkins, 2010, pp 249–251.

▶ Lai WW, Mertens LL, Cohen MS, et al (eds): *Echocardiography in Pediatric and Congenital Heart Disease: From Fetus to Adult*, 2nd edition. Chichester, UK, Wiley-Blackwell, 2016, pp 709–713.

85. A. During inspiration mitral valve inflow decreases.

During inspiration intrathoracic pressure decreases, and this increases systemic venous connection to the right atrium. At the same time, the lungs expand and pulmonary venous return to the left atrium decreases. During expiration the opposite occurs. With tamponade physiology respiration will produce more significant changes in tricuspid and mitral valve inflow due to increased intrapericardial pressure. Also, left ventricular and right ventricular relaxation is limited; tamponade physiology exaggerates ventricular interdependence. With tamponade physiology mitral valve inflow will usually change more than 30% during respiration, and tricuspid valve inflow will usually change more than 50%.

▶ Appleton CP et al: Relation of transmitral flow velocity patterns to left ventricular diastolic function: new insights from a combined hemodynamic and Doppler echocardiographic study. J Am Coll Cardiol 12:426–440, 1988.

▶ Armstrong WF, Ryan T: *Feigenbaum's Echocardiography*, 7th edition. Philadelphia, Lippincott Williams & Wilkins, 2010, pp 249–251.

▶ Klein AL, Cohen GI: Doppler echocardiographic assessment of constrictive pericarditis, cardiac amyloidosis and cardiac tamponade. Cleve Clin J Med 59:278–290, 1992.

▶ Lai WW, Mertens LL, Cohen MS, et al (eds): *Echocardiography in Pediatric and Congenital Heart Disease: From Fetus to Adult*, 2nd edition. Chichester, UK, Wiley-Blackwell, 2016, pp 711–713.

86. A. Right ventricular free wall collapse in early diastole.

Right ventricular (RV) free wall collapse in early diastole is the first sign of cardiac tamponade due to intrapericardial pressure that is greater than RV pressure, but if the patient has pulmonary hypertension or any other cause of increased

RV pressure, the sensitivity of RV free wall collapse will be reduced. Usually, due to high RV pressure, the RV free wall will not be collapsed in systole. Right atrial (RA) wall collapse occurs in late diastole in tamponade, but it happens after RV free wall collapse and the sensitivity of RA wall collapse is only 55%, with a specificity of 90%. The patient may have a large pericardial effusion without tamponade physiology, but eventually tamponade physiology will develop.

- Lai WW, Mertens LL, Cohen MS, et al (eds): *Echocardiography in Pediatric and Congenital Heart Disease: From Fetus to Adult*, 2nd edition. Chichester, UK, Wiley-Blackwell, 2016, p 710.
- Schiller NB, Botvinick EH: Right ventricular compression as a sign of cardiac tamponade: an analysis of echocardiographic ventricular dimensions and their clinical implications. Circulation 56:774–779, 1977.

87. D. Respiratory variation in mitral inflow E-wave velocity greater than 25%.

Constrictive pericarditis is characterized by pericardial thickening, leading to impaired right ventricular (RV) and left ventricular (LV) filling because of the rigid, noncompliant pericardium. With this condition, typically the E/A ratio is greater than 1, there is decreased mitral inflow deceleration time, and the E/e′ ratio (by tissue Doppler imaging) is less than 15. In the presence of constrictive pericarditis, changes in the mitral inflow E-wave velocity between inspiration and expiration are greater than 25%, so the correct choice is D.

- Lai WW, Mertens LL, Cohen MS, et al (eds): *Echocardiography in Pediatric and Congenital Heart Disease: From Fetus to Adult*, 2nd edition. Chichester, UK, Wiley-Blackwell, 2016, p 695.

88. B. Patients with an artificial mitral valve.

Patients at the highest risk for infective endocarditis include those with an artificial valve such as a bioprosthetic or homograft valve, those with cyanotic congenital heart disease, those who have heart devices like pacemakers, those with congenital heart disease status post repair with residual shunts, immunosuppressed patients, and intravenous drug abusers. All of these groups are at higher risk for the primary cause of infective endocarditis, which is bacterial infection of the endocardium.

- Lai WW, Mertens LL, Cohen MS, et al (eds): *Echocardiography in Pediatric and Congenital Heart Disease: From Fetus to Adult*, 2nd edition. Chichester, UK, Wiley-Blackwell, 2016, pp 763–765.

Refer to video PER-Q89.

89. A. Endocarditis.

The Melody valve is a bioprosthetic stented valve (taken from a cow's vein and attached to a wire frame) that is generally placed in the pulmonary position during a cardiac catheterization. Patients who have undergone Melody valve implantation are at increased risk for developing endocarditis on the valve. With a history of fever and fatigue, along with findings of a prominent mass on the Melody valve seen by echocardiography in video PER-Q89, it appears most likely that this patient has developed endocarditis on the Melody valve.

▶ Lai WW, Mertens LL, Cohen MS, et al (eds): *Echocardiography in Pediatric and Congenital Heart Disease: From Fetus to Adult*, 2nd edition. Chichester, UK, Wiley-Blackwell, 2016, pp 763–769.

90. C. Mitral valve regurgitation.

Rheumatic fever is an acute inflammatory disease that may affect several organs in the body, including the joints, kidney, and heart. It can cause permanent damage to heart valves. The mitral and aortic valves are usually affected first, and the damage can appear as regurgitation, stenosis, or both.

▶ Lai WW, Mertens LL, Cohen MS, et al (eds): *Echocardiography in Pediatric and Congenital Heart Disease: From Fetus to Adult*, 2nd edition. Chichester, UK, Wiley-Blackwell, 2016, pp 750–760.

91. C. Anthracyclines.

The best answer to this question is anthracyclines; none of the other choices—elevated high-density lipoprotein (HDL), radiation for a brain tumor, or dialysis—has a direct cardio-toxic effect. Many cardiotoxic agents can cause ventricular dysfunction. These include alcohol, chemotherapy drugs (such as anthracyclines), radiation to the chest near the heart, iron overload (related to chronic blood transfusion), and lead.

▶ Lai WW, Mertens LL, Cohen MS, et al (eds): *Echocardiography in Pediatric and Congenital Heart Disease: From Fetus to Adult*, 2nd edition. Chichester, UK, Wiley-Blackwell, 2016, p 654.

92. A. A patient who received doxorubicin (Adriamycin).

Doxorubicin (sold under the trade name Adriamycin and others) is an anthracycline used for chemotherapy. Patients who receive anthracycline therapy and/or chest radiation are at higher risk for cardiac toxicity. None of the other medications mentioned is associated with an increased risk of cardiac toxicity.

▶ Lai WW, Mertens LL, Cohen MS, et al (eds): *Echocardiography in Pediatric and Congenital Heart Disease: From Fetus to Adult*, 2nd edition. Chichester, UK, Wiley-Blackwell, 2016, pp 653–654.

93. C. Echodense ridge at the mid-left atrial level.

Following heart transplantation, the pulmonary veins and left atrium of the recipient heart are anastomosed to the left atrium of the donor heart. This creates a larger appearance of the left atrium with the potential for an echodense ridge in the mid-left atrium. The donor and recipient main pulmonary artery are anastomosed, but normally there is at most mild narrowing of this area, resulting in mild supravalvular pulmonary stenosis. The E/A ratio should be normal if there is no evidence of rejection. Worsening of mitral valve insufficiency should not be seen and, if present, suggests additional pathology.

- Lai WW, Mertens LL, Cohen MS, et al (eds): *Echocardiography in Pediatric and Congenital Heart Disease: From Fetus to Adult*, 2nd edition. Chichester, UK, Wiley-Blackwell, 2016, pp 138–139.
- Mondillo S, Maccherini M, Galderisi M: Usefulness and limitations of transthoracic echocardiography in heart transplantation recipients. Cardiovascular Ultrasound 6:1–12, 2008.
- Sun JP, Abdalla IA, Greenberg NL, et al: Non-invasive evaluation of orthotopic heart transplant rejection by echocardiography. J Heart Lung Transplant 24:160–165, 2005.

94. D. Pulsed-wave tissue Doppler imaging of the lateral mitral annulus.

Heart biopsy is the gold standard to detect heart rejection, but echocardiography is still a useful noninvasive tool to evaluate evidence of rejection. In early rejection ventricular systolic function may appear normal, while diastolic function may be more sensitive in detecting early graft abnormality. Other symptoms of heart rejection include pericardial effusion, increased mitral and tricuspid regurgitation, and arrhythmia. Assessment of left ventricular (LV) diastolic function is important for evaluating a heart transplant. LV diastolic function parameters that can be assessed using echocardiography include mitral valve inflow, E/A ratio, mitral valve pressure half-time, tissue Doppler imaging of the lateral mitral valve annulus, pulmonary venous flow pattern, and isovolumic relaxation time.

- Mondillo S, Maccherini M, Galderisi M: Usefulness and limitations of transthoracic echocardiography in heart transplantation recipients. Cardiovascular Ultrasound 6:1–12, 2008.

95. D. Atrioventricular canal defect.

Cardiac defects are found in 50% of Down syndrome patients. The most common lesion is an atrioventricular canal defect (AVCD), which is seen in about 40% of Down patients. This lesion is also known as an endocardial cushion defect (ECD) or atrioventricular septal defect (AVSD).

▶ Ko JM: Genetic syndromes associated with congenital heart disease. Korean Circ J 45:357–361, 2015.

▶ Lai WW, Mertens LL, Cohen MS, et al (eds): *Echocardiography in Pediatric and Congenital Heart Disease: From Fetus to Adult*, 2nd edition. Chichester, UK, Wiley-Blackwell, 2016, p 259.

96. A. Down syndrome.

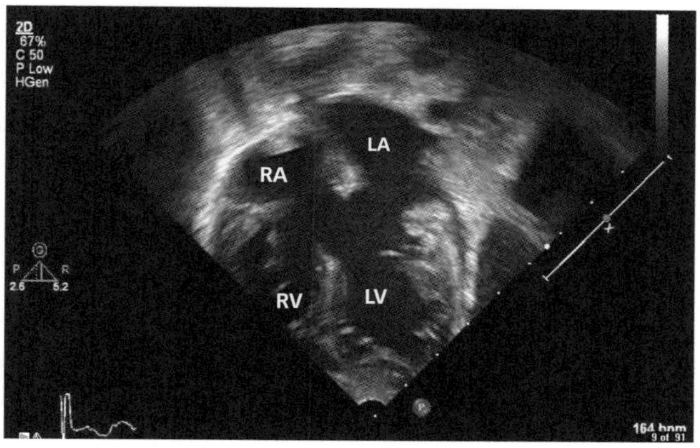

This four-chamber view shows a typical atrioventricular canal defect, with large atrial and ventricular communications and a common atrioventricular valve orifice. Atrioventricular canal defects are commonly seen in patients with Down syndrome. Noonan syndrome is most often associated with pulmonary valve stenosis, atrial septal defects, and hypertrophic cardiomyopathy. Williams syndrome is most often associated with supravalvular aortic stenosis as well as branch pulmonary artery stenosis. As originally reported, Shone syndrome (also known as Shone complex) refers to the association of a supravalvular mitral ring, parachute mitral valve, subaortic stenosis, and coarctation of the aorta (CoA). More recently the term "Shone syndrome" has been generalized to patients who have varying degrees of hypoplasia and stenosis of more than one left-sided cardiac structure (such as mitral stenosis with left ventricular outflow tract obstruction). RA = right atrium, LA = left atrium, RV = right ventricle, LV = left ventricle.

▶ Ko JM: Genetic syndromes associated with congenital heart disease. Korean Circ J 45:357–361, 2015.

▶ Lai WW, Mertens LL, Cohen MS, et al (eds): *Echocardiography in Pediatric and Congenital Heart Disease: From Fetus to Adult*, 2nd edition. Chichester, UK, Wiley-Blackwell, 2016, p 259.

97. B. Trisomy 21.

Trisomy 21 is also known as Down syndrome. 22q11 deletion syndrome is also called DiGeorge syndrome. Trisomy 18 is also known as Edwards syndrome, and trisomy 13 is also known as Patau syndrome.

- Ko JM: Genetic syndromes associated with congenital heart disease. Korean Circ J 45:357–361, 2015.
- Lai WW, Mertens LL, Cohen MS, et al (eds): *Echocardiography in Pediatric and Congenital Heart Disease: From Fetus to Adult*, 2nd edition. Chichester, UK, Wiley-Blackwell, 2016, p 259.

98. A. Aortic isthmus.

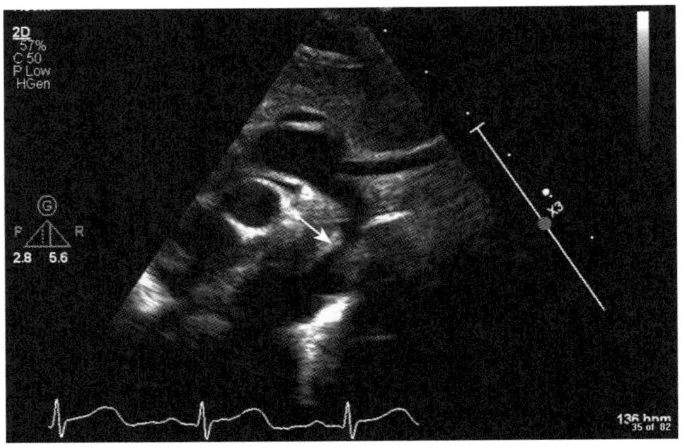

In this image, the patient appears to have coarctation of the aorta. The arrow is pointing to the aortic isthmus, which is often the site of narrowing in coarctation of the aorta.

- Lai WW, Mertens LL, Cohen MS, et al (eds): *Echocardiography in Pediatric and Congenital Heart Disease: From Fetus to Adult*, 2nd edition. Chichester, UK, Wiley-Blackwell, 2016, pp 382–383.

99. D. Coarctation of the aorta (CoA).

In Turner syndrome, the most commonly associated cardiac lesions include bicuspid aortic valve, coarctation of the aorta, mitral valve anomalies, and partial anomalous pulmonary venous connection. Supravalvular aortic stenosis and branch pulmonary artery stenosis are defects associated with Williams syndrome. Primum atrial septal defects (partial atrioventricular canal defects) are associated with Down syndrome.

- Allen HD, Driscoll DJ, Shaddy RE, et al: *Moss and Adams' Heart Disease in Infants, Children, and Adolescents: Including the Fetus and Young Adult*, 8th edition. Philadelphia, Lippincott Williams & Wilkins, 2013, p 619.
- Bechtold SM, Dalla Pozza R, Becker A, et al: Partial anomalous pulmonary vein connection: an underestimated cardiovascular defect in Ullrich-Turner syndrome. Eur J Pediatr 163:158–162, 2004.
- Ko JM: Genetic syndromes associated with congenital heart disease. Korean Circ J 45:357–361, 2015.

100. A. Tetralogy of Fallot.

Tetralogy of Fallot can be found in up to 35% of DiGeorge syndrome patients who have congenital heart disease. The other cardiac defects listed in the question—supramitral valve ring, pulmonary venous abnormality, and levoatrial cardinal vein—are not associated with DiGeorge syndrome.

- Allen HD, Driscoll DJ, Shaddy RE, et al: *Moss and Adams' Heart Disease in Infants, Children, and Adolescents: Including the Fetus and Young Adult*, 8th edition. Philadelphia, Lippincott Williams & Wilkins, 2013, p 627.
- Ko JM: Genetic syndromes associated with congenital heart disease. Korean Circ J 45:357–361, 2015.
- Lai WW, Mertens LL, Cohen MS, et al (eds): *Echocardiography in Pediatric and Congenital Heart Disease: From Fetus to Adult*, 2nd edition. Chichester, UK, Wiley-Blackwell, 2016, pp 407–408.

101. B. DiGeorge syndrome.

Common cardiac abnormalities found in patients with DiGeorge syndrome include truncus arteriosus, tetralogy of Fallot, pulmonary atresia with ventricular septal defect, and interrupted aortic arch type B. At least 50% of patients with interrupted aortic arch type B have DiGeorge syndrome. One-third of patients with truncus arteriosus have DiGeorge syndrome. Ehlers-Danlos syndrome affects the connective tissues, similar to Marfan syndrome. Ehlers-Danlos can produce aortic root dilatation and mitral valve prolapse, but neither it nor Marfan syndrome is associated with truncus arteriosus. Holt-Oram syndrome is associated with other cardiac defects, including atrial septal defects and ventricular septal defects, as well as partial anomalous pulmonary venous connection.

- Allen HD, Driscoll DJ, Shaddy RE, et al: *Moss and Adams' Heart Disease in Infants, Children, and Adolescents: Including the Fetus and Young Adult*, 8th edition. Philadelphia, Lippincott Williams & Wilkins, 2013, pp 621–627.
- Ko JM: Genetic syndromes associated with congenital heart disease. Korean Circ J 45:357–361, 2015.
- Lai WW, Mertens LL, Cohen MS, et al (eds): *Echocardiography in Pediatric and Congenital Heart Disease: From Fetus to Adult*, 2nd edition. Chichester, UK, Wiley-Blackwell, 2016, pp 433–434.

102. D. Left-sided cardiac lesion.

Shone syndrome, also known as Shone complex, was originally used to describe the following group of cardiac defects:

- *supravalvular mitral membrane ring*
- *parachute mitral valve and mitral valve stenosis*
- *subaortic stenosis*
- *coarctation of the aorta*

More recently the term "Shone syndrome" has been generalized to patients who have varying degrees of hypoplasia/stenosis of more than one left-sided cardiac structure, such as mitral stenosis with left ventricular outflow tract obstruction.

▶ Popescu BA, Jurcut R, Serban M, et al: Shone's syndrome diagnosed with echocardiography and confirmed at pathology. Eur J Echocardiogr 9:865–867, 2008.

103. B. Trisomy 18.

At least 99% of patients with trisomy 18 (Edwards syndrome) will have some cardiac defects. In contrast, the incidence of cardiac defects seen with Down syndrome patients is approximately 50%. With Alagille syndrome the incidence is about 90%, and with Noonan syndrome it is about 80%.

▶ Yagel S, Silverman NH, Gembruch U (eds): *Fetal Cardiology: Embryology, Genetics, Physiology, Echocardiographic Evaluation, Diagnosis and Perinatal Management of Cardiac Diseases*, 2nd edition. New York, Taylor & Francis, 2009, p 610.

104. A. Turner syndrome.

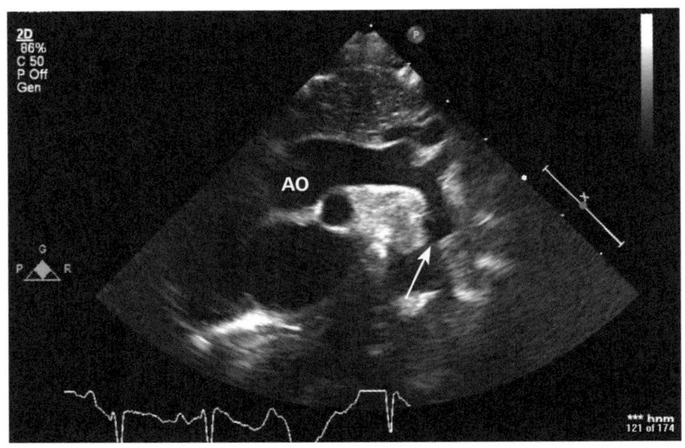

The arrow in this image points to coarctation of the aorta. In Turner syndrome, the most common cardiac lesions are bicuspid aortic valve and coarctation of the aorta. None of the other syndromes has a known association with coarctation. AO = aorta.

▶ Ko JM: Genetic syndromes associated with congenital heart disease. Korean Circ J 45:357–361, 2015.

105. B. IAA type B.

Patients with DiGeorge syndrome are at higher risk of having an interrupted aortic arch (IAA). The most common is type B.

▶ Ko JM: Genetic syndromes associated with congenital heart disease. Korean Circ J 45:357–361, 2015.

▶ Lai WW, Mertens LL, Cohen MS, et al (eds): *Echocardiography in Pediatric and Congenital Heart Disease: From Fetus to Adult*, 2nd edition. Chichester, UK, Wiley-Blackwell, 2016, p 394.

106. D. Partial anomalous pulmonary venous connection.

Scimitar syndrome is characterized by hypoplasia of the right lung and right pulmonary artery. The right-sided pulmonary veins (one or more) will drain anomalously below the diaphragm into the inferior vena cava (IVC). The crescent shape of the anomalously draining pulmonary vein on x-ray resembles the shape of a scimitar (a type of sword with a curved blade)—hence the name Scimitar syndrome.

▶ Lai WW, Mertens LL, Cohen MS, et al (eds): *Echocardiography in Pediatric and Congenital Heart Disease: From Fetus to Adult*, 2nd edition. Chichester, UK, Wiley-Blackwell, 2016, p 160.

107. B. Tetralogy of Fallot.

Ectopia cordis is a midline defect; in this condition, the heart is located partially or completely outside of the thorax. Cardiac defects that are often associated with ectopia cordis include tetralogy of Fallot, transposition of the great arteries, tricuspid atresia, and double-outlet right ventricle.

▶ Allen HD, Driscoll DJ, Shaddy RE, et al: *Moss and Adams' Heart Disease in Infants, Children, and Adolescents: Including the Fetus and Young Adult*, 8th edition. Philadelphia, Lippincott Williams & Wilkins, 2013, p 1214.

▶ Lai WW, Mertens LL, Cohen MS, et al (eds): *Echocardiography in Pediatric and Congenital Heart Disease: From Fetus to Adult*, 2nd edition. Chichester, UK, Wiley-Blackwell, 2016, p 35.

108. A. Turner syndrome.

Turner syndrome has the highest incidence of partial anomalous pulmonary venous connection. The most common cardiac defect in Down syndrome is an atrioventricular canal defect. Alagille syndrome is associated with cardiac defects such as ventricular septal defect, tetralogy of Fallot, and pulmonary stenosis. Williams syndrome is associated with aortic valve stenosis and supravalvular aortic stenosis, as well as pulmonary artery branch stenosis.

▶ Allen HD, Driscoll DJ, Shaddy RE, et al: *Moss and Adams' Heart Disease in Infants, Children, and Adolescents: Including the Fetus and Young Adult*, 8th edition. Philadelphia, Lippincott Williams & Wilkins, 2013, pp 619–621.

109. D. Aortic dissection.

Marfan syndrome is an autosomal dominant connective tissue disease. Major echocardiographic findings include mitral valve prolapse, dilatation of the ascending and descending aorta, and main pulmonary artery dilatation. Progressive aortic dilatation can lead to dissection of the ascending and descending aorta, which can cause severe chest and abdominal pain. In some instances, this complication can be life-threatening.

▶ Lai WW, Mertens LL, Cohen MS, et al (eds): *Echocardiography in Pediatric and Congenital Heart Disease: From Fetus to Adult*, 2nd edition. Chichester, UK, Wiley-Blackwell, 2016, pp 627–630.

110. A. Connective tissue disorders.

Vascular Ehlers-Danlos syndrome, Loeys-Dietz syndrome, arterial tortuosity syndrome, and Marfan syndrome are all heritable connective tissue disorders. Takayasu's syndrome is a specific arteritis that leads to stenosis of the large and medium-sized arteries.

▶ Lai WW, Mertens LL, Cohen MS, et al (eds): *Echocardiography in Pediatric and Congenital Heart Disease: From Fetus to Adult*, 2nd edition. Chichester, UK, Wiley-Blackwell, 2016, pp 632–634.

111. B. Marfan syndrome.

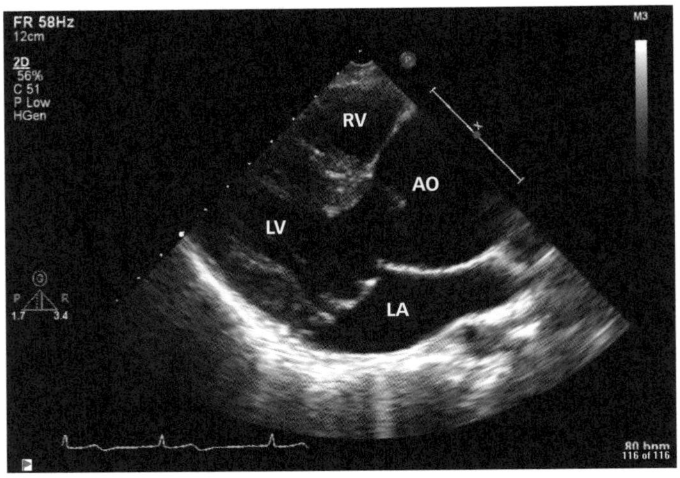

The echocardiographic image shows aortic root dilatation as well as mitral valve prolapse. These are findings characteristic of Marfan syndrome. In Noonan syndrome, the most frequent anomalies are pulmonary stenosis, hypertrophic cardiomyopathy, and secundum atrial septal defects. Alagille syndrome affects the liver, heart, and kidneys. The major congenital heart defects are tetralogy of Fallot, pulmonary valve stenosis, and ventricular septal defects. Holt-Oram syndrome is also

called heart-hand syndrome; the most commonly associated heart defects are atrial septal and ventricular septal defects. RV = right ventricle, LV = left ventricle, LA = left atrium, AO = aorta.

▶ Allen HD, Driscoll DJ, Shaddy RE, et al: *Moss and Adams' Heart Disease in Infants, Children, and Adolescents: Including the Fetus and Young Adult*, 8th edition. Philadelphia, Lippincott Williams & Wilkins, 2013, pp 619–621.

▶ Ko JM: Genetic syndromes associated with congenital heart disease. Korean Circ J 45:357–361, 2015.

112. A. Hypertrophic cardiomyopathy.

The most common cardiac abnormality seen in babies born to mothers with diabetes is hypertrophic cardiomyopathy. The child's condition generally improves after birth.

▶ Tabib A, Shirzad N, Sheikhbahaei S, et al: Cardiac malformations in fetuses of gestational and pre gestational diabetic mothers. Iranian J Pediatr 23:664–668, 2013.

113. B. Lithium.

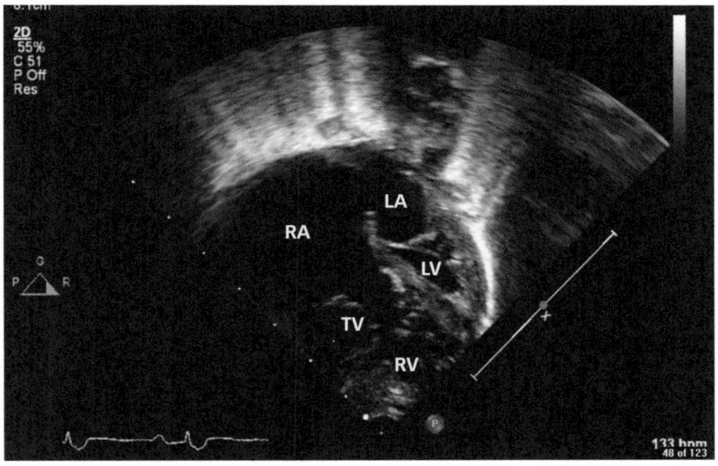

The echocardiographic image shows Ebstein anomaly of the tricuspid valve. Maternal use of lithium during the first trimester is associated with an increased risk of cardiac malformation, particularly Ebstein anomaly. None of the other medications listed, when taken during pregnancy, is associated with Ebstein anomaly. Fetuses exposed to thalidomide in utero have been born with malformed limbs as well as other congenital defects. RA = right atrium, LA = left atrium, RV = right ventricle, LV = left ventricle, TV = tricuspid valve.

▶ Callen PW: *Ultrasonography in Obstetrics and Gynecology*, 5th edition. Philadelphia, Saunders Elsevier, 2008, pp 39–40, 1203.

▶ Patorno E, Huybrechts KF, Bateman BT, et al: Lithium use in pregnancy and the risk of cardiac malformations. N Engl J Med 376:2245–2254, 2017.

114. C. Omphalocele.

Fetuses suspected to have hydrocephalus, microcephaly, holoprosencephaly, agenesis of the corpus callosum, Meckel-Gruber syndrome, esophageal atresia, duodenal atresia, diaphragmatic hernia, omphalocele, or renal dysplasia can have associated cardiac defects. Echocardiography is recommended for evaluation. Gastroschisis, bronchus suis, and Ogilvie syndrome are not associated with an increased risk of cardiac defects. It is important to note, however, that patients with gastroschisis also often have omphalocele, and these patients are at higher risk for having cardiac defects.

▶ Copel JA, Pilu G, Kleinman CS: Congenital heart disease and extra cardiac anomalies: associations and indications for fetal echocardiography. Am J Obstet Gynecol 154:1121–1132, 1986.

▶ Yagel S, Silverman NH, Gembruch U (eds): *Fetal Cardiology: Embryology, Genetics, Physiology, Echocardiographic Evaluation, Diagnosis and Perinatal Management of Cardiac Diseases*, 2nd edition. New York, Taylor & Francis, 2009, p 637.

115. A. Tetralogy of Fallot.

Conotruncal abnormalities such as tetralogy of Fallot and double-outlet right ventricle are more prevalent in children of diabetic mothers.

▶ Narchi H, Kulaylat N: Heart disease in infants of diabetic mothers. Images Paediatr Cardiol 2:17–23, 2000.

▶ Tabib A, Shirzad N, Sheikhbahaei S, et al: Cardiac malformations in fetuses of gestational and pre gestational diabetic mothers. Iranian J Pediatr 23:664–668, 2013.

116. B. Pulmonary valve stenosis.

An infected fetus may have eye, ear, and heart defects. The common cardiac defects include branch pulmonary stenosis, pulmonary valve stenosis, and patent ductus arteriosus (PDA).

▶ Lai WW, Mertens LL, Cohen MS, et al (eds): *Echocardiography in Pediatric and Congenital Heart Disease: From Fetus to Adult*, 2nd edition. Chichester, UK, Wiley-Blackwell, 2016, p 281.

▶ Mekonnen D: Clinically confirmed congenital rubella syndrome: the role of echocardiography. Ethiop J Health Sci 27:197–202, 2017.

117. C. Coarctation of the aorta.

The cardiac defect that most commonly leads to systemic hypertension is coarctation of the aorta (CoA). Echocardiography is the best tool to evaluate the aortic arch to rule out CoA. During the echocardiographic examination, it is important not only to evaluate the aortic arch but also to evaluate the abdominal aortic flow profile. This is especially true in young adults, because their suprasternal notch view can be difficult. It is important to note that systemic hypertension can be primary, or it can be the result of some other systemic processes such as renal or renovascular disease, obesity, endocrine disease, mental stress, and medications, in which case it is known as secondary hypertension. If the secondary disease is treated effectively, the systemic hypertension will usually improve or resolve.

▸ Baykan A, Argun M, Ozyurt A, et al: Hypertension associated with coarctation of aorta revisited: case-based update from experience of three children. Case Rep Pediatr, article 716438, 2013.

▸ Flynn JT, Kaelber DC, Baker-Smith CM, et al: Clinical practice guideline for screening and management of high blood pressure in children and adolescents. Pediatrics 140:e20171904, 2017.

118. D. Coarctation of the aorta.

With coarctation of the aorta, the narrowing of the distal aortic arch produces a difference in upper and lower extremity blood pressures. Thus the leg blood pressures will be lower than pressures in the upper extremities. The other cardiac defects listed—aortopulmonary window, hypertrophic cardiomyopathy, and aortic valve stenosis—do not produce this type of discrepancy in blood pressures.

▸ Park MK: *Park's Pediatric Cardiology for Practitioners*, 6th edition. Philadelphia, Saunders, 2014, pp 200–201.

119. B. Concentric left ventricular hypertrophy.

Untreated systemic hypertension typically causes concentric left ventricular hypertrophy with a small left ventricular cavity. Diastolic function can be impaired, while systolic function is normal in the early stage.

▸ Inouye I, Massie B, Loge D, et al: Abnormal left ventricular filling: an early finding in mild to moderate systemic hypertension. Am J Cardiol 53:120–126, 1984.

▸ Verdecchia P, Schillaci G, Borgioni C, et al: Prognostic value of left ventricular mass and geometry in systemic hypertension with left ventricular hypertrophy. Am J Cardiol 15:197–202, 1996.

ANSWERS

120. A. Patients after a Fontan procedure.

Patients who have undergone a Fontan procedure are at a high risk for systemic venous thrombosis, with an overall incidence of 3%–33% based on different studies. None of the other cardiac defects mentioned is associated with as high an incidence of thrombosis.

▶ Allen HD, Driscoll DJ, Shaddy RE, et al: *Moss and Adams' Heart Disease in Infants, Children, and Adolescents: Including the Fetus and Young Adult*, 8th edition. Philadelphia, Lippincott Williams & Wilkins, 2013, p 1600.

121. B. Right ventricle.

The right ventricle (RV) is located anteriorly, nearest to the chest wall, making it more prone to cardiac contusion. When a cardiac contusion occurs to the RV, the RV anterior wall can manifest wall motion abnormalities. RV rupture is more common than left ventricle rupture.

▶ Allen HD, Driscoll DJ, Shaddy RE, et al: *Moss and Adams' Heart Disease in Infants, Children, and Adolescents: Including the Fetus and Young Adult*, 8th edition. Philadelphia, Lippincott Williams & Wilkins, 2013, pp 552–554.

122. B. Thrombosis.

A long-term indwelling central line places this patient at high-risk for thrombosis. Central venous lines in the right chest will likely be in the innominate (brachiocephalic) vein or superior vena cava (SVC), and development of thrombus can partially or completely block the innominate vein or SVC blood flow and cause an increase in jugular venous pressure and facial swelling.

▶ Allen HD, Driscoll DJ, Shaddy RE, et al: *Moss and Adams' Heart Disease in Infants, Children, and Adolescents: Including the Fetus and Young Adult*, 8th edition. Philadelphia, Lippincott Williams & Wilkins, 2013, p 1598.

Refer to video PER-Q123.

123. C. Thrombus.

The patient in video PER-Q123 had a Fontan procedure. The circular structure to the right is the Fontan conduit (in cross section). The echogenic mass inside the conduit represents a thrombus.

▶ Allen HD, Driscoll DJ, Shaddy RE, et al: *Moss and Adams' Heart Disease in Infants, Children, and Adolescents: Including the Fetus and Young Adult*, 8th edition. Philadelphia, Lippincott Williams & Wilkins, 2013, p 1600.

124. D. All of the above.

Asplenia and polysplenia syndromes are also known as heterotaxy syndromes, which are disorders of laterality or sidedness. These abnormalities affect a number of organs in the body that tend to "lateralize" (those that are normally located on one or the other side of midline), such as the liver, spleen, lungs, and heart. Cardiac defects are often complex and include atrioventricular canal defects (AVCDs), pulmonary atresia, transposition of the great arteries, interrupted inferior vena cava, bilateral superior vena cava, and total anomalous pulmonary venous connection (TAPVC). Some cardiac abnormalities are seen with both syndromes, such as dextrocardia and AVCDs, but some anatomic/echocardiographic findings will be found in one more than the other. For example, asplenia syndrome is frequently associated with a midline liver, intact inferior vena cava, and TAPVC. Patients with polysplenia syndrome may have an interrupted inferior vena cava and ipsilateral pulmonary venous return.

▶ Ezon DS, Goldberg JF, Kyle WB: *Atlas of Congenital Heart Disease Nomenclature: An Illustrated Guide to the Van Praagh and Anderson Approaches to Describing Congenital Cardiac Pathology*. Houston, Ezon Educational Services/CreateSpace, 2015, pp 20–26, 44.

▶ Lai WW, Mertens LL, Cohen MS, et al (eds): *Echocardiography in Pediatric and Congenital Heart Disease: From Fetus to Adult*, 2nd edition. Chichester, UK, Wiley-Blackwell, 2016, pp 563–580.

125. D. All of the above.

See the answer to question 124.

▶ Ezon DS, Goldberg JF, Kyle WB: *Atlas of Congenital Heart Disease Nomenclature: An Illustrated Guide to the Van Praagh and Anderson Approaches to Describing Congenital Cardiac Pathology*. Houston, Ezon Educational Services/CreateSpace, 2015, pp 20–26.

▶ Lai WW, Mertens LL, Cohen MS, et al (eds): *Echocardiography in Pediatric and Congenital Heart Disease: From Fetus to Adult*, 2nd edition. Chichester, UK, Wiley-Blackwell, 2016, pp 563–580.

126. A. Polysplenia.

See Color Plate 8 on page xxiii.

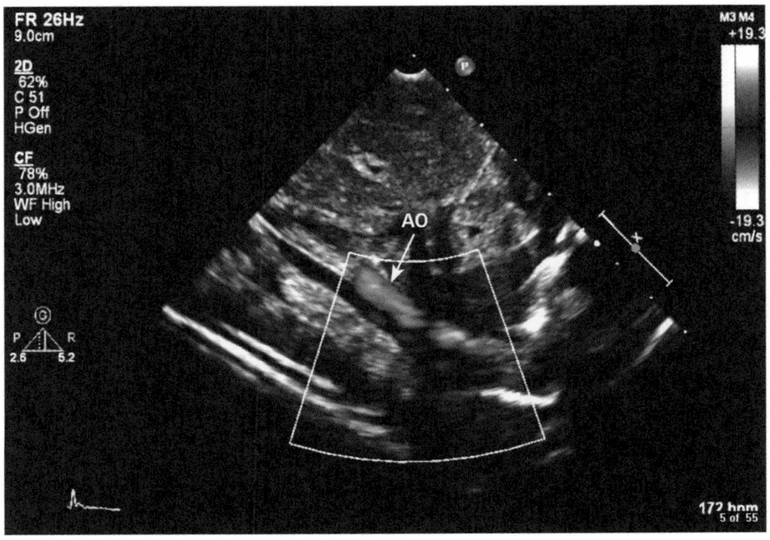

In this image the anterior vessel is the aorta, there is no inferior vena cava (IVC) seen in the liver, and the posterior vessel is a prominent azygos vein, which is also suggestive of an interrupted IVC. Most of the patients with polysplenia syndrome have an interrupted hepatic portion of the IVC with the lower-body venous blood returning above the diaphragm to the superior vena cava (SVC) by way of a large azygos vein, which is why the azygos vein is so prominent in these patients. AO = aorta.

- Ezon DS, Goldberg JF, Kyle WB: *Atlas of Congenital Heart Disease Nomenclature: An Illustrated Guide to the Van Praagh and Anderson Approaches to Describing Congenital Cardiac Pathology*. Houston, Ezon Educational Services/CreateSpace, 2015, pp 20–26.
- Lai WW, Mertens LL, Cohen MS, et al (eds): *Echocardiography in Pediatric and Congenital Heart Disease: From Fetus to Adult*, 2nd edition. Chichester, UK, Wiley-Blackwell, 2016, pp 563–580.

127. D. Asplenia syndrome (right atrial isomerism).

As evidenced by the midline liver and dextrocardia, this patient most likely has a disorder of laterality or sidedness known as heterotaxy. Heterotaxy is divided into two basic types: asplenia, also known as right atrial isomerism, and polysplenia, also known as left atrial isomerism. Each group has complex cardiac defects. Some cardiac defects are common to both syndromes, such as dextrocardia, atrioventricular canal, common atrium, and often bilateral superior vena cava, but some findings will indicate one or another. For example, most patients with polysplenia syndrome have an interrupted inferior vena cava (IVC), normally related great arteries, pulmonary veins that drain to the back of a common atrium, and a complete atrioventricular (AV) block. Patients with asplenia syndrome will often have an intact IVC, total anomalous pulmonary venous connection (TAPVC), pulmonary stenosis/atresia, an unroofed coronary sinus, and an unbalanced AV canal. In the example here, the baby has cardiac defects that are most consistent with asplenia.

- Ezon DS, Goldberg JF, Kyle WB: *Atlas of Congenital Heart Disease Nomenclature: An Illustrated Guide to the Van Praagh and Anderson Approaches to Describing Congenital Cardiac Pathology*. Houston, Ezon Educational Services/CreateSpace, 2015, pp 20–26.
- Lai WW, Mertens LL, Cohen MS, et al (eds): *Echocardiography in Pediatric and Congenital Heart Disease: From Fetus to Adult*, 2nd edition. Chichester, UK, Wiley-Blackwell, 2016, pp 563–570.

PART 3

Congenital Anomalies

128. C. Interruption after the left subclavian artery.

With a type A interrupted aortic arch (IAA), the interruption is located after the left subclavian artery. With a type B IAA the interruption occurs between the left common carotid artery and the left subclavian artery; a type B IAA is also often associated with a posterior malalignment ventricular septal defect and aberrant origin of the right subclavian artery. With a type C IAA the interruption occurs between the right and left common carotid arteries.

▸ Lai WW, Mertens LL, Cohen MS, et al (eds): *Echocardiography in Pediatric and Congenital Heart Disease: From Fetus to Adult*, 2nd edition. Chichester, UK, Wiley-Blackwell, 2016, p 395.

129. B. Type B.

About 62%–70% of interrupted aortic arch (IAA) cases are type B. About 30%–37% of IAA cases are type A, and 1% or less are type C. Most references classify IAA into these three types (as defined by Celoria and Patton). No IAA type D exists.

▸ Lai WW, Mertens LL, Cohen MS, et al (eds): *Echocardiography in Pediatric and Congenital Heart Disease: From Fetus to Adult*, 2nd edition. Chichester, UK, Wiley-Blackwell, 2016, p 395.

130. A. Aberrant left subclavian artery.

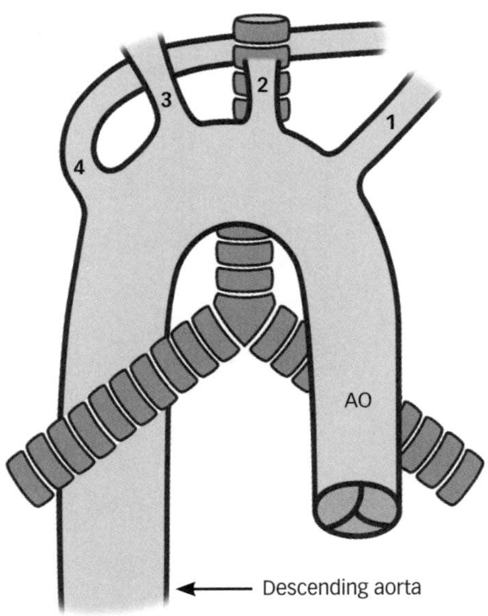

Because it is a right arch, the first branch should be the left innominate (brachiocephalic) artery, the second branch should be the right common carotid artery, and the third

branch should be the right subclavian artery. However, there is no bifurcation of the first branch of head vessels into left subclavian and left carotid arteries, which implies that the left subclavian artery arises aberrantly from the descending aorta. In this schematic 1 = left carotid artery, 2 = right carotid artery, 3 = right subclavian artery, 4 = aberrant left subclavian artery, AO = aorta.

▸ Lai WW, Mertens LL, Cohen MS, et al (eds): *Echocardiography in Pediatric and Congenital Heart Disease: From Fetus to Adult*, 2nd edition. Chichester, UK, Wiley-Blackwell, 2016, p 611.

ANSWERS

131. A. Type A interrupted aortic arch (IAA).

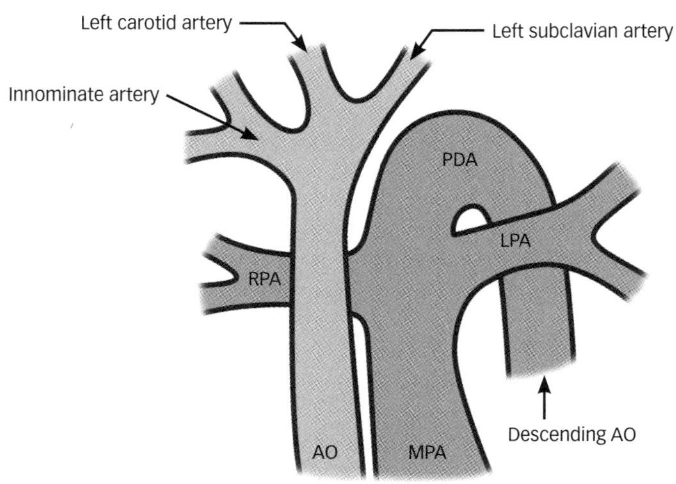

In this schematic PDA = patent ductus arteriosus, LPA = left pulmonary artery, RPA = right pulmonary artery, AO = aorta, PA = main pulmonary artery.

▸ Lai WW, Mertens LL, Cohen MS, et al (eds): *Echocardiography in Pediatric and Congenital Heart Disease: From Fetus to Adult*, 2nd edition. Chichester, UK, Wiley-Blackwell, 2016, p 395.

132. B. Type B IAA.

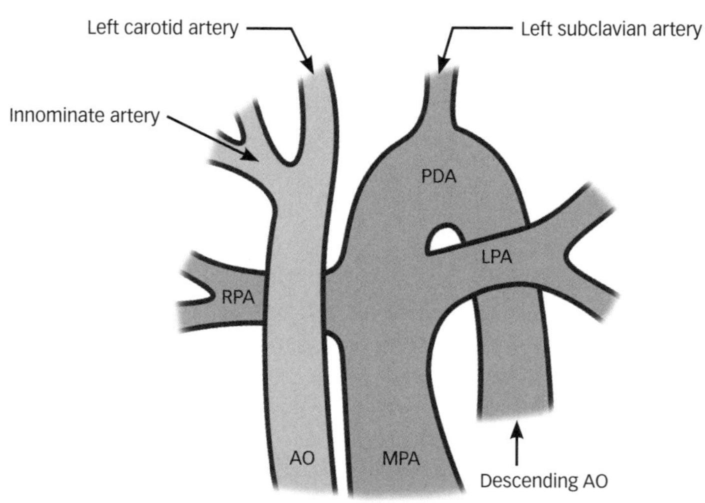

In this schematic PDA = patent ductus arteriosus, LPA = left pulmonary artery, RPA = right pulmonary artery, AO = aorta, MPA = main pulmonary artery.

▶ Lai WW, Mertens LL, Cohen MS, et al (eds): *Echocardiography in Pediatric and Congenital Heart Disease: From Fetus to Adult*, 2nd edition. Chichester, UK, Wiley-Blackwell, 2016, pp 395–396.

133. B. Coarctation of the aorta (CoA).

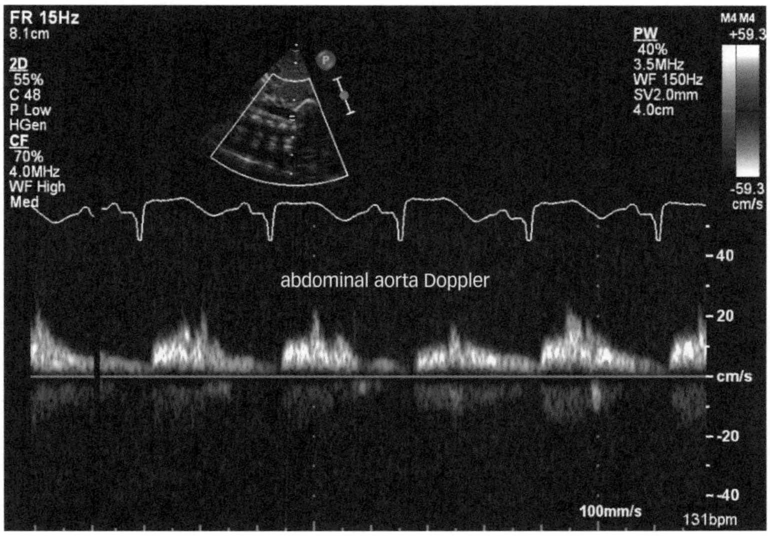

In a normal person, the abdominal aortic flow profile is a pulsatile pattern seen in systole. When there is a coarctation of the aorta (CoA), the abdominal aortic flow is dampened, with a lack of a high peak velocity in systole; instead, the Doppler waveform appears more like a "sawtooth." If CoA is severe, the peak velocity in the abdominal aorta will be very low, with antegrade flow in diastole and minimal phasic variation, as seen in this spectral waveform. It is important to note that if a large aortopulmonary (AP) collateral or a patent ductus arteriosus (PDA) coexists with CoA, the abdominal aortic waveform can appear normal.

▶ Lai WW, Mertens LL, Cohen MS, et al (eds): *Echocardiography in Pediatric and Congenital Heart Disease: From Fetus to Adult*, 2nd edition. Chichester, UK, Wiley-Blackwell, 2016, pp 388–391.

134. A. PDA flow shunts right to left in systole and left to right in diastole.

When a patient has a significant coarctation of the aorta combined with pulmonary hypertension, the PDA flow is typically bidirectional. In systole, the blood flow is from the

ANSWERS

pulmonary artery to the descending aorta (right to left), and in diastole the blood flow can be from the descending aorta to the pulmonary artery (left to right).

▸ Lai WW, Mertens LL, Cohen MS, et al (eds): *Echocardiography in Pediatric and Congenital Heart Disease: From Fetus to Adult*, 2nd edition. Chichester, UK, Wiley-Blackwell, 2016, pp 386–389.

135. A. Right aortic arch with a retroesophageal left subclavian artery and a left ductal ligament.

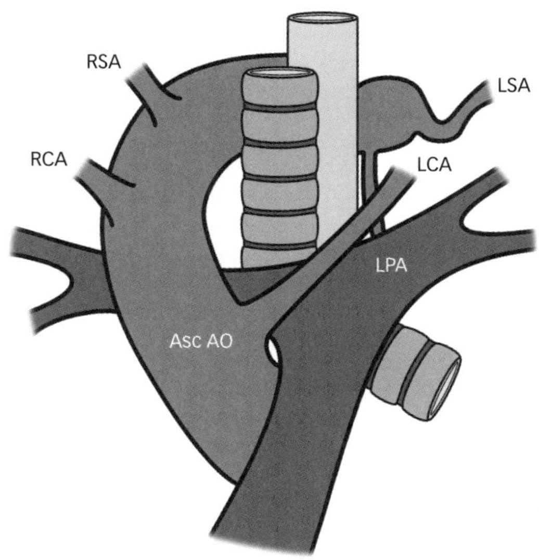

A vascular ring is formed by vascular structures that completely encircle the trachea and the esophagus. A left aortic arch with normal branching and a left ductal ligament is a normal finding and does not produce a vascular ring. Similarly, a right aortic arch with mirror-image branching does not cause a vascular ring. A left aortic arch with an aberrant right subclavian artery is not a vascular ring, due to the left ductal ligament. A vascular ring is formed when the right aortic arch with a retroesophageal left subclavian artery gives rise to a left ductal ligament originating from the base of the left subclavian artery (the diverticulum of Kommerell) that courses leftward and anteriorly to insert into the main or left pulmonary artery. Asc AO = ascending aorta, RCA = right coronary artery, RSA = right subclavian artery, LSA = left subclavian artery, LCA = left coronary artery, LPA = left pulmonary artery.

▸ Allen HD, Driscoll DJ, Shaddy RE, et al: *Moss and Adams' Heart Disease in Infants, Children, and Adolescents: Including the Fetus and Young Adult*, 8th edition. Philadelphia, Lippincott Williams & Wilkins, 2013, p 767.

▸ Lai WW, Mertens LL, Cohen MS, et al (eds): *Echocardiography in Pediatric and Congenital Heart Disease: From Fetus to Adult*, 2nd edition. Chichester, UK, Wiley-Blackwell, 2016, p 611.

136. D. The double aortic arch is a type of vascular ring.

Early in normal cardiac development in the embryo, a double aortic arch is present, but involution of the right dorsal aorta leads to development of the normal left aortic arch. When both the embryonic right and left fourth arches and both right and left dorsal aortae persist, a double aortic arch remains present. When a double aortic arch remains present, usually the right-sided arch is larger than the left-sided arch, and in some cases the left-sided arch can be quite hypoplastic or even have an atretic portion. The right and left arches pass around the trachea and esophagus on opposite sides, joining just below the level of the arches to form the descending thoracic aorta. This completes the vascular ring.

▶ Allen HD, Driscoll DJ, Shaddy RE, et al: *Moss and Adams' Heart Disease in Infants, Children, and Adolescents: Including the Fetus and Young Adult*, 8th edition. Philadelphia, Lippincott Williams & Wilkins, 2013, pp 778–781.

▶ Lai WW, Mertens LL, Cohen MS, et al (eds): *Echocardiography in Pediatric and Congenital Heart Disease: From Fetus to Adult*, 2nd edition. Chichester, UK, Wiley-Blackwell, 2016, p 610.

137. C. Abnormal origin of the left pulmonary artery from the right pulmonary artery.

An abnormal origin of the left pulmonary artery from the right pulmonary artery is also known as a pulmonary artery sling. The left pulmonary artery arises from the right pulmonary artery and travels posterior to the trachea and anterior to the esophagus to reach the left lung hilum. This left pulmonary artery course can compress the trachea and cause airway obstruction. More important, many cases of left pulmonary artery sling also have associated complete tracheal rings that can result in airway narrowing and stridor. The other options—pulmonary valve stenosis, right aortic arch with mirror-image branching, and a large patent ductus arteriosus—do not result in a vascular ring and will not cause stridor secondary to airway obstruction.

▶ Allen HD, Driscoll DJ, Shaddy RE, et al: *Moss and Adams' Heart Disease in Infants, Children, and Adolescents: Including the Fetus and Young Adult*, 8th edition. Philadelphia, Lippincott Williams & Wilkins, 2013, p 786.

▶ Lai WW, Mertens LL, Cohen MS, et al (eds): *Echocardiography in Pediatric and Congenital Heart Disease: From Fetus to Adult*, 2nd edition. Chichester, UK, Wiley-Blackwell, 2016, pp 618–619.

Refer to video PER-Q138.

138. B. Pulmonary artery sling.

This video clip is demonstrating a pulmonary artery sling. Note that the normal echocardiographic appearance of the branch pulmonary arteries and their takeoffs is not seen in this video clip. Instead, the left pulmonary artery arises from the right pulmonary artery and courses posterior to the trachea (which is difficult to visualize in this study) and to the left.

▸ Lai WW, Mertens LL, Cohen MS, et al (eds): *Echocardiography in Pediatric and Congenital Heart Disease: From Fetus to Adult*, 2nd edition. Chichester, UK, Wiley-Blackwell, 2016, pp 618–619.

139. B. Right arch with mirror-image branching and a ductus arteriosus arising anteriorly from the left innominate artery.

A vascular ring occurs when there are vascular structures that completely encircle the trachea and esophagus, potentially causing narrowing of both structures. Of the four options listed, only choice B—right arch with mirror-image branching and a ductus arteriosus arising anteriorly from the left innominate (brachiocephalic) artery—does not have vascular structures on all sides of the trachea and esophagus and can therefore occur without a vascular ring.

▸ Allen HD, Driscoll DJ, Shaddy RE, et al: *Moss and Adams' Heart Disease in Infants, Children, and Adolescents: Including the Fetus and Young Adult*, 8th edition. Philadelphia, Lippincott Williams & Wilkins, 2013, pp 758–796.

▸ Lai WW, Mertens LL, Cohen MS, et al (eds): *Echocardiography in Pediatric and Congenital Heart Disease: From Fetus to Adult*, 2nd edition. Chichester, UK, Wiley-Blackwell, 2016, pp 609–618.

140. D. Type C interrupted aortic arch with a closing ductus arteriosus.

A differential carotid pulse occurs because the right carotid artery is proximal to the interruption and the left carotid artery is distal to the interruption. A double aortic arch, coarctation of the aorta, and type B interrupted aortic arch (IAA) will be associated with pulses of the same strength on both sides of the carotid arteries. In the case of coarctation and type B IAA, the narrowing or interruption of the aortic arch occurs distal to the takeoff of both carotid arteries; hence there might be a difference between arm and leg pulses, but there will be no difference between carotid pulses.

▸ Lai WW, Mertens LL, Cohen MS, et al (eds): *Echocardiography in Pediatric and Congenital Heart Disease: From Fetus to Adult*, 2nd edition. Chichester, UK, Wiley-Blackwell, 2016, pp 395–396.

ANSWERS

141. C. Left aortic arch with right descending aorta and right ductus arteriosus.

Of the four options, only choice C has the anatomy that can produce a vascular ring. A common brachiocephalic trunk (choice A) is a normal variant of aortic arch branching. A left aortic arch with aberrant right subclavian artery (choice B) and a right arch with mirror-image branching (choice D) are abnormal arches, but they are not vascular structures that completely encircle the trachea and esophagus. Hence these options do not have an anatomic setup for a vascular ring, and no surgery is needed.

▸ Allen HD, Driscoll DJ, Shaddy RE, et al: *Moss and Adams' Heart Disease in Infants, Children, and Adolescents: Including the Fetus and Young Adult,* 8th edition. Philadelphia, Lippincott Williams & Wilkins, 2013, pp 758–796.

142. B. Left aortic arch with anomalous right subclavian artery.

The most common anatomic variant found with aortic arch development is a left aortic arch with an anomalous origin of the right subclavian artery, and no surgery is needed to correct it. This variant is often found by routine echocardiography ordered for another reason. The incidence of this variant is high in patients with trisomy 21 (Down syndrome) accompanied by a congenital heart defect.

▸ Allen HD, Driscoll DJ, Shaddy RE, et al: *Moss and Adams' Heart Disease in Infants, Children, and Adolescents: Including the Fetus and Young Adult,* 8th edition. Philadelphia, Lippincott Williams & Wilkins, 2013, p 760.

143. D. Bicuspid aortic valve.

Some studies show that up to 85% of patients with coarctation also have a bicuspid aortic valve. Ventricular septal defects can coexist with CoA, but the incidence of VSDs is not as high as the incidence of bicuspid aortic valves.

▸ Allen HD, Driscoll DJ, Shaddy RE, et al: *Moss and Adams' Heart Disease in Infants, Children, and Adolescents: Including the Fetus and Young Adult,* 8th edition. Philadelphia, Lippincott Williams & Wilkins, 2013, p 1044.

144. A. The conal septum is deviated anteriorly, creating the VSD.

Classic tetralogy of Fallot (TOF) has a ventricular septal defect (VSD) due to anterior and leftward rotation of the conal (infundibular) septum. This malposition of the conal septum prevents it from fusing with the trabecular septum, resulting in a large gap that enables interventricular communication. Another name for this type of defect is a malalignment VSD.

- Lai WW, Mertens LL, Cohen MS, et al (eds): *Echocardiography in Pediatric and Congenital Heart Disease: From Fetus to Adult*, 2nd edition. Chichester, UK, Wiley-Blackwell, 2016, p 409.
- Van Praagh R, Geva T, Kreutzer J: Ventricular septal defects: how shall we describe, name and classify them? J Am Coll Cardiol 4:1298–1299, 1989.

145. C. Mitral valve to aortic valve fibrous continuity.

Almost all cases of tetralogy of Fallot (TOF) have mitral valve to aortic valve fibrous continuity. Typically patients with TOF have right ventricular hypertrophy because the right ventricle pumps at high pressure due to pulmonary stenosis, but patients with TOF rarely have right ventricular dilatation. Patients with TOF do not always need a patent ductus arteriosus (PDA) to survive, so a PDA is not present in all cases. Shunting through a ventricular septal defect (VSD) is usually either bidirectional or right-to-left, not left-to-right. In some cases of TOF the subpulmonary and pulmonary valve stenoses are mild, resulting in a left-to-right shunt across the VSD, normal or excessive flow into the pulmonary arteries, and normal systemic arterial oxygen saturations. This clinical presentation is sometimes known as "pink TOF."

- Howell CE et al: Variations within the fibrous skeleton and ventricular outflow tracts in tetralogy of Fallot. Ann Thorac Surg 50:450–457, 1990.
- Lai WW, Mertens LL, Cohen MS, et al (eds): *Echocardiography in Pediatric and Congenital Heart Disease: From Fetus to Adult*, 2nd edition. Chichester, UK, Wiley-Blackwell, 2016, pp 407–409.

146. A. 88%.

With tetralogy of Fallot (TOF), 88% of patients have normal coronary artery origins, 6.4% have normal coronary arteries but also have a large conal branch, 3% have a left anterior descending artery (LAD) arising from the right coronary artery, and 1.8% have dual LADs. Other rare coronary artery variations in TOF include a single right or left coronary artery.

- Lai WW, Mertens LL, Cohen MS, et al (eds): *Echocardiography in Pediatric and Congenital Heart Disease: From Fetus to Adult*, 2nd edition. Chichester, UK, Wiley-Blackwell, 2016, p 413.
- Need LR, Powell AJ, del Nido P, et al: Coronary echocardiography in tetralogy of Fallot: diagnostic accuracy, resource utilization and surgical implications over 13 years. J Am Coll Cardiol 36:1371–1377, 2000.

147. D. Large conal branch arising from the right coronary artery.

See the answer to question 146. A large conal branch arising from the right coronary artery and crossing the right ventricular outflow tract is commonly seen in patients with tetralogy of Fallot, and this can be demonstrated by echocardiography using the parasternal short-axis view. Of note, dual left anterior descending coronary arteries can present a similar echocardiographic appearance, and sometimes it can be difficult to distinguish between the two. These two types of coronary artery patterns can affect surgical strategy.

▶ Lai WW, Mertens LL, Cohen MS, et al (eds): *Echocardiography in Pediatric and Congenital Heart Disease: From Fetus to Adult*, 2nd edition. Chichester, UK, Wiley-Blackwell, 2016, p 413.

▶ Need LR, Powell AJ, del Nido P, et al: Coronary echocardiography in tetralogy of Fallot: diagnostic accuracy, resource utilization and surgical implications over 13 years. J Am Coll Cardiol 36:1371–1377, 2000.

148. A. Atrial septal defect.

The four primary anomalies associated with tetralogy of Fallot (TOF) are a ventricular septal defect (VSD), overriding aorta, pulmonary stenosis, and right ventricular hypertrophy. In addition, about 86% of patients with TOF have an atrial septal defect (ASD) or a patent foramen ovale (PFO), and in 25% of cases the patient has a right aortic arch. In about 12% of TOF cases patients have an abnormal coronary artery. Coarctation of the aorta associated with TOF is very rare.

▶ Lai WW, Mertens LL, Cohen MS, et al (eds): *Echocardiography in Pediatric and Congenital Heart Disease: From Fetus to Adult*, 2nd edition. Chichester, UK, Wiley-Blackwell, 2016, p 416.

▶ Rao BN, Anderson RC, Edwards JE, et al: Anatomic variations in the tetralogy of Fallot. Am Heart J 81:361–371, 1971.

149. D. Large patent ductus arteriosus.

Key features of tetralogy of Fallot with absent pulmonary valve include enlarged, aneurysmally dilated main and branch pulmonary arteries. In such cases the pulmonary valve might be completely absent, or there can be rudimentary valve leaflets resulting in mild right ventricular outflow tract obstruction and severe pulmonary regurgitation. Overriding aorta is always one of the key features of TOF. However, a patent ductus arteriosus (PDA) is usually not *present in TOF with absent pulmonary valve.*

▸ Allen HD, Driscoll DJ, Shaddy RE, et al: *Moss and Adams' Heart Disease in Infants, Children, and Adolescents: Including the Fetus and Young Adult*, 8th edition. Philadelphia, Lippincott Williams & Wilkins, 2013, p 975.

▸ Lai WW, Mertens LL, Cohen MS, et al (eds): *Echocardiography in Pediatric and Congenital Heart Disease: From Fetus to Adult*, 2nd edition. Chichester, UK, Wiley-Blackwell, 2016, p 425.

150. B. Tetralogy of Fallot with a common atrioventricular canal defect.

A

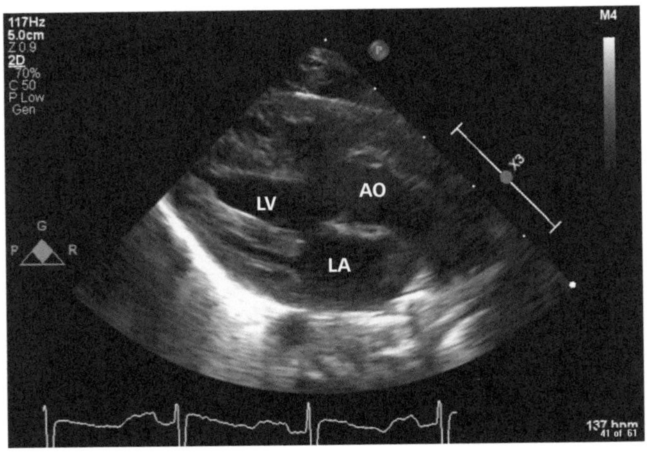

B

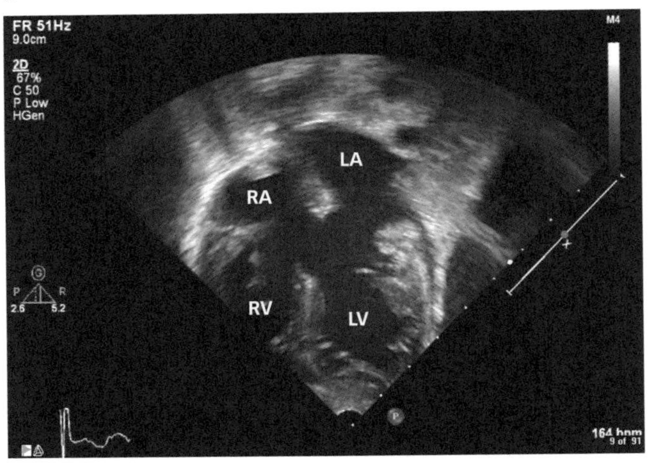

This patient has the overriding aorta (image ***A****) that typifies tetralogy of Fallot (TOF), and the apical view (image* ***B****) shows the typical echocardiographic features of a common atrioventricular canal defect (CAVC), also known as an atrioventricular septal defect (AVSD). TOF with a CAVC is often associated with Down syndrome patients. Conversely, transposition of*

the great arteries is not found in these patients. AO = aorta, RA = right atrium, LA = left atrium, RV = right ventricle, LV = left ventricle.

▶ Lai WW, Mertens LL, Cohen MS, et al (eds): *Echocardiography in Pediatric and Congenital Heart Disease: From Fetus to Adult*, 2nd edition. Chichester, UK, Wiley-Blackwell, 2016, pp 425–426.

151. B. Rastelli type B.

The Rastelli classification of complete common atrioventricular canal defect (CAVC) divides the common atrioventricular valve into three types, based on the morphology of the anterior (superior) bridging leaflet:

- *Type A: The anterior-superior common AV valve leaflet is divided into two, one mitral valve portion and one tricuspid valve portion, with medial attachments to the crest of the interventricular septum.*
- *Type B: The anterior-superior leaflet is partially divided and has some attachments onto a papillary muscle in the right ventricle.*
- *Type C: The anterior-superior leaflet is undivided and free-floating.*

Of these three types, the least common is Rastelli type B, whether tetralogy of Fallot is present or not.

▶ Ezon DS, Goldberg JF, Kyle WB: *Atlas of Congenital Heart Disease Nomenclature: An Illustrated Guide to the Van Praagh and Anderson Approaches to Describing Congenital Cardiac Pathology*. Houston, Ezon Educational Services/CreateSpace, 2015, p 62.

▶ Lai WW, Mertens LL, Cohen MS, et al (eds): *Echocardiography in Pediatric and Congenital Heart Disease: From Fetus to Adult*, 2nd edition. Chichester, UK, Wiley-Blackwell, 2016, pp 261–264, 425–426.

152. A. Tricuspid valve.

In truncus arteriosus, a tricuspid (trileaflet) valve is found in about 65%–70% of cases, a quadricuspid valve in about 9%–24% of cases, and a bicuspid valve in about 6%–23% of cases. In rare cases a unicuspid valve is found.

▶ Lai WW, Mertens LL, Cohen MS, et al (eds): *Echocardiography in Pediatric and Congenital Heart Disease: From Fetus to Adult*, 2nd edition. Chichester, UK, Wiley-Blackwell, 2016, p 434.

▶ Van Praagh R, Van Praagh S: The anatomy of common aorticopulmonary trunk (truncus arteriosus communis) and its embryologic implications: a study of 57 necropsy cases. Am J Cardiol 16:406–425, 1965.

ANSWERS

153. D. Origin of the pulmonary arteries.

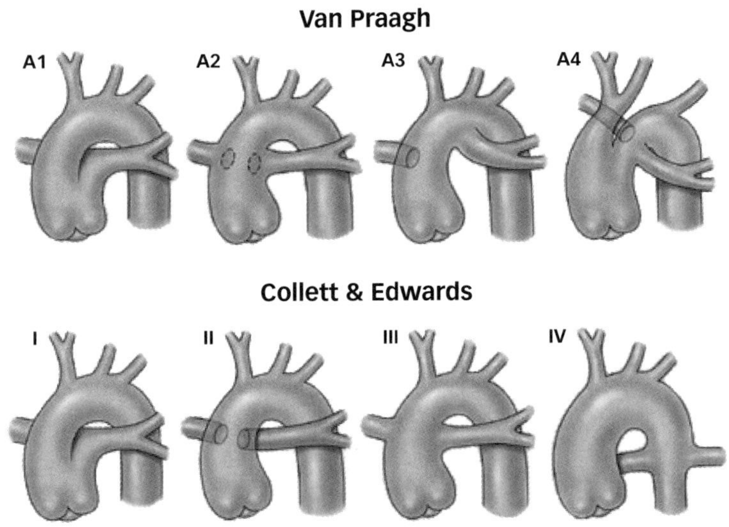

Source: Adapted from Children's Hopsital Boston, https://apps.childrenshospital.org/MML/index.cfm?CAT=media&MEDIA_ID=2027. Reprinted with permission.

The truncus arteriosus (TA) classification systems of Van Praagh and Collett and Edwards use different origins of the pulmonary arteries to classify TA into anatomic subtypes. Each classification system uses four subtypes (see the references listed below). Of note, Collett and Edwards' TA type IV is no longer thought to be truncus arteriosus but is now considered to be tetralogy of Fallot with pulmonary atresia and aortopulmonary collateral vessels.

Van Praagh system:

- *Type A1: Both aorta and main pulmonary artery arise from a common trunk.*
- *Type A2: Separate origins of the branch pulmonary arteries from the common trunk.*
- *Type A3: Origin of one branch pulmonary artery (usually the right) from the common trunk, with the other lung supplied either by collaterals or by a pulmonary artery arising from the aortic arch.*
- *Type A4: Presence of an associated interrupted aortic arch.*

Collett and Edwards system:

- *Type I (most common): Identical to Van Praagh type A1.*
- *Type II: Pulmonary arteries arise separately from the posterior aspect of the trunk, close to each other just above the truncal valve (negligible main pulmonary artery segment).*
- *Type III (least common): Pulmonary arteries arise independently from either side of the trunk.*

- *Type IV: Neither pulmonary arterial branch arises from the common trunk (pseudotruncus); the pulmonary circulation is supplied by collaterals from the descending aorta. Currently considered a form of pulmonary atresia with a VSD.*

▶ Ezon DS, Goldberg JF, Kyle WB: *Atlas of Congenital Heart Disease Nomenclature: An Illustrated Guide to the Van Praagh and Anderson Approaches to Describing Congenital Cardiac Pathology*. Houston, Ezon Educational Services/CreateSpace, 2015, pp 76–77.

▶ Lai WW, Mertens LL, Cohen MS, et al (eds): *Echocardiography in Pediatric and Congenital Heart Disease: From Fetus to Adult*, 2nd edition. Chichester, UK, Wiley-Blackwell, 2016, p 434.

▶ Van Praagh R, Van Praagh S: The anatomy of common aorticopulmonary trunk (truncus arteriosus communis) and its embryologic implications: a study of 57 necropsy cases. Am J Cardiol 16:406–425, 1965.

154. A. Posterior-left common trunk with short main pulmonary artery.

For truncus arteriosus, a posterior-left common trunk with a short main pulmonary artery (type 1) is the most common type, accounting for 48%–68% of cases. Posterior-left common trunk with separate pulmonary artery origins (type 2) is the second most common type, with 29%–48% of cases.

▶ Allen HD, Driscoll DJ, Shaddy RE, et al: *Moss and Adams' Heart Disease in Infants, Children, and Adolescents: Including the Fetus and Young Adult*, 8th edition. Philadelphia, Lippincott Williams & Wilkins, 2013, p 991.

▶ Bharati S, McAllister HA, Rosenquist GC, et al: The surgical anatomy of truncus arteriosus communis. J Thorac Cardiovasc Surg 67:501–510, 1974.

▶ Lai WW, Mertens LL, Cohen MS, et al (eds): *Echocardiography in Pediatric and Congenital Heart Disease: From Fetus to Adult*, 2nd edition. Chichester, UK, Wiley-Blackwell, 2016, p 434.

155. C. Pulmonary arteries arising from the arterial trunk.

The definition of truncus arteriosus (TA) is a single arterial trunk that gives rise to the ascending aorta, descending aorta (except in the TA subtype with interrupted aortic arch), and pulmonary arteries. Usually TA is found without a patent ductus arteriosus (PDA), except in Van Praagh type A4 (the TA subtype with interrupted aortic arch). In tetralogy of Fallot (TOF) with pulmonary atresia, the pulmonary arteries do not arise directly from the aorta but instead are supplied by a PDA or systemic aortopulmonary collateral arteries. In both TA and TOF with pulmonary atresia, a semilunar valve overrides the ventricular septum and there is a large ventricular septal defect.

▶ Lai WW, Mertens LL, Cohen MS, et al (eds): *Echocardiography in Pediatric and Congenital Heart Disease: From Fetus to Adult*, 2nd edition. Chichester, UK, Wiley-Blackwell, 2016, p 434.

156. D. Type A4.

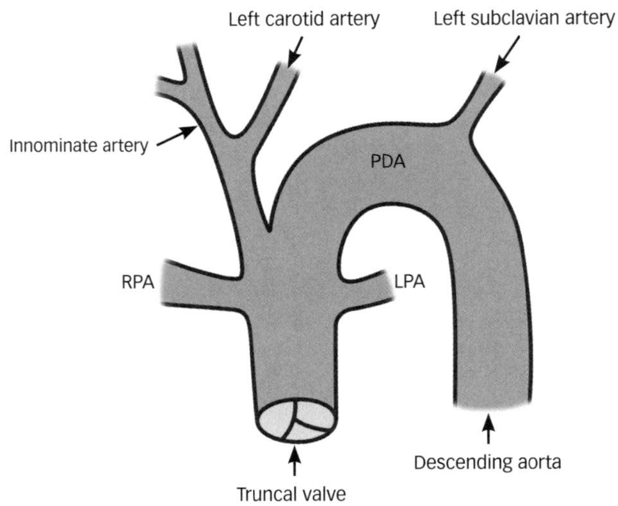

This diagram shows TA with an interrupted aortic arch, Van Praagh classification type A4. Most authorities use the Collett and Edwards and/or Van Praagh schemes to classify truncus arteriosus (TA). Each classification scheme identifies four types of TA, but there are important differences between the Collett and Edwards and Van Praagh systems—see the answer to question 153. PDA = patent ductus arteriosus, RPA = right pulmonary artery, LPA = left pulmonary artery.

- Allen HD, Driscoll DJ, Shaddy RE, et al: *Moss and Adams' Heart Disease in Infants, Children, and Adolescents: Including the Fetus and Young Adult*, 8th edition. Philadelphia, Lippincott Williams & Wilkins, 2013, p 992.
- Lai WW, Mertens LL, Cohen MS, et al (eds): *Echocardiography in Pediatric and Congenital Heart Disease: From Fetus to Adult*, 2nd edition. Chichester, UK, Wiley-Blackwell, 2016, p 434.

157. C. Subaortic VSD.

The incidence of ventricular septal defects (VSDs) by type, when double-outlet right ventricle (DORV) is present, is as follows:

Type of VSD	***Percentage of VSD Cases***
Subaortic	*42%–57%*
Subpulmonary	*24%–37%*
Doubly committed	*3%–12%*
Noncommitted	*9%–19%*

- Anderson RH, McCarthy K, Cook AC: Double outlet right ventricle. Cardiol Young 11:329–344, 2001.
- Lai WW, Mertens LL, Cohen MS, et al (eds): *Echocardiography in Pediatric and Congenital Heart Disease: From Fetus to Adult*, 2nd edition. Chichester, UK, Wiley-Blackwell, 2016, pp 468–469.
- Van Praagh R, Pérez-Trevino C, Reynolds JL, et al: Double outlet right ventricle (S,D,L) with subaortic ventricular septal defect and pulmonary stenosis. Am J Cardiol 35:42–53, 1975.

158. A. Aorta to the right of the pulmonary artery.

The most common type of great artery relationship in DORV is the aorta to the right of the pulmonary artery, either side-by-side or with the aorta rightward and anterior to the pulmonary artery. The other choices—aorta directly anterior to the pulmonary artery, aorta leftward and posterior to the pulmonary artery, and aorta leftward and anterior to the pulmonary artery—can occur but are much less common.

▶ Lai WW, Mertens LL, Cohen MS, et al (eds): *Echocardiography in Pediatric and Congenital Heart Disease: From Fetus to Adult*, 2nd edition. Chichester, UK, Wiley-Blackwell, 2016, p 473.

159. D. Double-outlet right ventricle.

When double-outlet right ventricle (DORV) is present, the aorta and pulmonary arteries are located more toward the right side of the heart, and leftward juxtaposition of the right atrial appendage is sometimes present. This anatomic variation of the atrial appendages is exceedingly rare with an atrioventricular canal defect, tetralogy of Fallot, or hypoplastic left heart syndrome.

▶ Lai WW, Mertens LL, Cohen MS, et al (eds): *Echocardiography in Pediatric and Congenital Heart Disease: From Fetus to Adult*, 2nd edition. Chichester, UK, Wiley-Blackwell, 2016, p 474.

▶ Lai WW, Ravishankar C, Gross RP, et al: Juxtaposition of the atrial appendages: a clinical series of 22 patients. Pediatric Cardiol 22:121–127, 2001.

160. B. Subpulmonary VSD, side-by-side great arteries, an unobstructed pulmonary outflow tract, and possible subaortic obstruction.

In 1949 Helen B. Taussig and Richard Bing for the first time described a heart with double-outlet right ventricle (DORV) as characterized by the following:

- *side-by-side great arteries*
- *a subpulmonary ventricular septal defect (VSD)*
- *bilateral conus*

In a large percentage of Taussig-Bing DORV cases, a prominent subaortic conus can produce subaortic narrowing associated with coarctation of the aorta or interrupted aortic arch.

▶ Ezon DS, Goldberg JF, Kyle WB: *Atlas of Congenital Heart Disease Nomenclature: An Illustrated Guide to the Van Praagh and Anderson Approaches to Describing Congenital Cardiac Pathology*. Houston, Ezon Educational Services/CreateSpace, 2015, p 80.

▶ Hayes DA, Jones S, Quaegebeur JM, et al: Primary arterial switch operation as a strategy for total correction of Taussig-Bing anomaly: a 21-year experience. Circulation 128:S194–S198, 2013.

▶ Lai WW, Mertens LL, Cohen MS, et al (eds): *Echocardiography in Pediatric and Congenital Heart Disease: From Fetus to Adult*, 2nd edition. Chichester, UK, Wiley-Blackwell, 2016, p 469.

▶ Taussig HB, Bing RJ: Complete transposition of the aorta and a levo-position of the pulmonary artery: clinical, physiological, and pathological findings. Am Heart J 37:551–559, 1949.

161. B. When the conal septum is deviated toward the subaortic outflow tract.

When the conal septum deviates to the subaortic area, it can cause subaortic stenosis, which is often associated with an aortic arch anomaly such as coarctation of the aorta or interrupted aortic arch.

▶ Lai WW, Mertens LL, Cohen MS, et al (eds): *Echocardiography in Pediatric and Congenital Heart Disease: From Fetus to Adult*, 2nd edition. Chichester, UK, Wiley-Blackwell, 2016, p 473.

162. B. DORV with a subpulmonary ventricular septal defect (VSD).

Of the choices given, double-outlet right ventricle (DORV) with subpulmonary VSD (often called Taussig-Bing anomaly) is most commonly associated with straddling mitral valve. Mitral valve chordae cross the subpulmonary ventricular septal defect (VSD) to insert into the right ventricle or the subpulmonary conus.

▶ Fraisse A, del Nido PJ, Guadart J, et al: Echocardiographic characteristics and outcome of straddling mitral valve. J Am Coll of Cardiology 38:819–826, 2011.

▶ Lai WW, Mertens LL, Cohen MS, et al (eds): *Echocardiography in Pediatric and Congenital Heart Disease: From Fetus to Adult*, 2nd edition. Chichester, UK, Wiley-Blackwell, 2016, p 469.

163. B. SMV is abnormal mitral valve chordae attaching to both the right and left ventricles.

The definition of a straddling mitral valve (SMV) is a mitral valve with chordae that attach to both sides of the ventricular septum by passing through a ventricular septal defect (VSD), which is always present and which makes this aberrant anatomy possible. An SMV can occur with an overriding mitral valve (OMV)—i.e., one that overrides the ventricular septum. However, an OMV can also exist without an SMV, since OMV anatomy can include the mitral valve chordae overriding the septum without actually straddling into the other ventricle.

▶ Allen HD, Driscoll DJ, Shaddy RE, et al: *Moss and Adams' Heart Disease in Infants, Children, and Adolescents: Including the Fetus and Young Adult*, 8th edition. Philadelphia, Lippincott Williams & Wilkins, 2013, pp 48–50.

▶ Lai WW, Mertens LL, Cohen MS, et al (eds): *Echocardiography in Pediatric and Congenital Heart Disease: From Fetus to Adult*, 2nd edition. Chichester, UK, Wiley-Blackwell, 2016, p 243.

164. C. Aortopulmonary window.

An aortopulmonary window (AP window) is easy to miss. In normal patients with no AP window, an echo "dropout" may manifest during a routine parasternal short-axis scan; however, with an AP window the absent portion of the wall between the aorta and the pulmonary artery (the most common site for an AP window) will also appear on the echocardiogram as an echo dropout. Hence, visualization of this echo dropout cannot automatically be dismissed as a normal finding. With an AP window, right ventricular pressure is elevated and a very low-velocity left-to-right shunt is seen on color flow Doppler. These subtle echocardiographic findings might easily escape notice, and the echocardiographer might not think to investigate further if ignoring the possibility of an AP window. Early clinical features of an AP window are similar to those of a large ventricular septal defect or patent ductus arteriosus, with high-volume pulmonary blood flow from a left-to-right shunt. In the scenario posed by the question, these defects were ruled out by the echocardiographer's study. However, reversal of flow is often seen with an AP window because of "steal" and runoff diastolic flow from the descending into the ascending aorta and then into the main pulmonary artery. If an AP window is not diagnosed early, patients can develop more significant pulmonary hypertension, leading to reduced left-to-right shunting across the AP window, in which case reversal of flow will be less significant or absent. An atrial septal defect (choice A) and anomalous left coronary artery from the pulmonary artery (choice B) will not produce aortic diastolic flow reversal, and transposition of the great arteries (choice D) should be readily apparent to both the echocardiographer and the cardiologist when a complete, comprehensive echocardiogram is performed.

▶ Allen HD, Driscoll DJ, Shaddy RE, et al: *Moss and Adams' Heart Disease in Infants, Children, and Adolescents: Including the Fetus and Young Adult*, 8th edition. Philadelphia, Lippincott Williams & Wilkins, 2013, pp 740–742.

▶ Lai WW, Mertens LL, Cohen MS, et al (eds): *Echocardiography in Pediatric and Congenital Heart Disease: From Fetus to Adult*, 2nd edition. Chichester, UK, Wiley-Blackwell, 2016, p 873.

ANSWERS

165. A. It is more common in males.

Approximately 70% of bicuspid aortic valves occur in males. Bicuspid aortic valve is one of the most common congenital heart defects, with a neonatal incidence of about 4.6 per 1000 live births.

- Lai WW, Mertens LL, Cohen MS, et al (eds): *Echocardiography in Pediatric and Congenital Heart Disease: From Fetus to Adult*, 2nd edition. Chichester, UK, Wiley-Blackwell, 2016, pp 336, 347.
- Nistri S, Basso C, Marzari C, et al: Frequency of bicuspid aortic valve in young male conscripts by echocardiogram. Am J Cardiol 96:718–721, 2005.
- Tutar E, Ekici F, Atalay S, et al: The prevalence of bicuspid aortic valve in newborns by echocardiographic screening. Am Heart J 150:513–515, 2005.

Refer to video PER-Q166.

166. A. Size of ascending aorta.

Video PER-Q166 demonstrates the bicuspid aortic valve anomaly. Ascending aortic dilatation is very common in bicuspid aortic valve patients, and the entire aorta should be interrogated since these patients are also at risk for coarctation and aortic hypoplasia. Unlike Marfan syndrome patients, who have primarily aortic root (sinuses of Valsalva) dilatation, bicuspid aortic valve patients can have progressive dilatation of the ascending aorta. Therefore careful follow-up by echocardiography is important.

- Lai WW, Mertens LL, Cohen MS, et al (eds): *Echocardiography in Pediatric and Congenital Heart Disease: From Fetus to Adult*, 2nd edition. Chichester, UK, Wiley-Blackwell, 2016, p 347.
- Warren AE, Boyd ML, O'Connell C, et al: Dilatation of the ascending aorta in paediatric patients with bicuspid aortic valve: frequency, rate of progression and risk factors. Heart 92:1496–1500, 2006.

167. B. Right coronary cusp.

The membranous ventricular septum is thin and fibrous, located at the posterior portion of the ventricular septum, which is adjacent to the septal leaflet of the tricuspid valve and beneath the right coronary cusp of the aortic valve. A membranous (also called perimembranous) ventricular septal defect (VSD) will be located in this area.

- Lai WW, Mertens LL, Cohen MS, et al (eds): *Echocardiography in Pediatric and Congenital Heart Disease: From Fetus to Adult*, 2nd edition. Chichester, UK, Wiley-Blackwell, 2016, p 217.

168. C. Aortic valve prolapse and regurgitation.

Because the right coronary cusp (RCC) is close to the membranous ventricular septal defect (VSD), the RCC can prolapse due to the Venturi effect from a high-velocity VSD jet, which can lead to aortic valve regurgitation. If an aortic valve cusp prolapses and aortic insufficiency results, surgical repair is indicated, even if the VSD shunt is small. In general, small VSDs will not cause congestive heart failure (choice A) or pulmonary hypertension (choice B). A patient with a VSD is not at high risk for endocarditis (choice D). Of note: Although choice C is the most correct answer to this question, the echocardiographer should not neglect to focus on all aspects of VSD evaluation, including VSD jet velocity, the morphology of the defect, atrioventricular and semilunar valves, other possible cardiac defects (such as atrial septal defects), and ventricular chamber size and function.

▶ Lai WW, Mertens LL, Cohen MS, et al (eds): *Echocardiography in Pediatric and Congenital Heart Disease: From Fetus to Adult*, 2nd edition. Chichester, UK, Wiley-Blackwell, 2016, pp 347–348.

▶ Park MK: *Park's Pediatric Cardiology for Practitioners*, 6th edition. Philadelphia, Saunders, 2014, pp 200–201.

169. C. Mitral valve annulus size.

In a newborn with critical aortic valve stenosis, there can be associated hypoplasia of other left-sided structures, such as the mitral valve, left ventricle, and ascending aorta or aortic arch. It is very important to measure all these structures, including the mitral valve annulus, mitral valve area, left ventricle in long axis, aortic valve annulus, and aortic arch diameters. All these measurements will affect the decision regarding whether to perform a two-ventricle repair or single-ventricle palliation—and if two-ventricle repair is indicated, whether a transcatheter or surgical approach should be attempted.

▶ Lai WW, Mertens LL, Cohen MS, et al (eds): *Echocardiography in Pediatric and Congenital Heart Disease: From Fetus to Adult*, 2nd edition. Chichester, UK, Wiley-Blackwell, 2016, p 342.

170. B. Right ventricle.

In a sinus of Valsalva aneurysm, the right coronary sinus is most commonly involved. Therefore, rupture of the right coronary sinus aneurysm results in blood flowing from the aorta into the right ventricle.

▶ Allen HD, Driscoll DJ, Shaddy RE, et al: *Moss and Adams' Heart Disease in Infants, Children, and Adolescents: Including the Fetus and Young Adult*, 8th edition. Philadelphia, Lippincott Williams & Wilkins, 2013, pp 755–756.

▶ Lai WW, Mertens LL, Cohen MS, et al (eds): *Echocardiography in Pediatric and Congenital Heart Disease: From Fetus to Adult*, 2nd edition. Chichester, UK, Wiley-Blackwell, 2016, p 349.

171. B. Interrogation with spectral Doppler.

Both a ventricular septal defect (VSD) and a right coronary sinus of Valsalva aneurysm rupture have a left-to-right shunt, which causes left ventricular dilatation, and both can have aortic valve prolapse. But with a VSD, the left-to-right shunt occurs only in systole; in sinus of Valsalva aneurysm rupture, spectral (and color flow) Doppler will demonstrate continuous left-to-right shunting throughout systole and diastole.

▶ Allen HD, Driscoll DJ, Shaddy RE, et al: *Moss and Adams' Heart Disease in Infants, Children, and Adolescents: Including the Fetus and Young Adult*, 8th edition. Philadelphia, Lippincott Williams & Wilkins, 2013, p 755.

172. C. Severe aortic valve regurgitation.

An aortico–left ventricular tunnel (ALVT) is an extracardiac tunnel-like connection between the left ventricle and the ascending aorta, with an opening located above the sinuses of Valsalva, passing in the aortic/left ventricular wall behind the right/left coronary cusps, and with another opening located in the ventricular septum, below the level of the aortic valve. The physiology of ALVT is the same as that found with severe aortic valve regurgitation, with aortic flow leaking back into the left ventricle during diastole, resulting in left ventricular volume overload. It can be difficult to differentiate this entity from aortic valve regurgitation because an ALVT is very rare. It is important to identify the precise location of aortic regurgitation. Mitral valve stenosis and aortic valve stenosis do not result in left ventricular volume overload. A ventricular septal defect (VSD) can produce left ventricular dilatation due to a significant left-to-right shunt; however, the echocardiographic appearance of the VSD shunt is significantly different from that of an ALVT.

▶ Allen HD, Driscoll DJ, Shaddy RE, et al: *Moss and Adams' Heart Disease in Infants, Children, and Adolescents: Including the Fetus and Young Adult*, 8th edition. Philadelphia, Lippincott Williams & Wilkins, 2013, pp 754–755.

▶ Lai WW, Mertens LL, Cohen MS, et al (eds): *Echocardiography in Pediatric and Congenital Heart Disease: From Fetus to Adult*, 2nd edition. Chichester, UK, Wiley-Blackwell, 2016, pp 350–352.

173. D. Interrupted aortic arch.

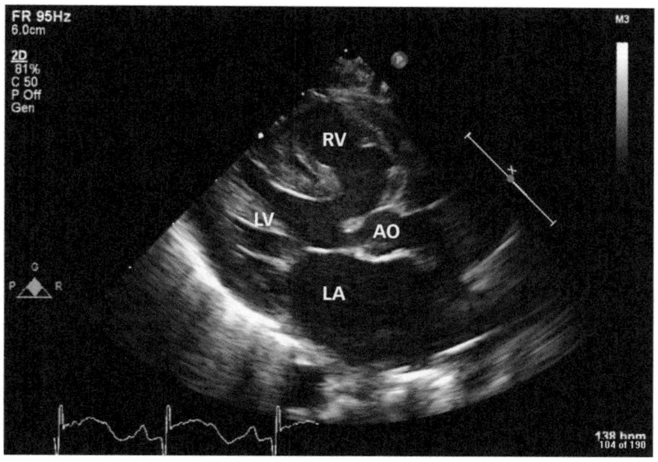

When posterior deviation of the conal septum occurs with a ventricular septal defect (VSD), as seen in this image, it causes the subaortic area to be small and potentially obstructed. It is also highly associated with a type B interrupted aortic arch (IAA) or coarctation of the aorta (CoA). LV = left ventricle, RV = right ventricle, AO = aorta, LA = left atrium.

▸ Lai WW, Mertens LL, Cohen MS, et al (eds): *Echocardiography in Pediatric and Congenital Heart Disease: From Fetus to Adult*, 2nd edition. Chichester, UK, Wiley-Blackwell, 2016, p 338.

Refer to video PER-Q174.

174. C. Echocardiography is required to determine whether the original lesion has recurred.

Subaortic membranes (seen in video PER-Q174) can regrow after surgical removal. One study (see Allen et al.) found a recurrence rate of 16% at 5 years and 30% at 10 years.

▸ Allen HD, Driscoll DJ, Shaddy RE, et al: *Moss and Adams' Heart Disease in Infants, Children, and Adolescents: Including the Fetus and Young Adult*, 8th edition. Philadelphia, Lippincott Williams & Wilkins, 2013, p 1468.

▸ Lai WW, Mertens LL, Cohen MS, et al (eds): *Echocardiography in Pediatric and Congenital Heart Disease: From Fetus to Adult*, 2nd edition. Chichester, UK, Wiley-Blackwell, 2016, p 337.

175. A. Mitral valve and pulmonary valve fibrous continuity.

There is a subaortic conus separating the aortic valve and the tricuspid valve in most cases of transposition of the great arteries (d-TGA). There is also mitral valve and pulmonary valve fibrous continuity.

▸ Allen HD, Driscoll DJ, Shaddy RE, et al: Moss and Adams' Heart Disease in Infants, Children, and Adolescents: Including the Fetus and Young Adult, 8th edition. Philadelphia, Lippincott Williams & Wilkins, 2013, p 1099.

▸ Lai WW, Mertens LL, Cohen MS, et al (eds): *Echocardiography in Pediatric and Congenital Heart Disease: From Fetus to Adult*, 2nd edition. Chichester, UK, Wiley-Blackwell, 2016, p 447.

176. D. Ventricular septal defect.

In 40%–45% of cases of transposition of the great arteries (d-TGA) there is an associated ventricular septal defect (VSD). In those patients with a VSD, the most common type (occurring about 30% of the time) is perimembranous (also called membranous) VSD, followed by a malalignment VSD (about 30% of cases) and a muscular VSD (about 25% of cases). VSDs that are found with d-TGA less frequently include outlet VSDs (doubly committed or subarterial) and inlet VSDs.

- Allen HD, Driscoll DJ, Shaddy RE, et al: *Moss and Adams' Heart Disease in Infants, Children, and Adolescents: Including the Fetus and Young Adult*, 8th edition. Philadelphia, Lippincott Williams & Wilkins, 2013, p 1101.
- Lai WW, Mertens LL, Cohen MS, et al (eds): *Echocardiography in Pediatric and Congenital Heart Disease: From Fetus to Adult*, 2nd edition. Chichester, UK, Wiley-Blackwell, 2016, p 447.

177. A. Left circumflex from right coronary.

In patients with transposition of the great arteries (d-TGA), about 67% have a "usual" coronary artery pattern, with the right coronary artery arising from the right-facing sinus and the left main coronary artery (giving rise to the left anterior descending and circumflex coronary arteries) arising from the left-facing sinus. In about 14% of d-TGA patients, the circumflex artery arises from the right coronary and left anterior descending arteries from the left-facing sinus. A single right coronary artery is found in approximately 7.5% of d-TGA patients, and a single left coronary artery is found in about 1.5% of d-TGA patients. An intramural left coronary artery is found in roughly 3%, an intramural right coronary artery in 0.75%, and inverted coronary artery origins in 2.6%.

- Lai WW, Mertens LL, Cohen MS, et al (eds): *Echocardiography in Pediatric and Congenital Heart Disease: From Fetus to Adult*, 2nd edition. Chichester, UK, Wiley-Blackwell, 2016, p 450.
- Pasquali SK, Hasselblad V, Li JS, et al: Coronary artery pattern and outcome of arterial switch operation for transposition of the great arteries: a meta-analysis. Circulation 106:2575–2580, 2002.

Refer to video PER-Q178.

178. B. Transposition of the great arteries.

Video PER-Q178 demonstrates two great arteries traveling in parallel, representing transposition of the great arteries (d-TGA). Tetralogy of Fallot (TOA) usually has normally related great arteries, and thus in the presence of TOF two parallel great arteries will not be seen in a parasternal long-axis view. Truncus arteriosus (TA) has only one semilunar (truncal) valve. The clip demonstrates that each ventricle has one outlet, so the clip does not represent double-outlet right ventricle (DORV).

Refer to video PER-Q179.

179. C. Restrictive atrial septal defect.

Based on the findings in video PER-Q179, the most likely diagnosis is transposition of the great arteries (d-TGA). In this defect, deoxygenated blood returning from the systemic veins is pumped back into the aorta via the right ventricle, and patients will therefore present with extremely low systemic oxygen saturations. At the same time, oxygenated blood returning from the lungs flows back through the pulmonary veins into the left ventricle and back into the lungs. This circulation is not compatible with survival unless some type of mixing is present to allow oxygenated blood returning from the lungs to mix with deoxygenated blood, thereby improving systemic arterial oxygen saturation. Shunting can occur through an atrial septal defect (ASD), ventricular septal defect (VSD), or patent ductus arteriosus (PDA). Of these, atrial shunting is the most crucial for adequate mixing of oxygenated and deoxygenated blood. When there is a restrictive ASD, atrial mixing is limited, and in such cases balloon atrial septostomy might be necessary to enlarge the ASD and enhance mixing. Note that the presence of a PDA by itself (without a good-sized ASD) might not improve systemic oxygenation, as PDA shunting in these patients is generally unidirectional: left-to-right from the aorta into the pulmonary arteries. Even with a good-sized VSD, ventricular-level shunting cannot be relied upon for adequate mixing due to streaming of the atrioventricular inflows to the respective outflows. A good-sized ASD might still be necessary to promote adequate mixing.

- Allen HD, Driscoll DJ, Shaddy RE, et al: *Moss and Adams' Heart Disease in Infants, Children, and Adolescents: Including the Fetus and Young Adult*, 8th edition. Philadelphia, Lippincott Williams & Wilkins, 2013, pp 1114–1116.
- Lai WW, Mertens LL, Cohen MS, et al (eds): *Echocardiography in Pediatric and Congenital Heart Disease: From Fetus to Adult*, 2nd edition. Chichester, UK, Wiley-Blackwell, 2016, pp 449–450.

180. A. Atrial situs solitus.

Of all cases of physiologically "corrected" (congenitally corrected) transposition of the great arteries (ccTGA), 94% have atrial situs solitus, with the segments (as described in the Van Praagh nomenclature) of {S, L, L}. The remaining 6% have atrial situs inversus with segments {I, D, D}.

- Allen HD, Driscoll DJ, Shaddy RE, et al: *Moss and Adams' Heart Disease in Infants, Children, and Adolescents: Including the Fetus and Young Adult*, 8th edition. Philadelphia, Lippincott Williams & Wilkins, 2013, p 1147.

▶ Ezon DS, Goldberg JF, Kyle WB: *Atlas of Congenital Heart Disease Nomenclature: An Illustrated Guide to the Van Praagh and Anderson Approaches to Describing Congenital Cardiac Pathology*. Houston, Ezon Educational Services/CreateSpace, 2015, pp 86–87.

▶ Lai WW, Mertens LL, Cohen MS, et al (eds): *Echocardiography in Pediatric and Congenital Heart Disease: From Fetus to Adult*, 2nd edition. Chichester, UK, Wiley-Blackwell, 2016, pp 489–492.

181. C. Ventricular septal defect.

Of all cases of physiologically "corrected" (congenitally corrected) transposition of the great arteries (ccTGA), 60%–80% have a ventricular septal defect (VSD). Other associated cardiac lesions include pulmonary outflow obstruction and an abnormal tricuspid valve.

▶ Allen HD, Driscoll DJ, Shaddy RE, et al: *Moss and Adams' Heart Disease in Infants, Children, and Adolescents: Including the Fetus and Young Adult*, 8th edition. Philadelphia, Lippincott Williams & Wilkins, 2013, p 1148.

▶ Lai WW, Mertens LL, Cohen MS, et al (eds): *Echocardiography in Pediatric and Congenital Heart Disease: From Fetus to Adult*, 2nd edition. Chichester, UK, Wiley-Blackwell, 2016, p 494.

182. D. Subpulmonary valve stenosis.

Of all cases of physiologically "corrected" transposition of the great arteries, 30%–50% have pulmonary outflow tract obstruction. The most common cause of pulmonary outflow obstruction originates from the subvalvular area, such as tissue tags from the atrioventricular valve(s), an aneurysm of the membranous ventricular septum, or bulging of a malaligned ventricular septum. Isolated pulmonary valve stenosis is not common. Branch pulmonary artery stenosis is uncommon and does not affect the pulmonary outflow tract. Given that the ventricular chamber connected to the pulmonary artery is the morphologic left ventricle (not the right ventricle), double-chambered right ventricle is incorrect.

▶ Allen HD, Driscoll DJ, Shaddy RE, et al: *Moss and Adams' Heart Disease in Infants, Children, and Adolescents: Including the Fetus and Young Adult*, 8th edition. Philadelphia, Lippincott Williams & Wilkins, 2013, p 1148.

▶ Lai WW, Mertens LL, Cohen MS, et al (eds): *Echocardiography in Pediatric and Congenital Heart Disease: From Fetus to Adult*, 2nd edition. Chichester, UK, Wiley-Blackwell, 2016, p 494.

183. B. D.

The letter "D" refers to D-looped ventricles. {I, D, D} is one of the physiologically "corrected" transposition arrangements. It is the mirror image of the usual physiologically "corrected" transposition of the great arteries, {S, L, L}.

▶ Lai WW, Mertens LL, Cohen MS, et al (eds): *Echocardiography in Pediatric and Congenital Heart Disease: From Fetus to Adult*, 2nd edition. Chichester, UK, Wiley-Blackwell, 2016, p 490.

184. D. 36 mmHg + atrial right pressure.

Because the patient has physiologically "corrected" transposition of the great arteries, the cardiac segmental arrangement will be atrial-ventricular discordance and ventricular-arterial discordance. The pulmonary artery therefore arises from the morphologic left ventricle, which in turn is connected to the morphologic right atrium. Because the type of atrioventricular valve (mitral or tricuspid) is always derived from the morphology of the ventricle, in this instance the pulmonary ventricle is the morphologic left ventricle. Therefore, the mitral valve is part of the pulmonary circulation. In the absence of pulmonary outflow tract obstruction, using the mitral valve regurgitation jet to calculate left ventricular pressure will directly indicate pulmonary artery systolic pressure.

185. B. Reduced right ventricular function.

Patients with physiologically "corrected" (congenitally corrected) transposition of the great arteries (ccTGA) may not have other associated lesions. Others may have minor lesions that may not have required surgical intervention when they were younger. However, as they age, these patients still face the risk of increased tricuspid valve regurgitation and right ventricular dysfunction. The right ventricle is the systemic pumping chamber, and patients can develop congestive heart failure if this ventricle fails. There are several theoretical reasons for right ventricular failure: The right ventricular muscle is not designed for systemic pressures, the systemic tricuspid valve may be abnormal (even exhibiting Ebstein-like anatomy), and the right ventricular myocardium is supplied by a single coronary artery (unlike the left ventricle).

▶ Allen HD, Driscoll DJ, Shaddy RE, et al: *Moss and Adams' Heart Disease in Infants, Children, and Adolescents: Including the Fetus and Young Adult*, 8th edition. Philadelphia, Lippincott Williams & Wilkins, 2013, pp 1147–1158.

▶ Lai WW, Mertens LL, Cohen MS, et al (eds): *Echocardiography in Pediatric and Congenital Heart Disease: From Fetus to Adult*, 2nd edition. Chichester, UK, Wiley-Blackwell, 2016, pp 491–495.

ANSWERS

186. A. Complete heart block.

Patients with congenitally corrected transposition of the great arteries (ccTGA) are at risk for complete heart block, also known as complete atrioventricular (AV) block: 4% of all patients with ccTGA have complete heart block at birth, and up to 30% of patients will develop complete heart block at some point during their lifetimes.

▶ Allen HD, Driscoll DJ, Shaddy RE, et al: *Moss and Adams' Heart Disease in Infants, Children, and Adolescents: Including the Fetus and Young Adult*, 8th edition. Philadelphia, Lippincott Williams & Wilkins, 2013, p 1150.

187. A. Apical four-chamber view.

Following the Mustard atrial switch operation, the superior vena caval (SVC) limb of the intra-atrial baffle is the area most likely to become obstructed, and the apical four-chamber view (with clockwise rotation) provides the best visualization of the SVC pathway to the intra-atrial Mustard baffle. Furthermore, from this window there is a favorable angle of insonation for color and spectral Doppler evaluation of SVC inflow. With counterclockwise rotation of the probe, the inferior vena cava (IVC) can also be visualized, although the angle of insonation is not as favorable for Doppler evaluation. The other choices listed for this question—the suprasternal notch, apical five-chamber, and parasternal short-axis views—are not as useful for the evaluation of the SVC pathway in pediatric patients and offer even poorer views in adults.

▶ Armstrong WF, Ryan T: *Feigenbaum's Echocardiography*, 7th edition. Philadelphia, Lippincott Williams & Wilkins, 2010, pp 617–620.

188. D. Double switch procedure.

The Mustard procedure and Senning repair are both intra-atrial procedures that redirect systemic and pulmonary venous blood to the opposite ventricle. These operations were previously used as physiologic corrections for transposition of the great arteries (d-TGA). In the current era, d-TGA is palliated with an arterial switch operation. This surgery restores the great arteries to the anatomically appropriate ventricles; hence this operation is known as an anatomic correction for d-TGA. When there is congenitally corrected transposition of the great arteries (ccTGA), both an atrial switch (Mustard or Senning procedure) and an arterial switch procedure are performed at the same time so that the left ventricle can serve as the systemic ventricle and the right ventricle can serve as the subpulmonary ventricle. This procedure is called the double switch operation.

▸ Allen HD, Driscoll DJ, Shaddy RE, et al: *Moss and Adams' Heart Disease in Infants, Children, and Adolescents: Including the Fetus and Young Adult*, 8th edition. Philadelphia, Lippincott Williams & Wilkins, 2013, pp 1122–1134, 1157–1158.

▸ Lai WW, Mertens LL, Cohen MS, et al (eds): *Echocardiography in Pediatric and Congenital Heart Disease: From Fetus to Adult*, 2nd edition. Chichester, UK, Wiley-Blackwell, 2016, p 497.

189. C. Subxiphoid long-axis view.

In both the subxiphoid/subcostal long-axis/coronal view and the subxiphoid/subcostal short-axis/sagittal view, the ultrasound beam is perpendicular to the atrial septum, which can help the echocardiographer to avoid false dropout artifacts that can be present in other views, such as the apical four-chamber and parasternal short-axis views. When available and of high quality, the high right parasternal view can also visualize the atrial septum well. However, in this view the lungs can affect image quality due to the sound beam's different propagation speed when it moves from tissue through the air-filled lung.

▸ Lai WW, Mertens LL, Cohen MS, et al (eds): *Echocardiography in Pediatric and Congenital Heart Disease: From Fetus to Adult*, 2nd edition. Chichester, UK, Wiley-Blackwell, 2016, pp 46–48.

Refer to video PER-Q190.

190. C. Bidirectional shunt.

Video PER-Q190 is a subcostal long-axis view showing an atrial septal defect with bidirectional shunting: left to right (red color) and right to left (blue color).

191. D. Subxiphoid sagittal (short-axis) view.

The subxiphoid (subcostal) sagittal (short-axis) view allows for visualization of the entire atrial septum, particularly the portion of the atrial septum just inferior to the right pulmonary artery at the level of the superior vena cava (SVC)/right atrial junction, where the most common form of sinus venosus atrial septal defect (ASD) is found. This view is also useful for visualizing the atrial septum at the level of the inferior vena cava (IVC)/right atrial junction, where the uncommon inferior sinus venosus ASD can be found.

▸ Lai WW, Mertens LL, Cohen MS, et al (eds): *Echocardiography in Pediatric and Congenital Heart Disease: From Fetus to Adult*, 2nd edition. Chichester, UK, Wiley-Blackwell, 2016, p 205.

ANSWERS

Refer to video PER-Q192.

192. B. Partial anomalous pulmonary venous connection.

Video PER-Q192 demonstrates a superior sinus venosus atrial septal defect (ASD). 87% of patients with a superior sinus venosus ASD have partial anomalous pulmonary venous connection (PAPVC), the right upper (and sometimes middle) pulmonary vein draining into the superior vena cava and right atrium.

▶ Lai WW, Mertens LL, Cohen MS, et al (eds): *Echocardiography in Pediatric and Congenital Heart Disease: From Fetus to Adult*, 2nd edition. Chichester, UK, Wiley-Blackwell, 2016, pp 199–200.

▶ Van Praagh S, Carrera ME, Sanders SP, et al: Sinus venosus defects: unroofing of the right pulmonary veins—anatomic and echocardiographic findings and surgical treatment. Am Heart J 128:365–379, 1994.

193. A. Cleft mitral valve.

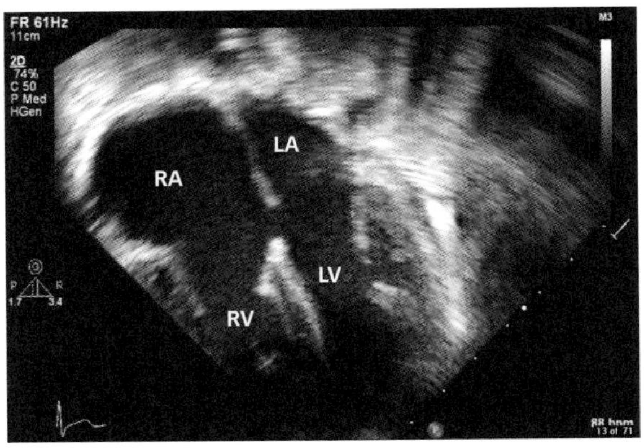

The image demonstrates an ostium primum atrial septal defect (ASD), which is also called a partial or incomplete atrioventricular canal defect (AVCD) or atrioventricular septal defect (AVSD). This type of defect is often accompanied by a cleft in the anterior leaflet of the left AV (mitral) valve. RA = right atrium, LA = left atrium, RV = right ventricle, LV = left ventricle.

▶ Allen HD, Driscoll DJ, Shaddy RE, et al: *Moss and Adams' Heart Disease in Infants, Children, and Adolescents: Including the Fetus and Young Adult*, 8th edition. Philadelphia, Lippincott Williams & Wilkins, 2013, pp 692, 1122–1134.

▶ Lai WW, Mertens LL, Cohen MS, et al (eds): *Echocardiography in Pediatric and Congenital Heart Disease: From Fetus to Adult*, 2nd edition. Chichester, UK, Wiley-Blackwell, 2016, p 262.

194. C. Right ventricle.

A moderate to large atrial septal defect (ASD) with an atrial left-to-right shunt causes volume overload of the right-sided chambers, leading to right atrial and right ventricular dilatation. The coronary sinus is not involved in this left-to-right shunt.

▶ Allen HD, Driscoll DJ, Shaddy RE, et al: *Moss and Adams' Heart Disease in Infants, Children, and Adolescents: Including the Fetus and Young Adult*, 8th edition. Philadelphia, Lippincott Williams & Wilkins, 2013, p 676.

195. B. Sinus venosus ASD.

Because 87%–90% of sinus venosus atrial septal defects (ASDs) also have partial anomalous right pulmonary venous drainage, device closure of the ASD in the catheterization laboratory would not be indicated. If a device closure is attempted, the anomalous right pulmonary venous drainage would not be addressed. Furthermore, sinus venosus ASDs typically have no superior rim on which to anchor a device. Therefore, surgical repair is indicated for this type of defect. A secundum ASD or patent foramen ovale is routinely closed in the catheterization laboratory. Some perimembranous VSDs can be closed in the catheterization laboratory, while others might still require referral for surgery.

- Allen HD, Shaddy RE, Penny DJ, et al: *Moss and Adams' Heart Disease in Infants, Children, and Adolescents, Including the Fetus and Young Adult*, 9th edition. Philadelphia, Wolters Kluwer, 2016, p 894.
- Wong PC, Miller-Hance WC (eds): *Transesophageal Echocardiography for Congenital Heart Disease*, London, Springer-Verlag, 2014, pp 438–442.

196. A. Dilated right atrium and right ventricle due to volume overload.

When a patient has a large atrial septal defect, the right side of the heart is dilated due to volume overload from a significant left-to-right shunt. This volume overload causes ventricular septal flattening during diastole. A 5-year-old would not be expected to have pulmonary hypertension from an isolated atrial shunt (septal flattening in systole or septal bowing into the left ventricle during systole).

- Allen HD, Driscoll DJ, Shaddy RE, et al: *Moss and Adams' Heart Disease in Infants, Children, and Adolescents: Including the Fetus and Young Adult*, 8th edition. Philadelphia, Lippincott Williams & Wilkins, 2013, p 678.

197. A. Posterior muscular VSD.

With a parasternal short-axis sweep of the left ventricle, a muscular ventricular septal defect (VSD) seen between 7 and 10 o'clock represents a posterior muscular VSD. Mid-muscular VSDs are located between 10 and 12 o'clock, and anterior muscular VSDs are seen between 12 and 2 o'clock. An apical muscular VSD is not visualized at the mid-left ventricular level.

- Lai WW, Mertens LL, Cohen MS, et al (eds): *Echocardiography in Pediatric and Congenital Heart Disease: From Fetus to Adult*, 2nd edition. Chichester, UK, Wiley-Blackwell, 2016, p 224.

Refer to video PER-Q198.

198. C. Anterior muscular VSD.

Video PER-Q198 is from the parasternal short-axis view. See the answer to question 197.

▶ Lai WW, Mertens LL, Cohen MS, et al (eds): *Echocardiography in Pediatric and Congenital Heart Disease: From Fetus to Adult*, 2nd edition. Chichester, UK, Wiley-Blackwell, 2016, p 224.

Refer to video PER-Q199.

199. D. Supracristal VSD.

Video PER-Q199 demonstrates a ventricular septal defect (VSD) directly below both the aortic and pulmonary valves; this type of defect is called a supracristal VSD. Other names used to describe this defect are "outlet VSD," "conal septal VSD," and "doubly committed subarterial VSD." Supracristal VSDs are often seen in the Asian population; they are also highly associated with aortic valve prolapse. Usually a supracristal VSD is located between the 12 and 2 o'clock positions when viewed from the parasternal short-axis view at the level of the aortic valve.

▶ Lai WW, Mertens LL, Cohen MS, et al (eds): *Echocardiography in Pediatric and Congenital Heart Disease: From Fetus to Adult*, 2nd edition. Chichester, UK, Wiley-Blackwell, 2016, p 219.

200. B. Atrioventricular canal type VSD.

With an atrioventricular canal type of ventricular septal defect (VSD), the mitral valve generally has a cleft. The other options—perimembranous VSD, outlet VSD, and supracristal VSD—are not associated with a mitral valve cleft.

▶ Lai WW, Mertens LL, Cohen MS, et al (eds): *Echocardiography in Pediatric and Congenital Heart Disease: From Fetus to Adult*, 2nd edition. Chichester, UK, Wiley-Blackwell, 2016, pp 260–264.

Refer to video PER-Q201.

201. A. Inlet VSD.

Video PER-Q201 demonstrates a defect between the mitral valve and the tricuspid valve, and both valves are seen at the same level. While the defect extends into the posterior muscular septum, there is no muscular rim between the defect and the atrioventricular valves. Usually this type of defect is called an inlet ventricular septal defect (VSD) or atrioventricular canal VSD, and it is strongly associated with a cleft mitral valve.

▶ Lai WW, Mertens LL, Cohen MS, et al (eds): *Echocardiography in Pediatric and Congenital Heart Disease: From Fetus to Adult*, 2nd edition. Chichester, UK, Wiley-Blackwell, 2016, pp 219–220, 225–226.

202. A. Doubly committed VSD.

A doubly committed ventricular septal defect (VSD) is also known as a supracristal or subpulmonary VSD, with an absent conal septum between the aortic and pulmonary valves, leading to fibrous continuity of the two semilunar valves. Without conal septal support, the right coronary cusp of the aortic valve can prolapse through the defect, and this can result in aortic valve regurgitation.

▶ Lai WW, Mertens LL, Cohen MS, et al (eds): *Echocardiography in Pediatric and Congenital Heart Disease: From Fetus to Adult*, 2nd edition. Chichester, UK, Wiley-Blackwell, 2016, p 219.

203. B. Aortic valve regurgitation.

See the answer to question 202.

▶ Lai WW, Mertens LL, Cohen MS, et al (eds): *Echocardiography in Pediatric and Congenital Heart Disease: From Fetus to Adult*, 2nd edition. Chichester, UK, Wiley-Blackwell, 2016, p 219.

204. B. Double-chambered right ventricle.

In 60%–90% of cases of double-chambered right ventricle, there is an associated ventricular septal defect (VSD), generally perimembranous. With a perimembranous VSD, anomalous muscle bundles in the right ventricle divide the chamber into two parts, with the VSD usually connected to the proximal chamber. Because the proximal chamber of the right ventricle has higher pressure due to the hypertrophied muscular bundles, it limits the left-to-right shunt and the velocity across the VSD is lower than might otherwise be expected. The subxiphoid (subcostal) views are very useful for diagnosing this type of cardiac defect.

▶ Allen HD, Driscoll DJ, Shaddy RE, et al: *Moss and Adams' Heart Disease in Infants, Children, and Adolescents: Including the Fetus and Young Adult*, 8th edition. Philadelphia, Lippincott Williams & Wilkins, 2013, pp 925–927.

205. C. Right upper pulmonary vein.

When a sinus venosus atrial septal defect (ASD) is associated with anomalous pulmonary venous return, the pulmonary vein involved most frequently (in 87% of cases) is the right upper pulmonary vein draining into the superior vena cava (SVC). The right middle pulmonary vein can also be involved. Rarely, the right lower pulmonary vein will drain anomalously.

▶ Lai WW, Mertens LL, Cohen MS, et al (eds): *Echocardiography in Pediatric and Congenital Heart Disease: From Fetus to Adult*, 2nd edition. Chichester, UK, Wiley-Blackwell, 2016, pp 204–206.

206. B. Rastelli B.

In the Rastelli classification, there are three common types of atrioventricular canal defects (AVCDs, also called atrioventricular septal defects or AVSDs): Rastelli types A, B, and C. See the answer to question 151. There is no Rastelli type D.

▶ Ezon DS, Goldberg JF, Kyle WB: *Atlas of Congenital Heart Disease Nomenclature: An Illustrated Guide to the Van Praagh and Anderson Approaches to Describing Congenital Cardiac Pathology*. Houston, Ezon Educational Services/CreateSpace, 2015, p 62.

▶ Lai WW, Mertens LL, Cohen MS, et al (eds): *Echocardiography in Pediatric and Congenital Heart Disease: From Fetus to Adult*, 2nd edition. Chichester, UK, Wiley-Blackwell, 2016, pp 262–263.

207. C. Partial AVCD.

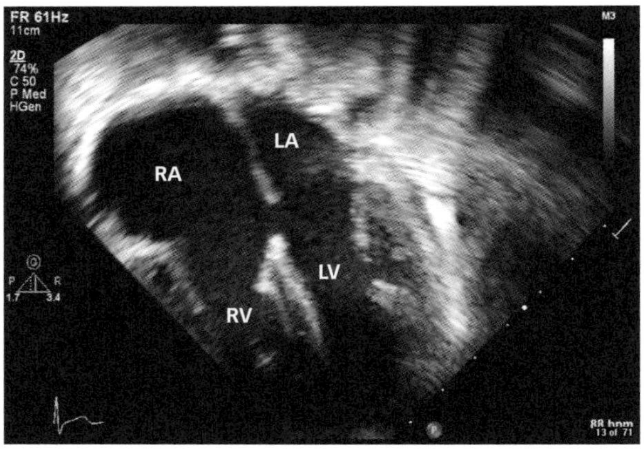

A complete atrioventricular canal defect (AVCD, also known as an atrioventricular septal defect or AVSD) has a common AV valve, along with an ostium primum type of atrial septal defect (ASD) and a large inlet (AV canal) ventricular septal defect (VSD). An incomplete or partial AVCD has only an ostium primum type of ASD with no VSD, and there is also a cleft mitral valve. A transitional AVCD has an ostium primum type of ASD and an AV canal VSD, but the VSD is small, with AV valve chordae attached to the crest of the ventricular septum. A dilated coronary sinus would be visualized more posteriorly and inferiorly, and often the AV valves will not be seen in the same plane. RA = right atrium, LA = left atrium, RV = right ventricle, LV = left ventricle.

▶ Ezon DS, Goldberg JF, Kyle WB: *Atlas of Congenital Heart Disease Nomenclature: An Illustrated Guide to the Van Praagh and Anderson Approaches to Describing Congenital Cardiac Pathology*. Houston, Ezon Educational Services/CreateSpace, 2015, p 63.

▶ Lai WW, Mertens LL, Cohen MS, et al (eds): *Echocardiography in Pediatric and Congenital Heart Disease: From Fetus to Adult*, 2nd edition. Chichester, UK, Wiley-Blackwell, 2016, pp 262–264.

208. D. 5.

▸ Lai WW, Mertens LL, Cohen MS, et al (eds): *Echocardiography in Pediatric and Congenital Heart Disease: From Fetus to Adult*, 2nd edition. Chichester, UK, Wiley-Blackwell, 2016, p 263.

209. B. Rotated counterclockwise.

In an atrioventricular canal defect (AVCD, also known as an atrioventricular septal defect or AVSD), the papillary muscles are rotated counterclockwise as compared to the papillary muscles in a normal heart.

▸ Allen HD, Driscoll DJ, Shaddy RE, et al: *Moss and Adams' Heart Disease in Infants, Children, and Adolescents: Including the Fetus and Young Adult*, 8th edition. Philadelphia, Lippincott Williams & Wilkins, 2013, p 692.

210. D. Left ventricular outflow tract obstruction.

An atrioventricular canal defect (AVCD, also called an atrioventricular septal defect or AVSD) often has an elongated left ventricular outflow tract (LVOT), also known as a "gooseneck deformity." In addition, abnormal AV valve chordal attachments and an abnormal left ventricular papillary muscle rotation can lead to LVOT obstruction before or after surgical repair.

▸ Allen HD, Driscoll DJ, Shaddy RE, et al: *Moss and Adams' Heart Disease in Infants, Children, and Adolescents: Including the Fetus and Young Adult*, 8th edition. Philadelphia, Lippincott Williams & Wilkins, 2013, pp 693–698.

211. A. Vertical vein.

This scenario describes obstructed total anomalous pulmonary venous connection (TAPVC) with a "vertical vein" coursing superiorly to the innominate (brachiocephalic) vein. Pulmonary venous connectors from a pulmonary vein confluence to a systemic vein run vertically but can also run in a left-right direction, such as TAPVC with a left-sided pulmonary vein confluence that drains into a right superior vena cava. The current scenario is of particular importance because the vertical vein courses posterior to the left pulmonary artery (LPA) and anterior to the left mainstem bronchus, and is considered a "hemodynamic vise"; obstruction of the vertical vein occurs due to the compression between the LPA and left mainstem bronchus. The phrenic and axillary veins would generally be too distant in this scenario to be correct choices. In most humans the azygos vein usually drains posteriorly into a right superior vena cava.

▸ Allen HD, Driscoll DJ, Shaddy RE, et al: *Moss and Adams' Heart Disease in Infants, Children, and Adolescents: Including the Fetus and Young Adult*, 8th edition. Philadelphia, Lippincott Williams & Wilkins, 2013, pp 824–825.

▸ Lai WW, Mertens LL, Cohen MS, et al (eds): *Echocardiography in Pediatric and Congenital Heart Disease: From Fetus to Adult*, 2nd edition. Chichester, UK, Wiley-Blackwell, 2016, p 182.

212. C. Supracardiac.

Studies have shown that the supracardiac type of total anomalous pulmonary venous connection (TAPVC) is most common (occurring in approximately 50% of cases), and mixed TAPVC is the least common.

▸ Lai WW, Mertens LL, Cohen MS, et al (eds): *Echocardiography in Pediatric and Congenital Heart Disease: From Fetus to Adult*, 2nd edition. Chichester, UK, Wiley-Blackwell, 2016, p 160.

213. A. Supracardiac total anomalous pulmonary venous connection.

With the usual type of supracardiac total anomalous pulmonary venous connection (supracardiac TAPVC), there is a significant amount of pulmonary venous blood flow returning into either the innominate (brachiocephalic) vein or the superior vena cava (SVC). This results in an excess of flow in the SVC returning to the right atrium. The SVC usually appears dilated, with a very prominent color Doppler signal. None of the other options produces excessive SVC return.

▸ Lai WW, Mertens LL, Cohen MS, et al (eds): *Echocardiography in Pediatric and Congenital Heart Disease: From Fetus to Adult*, 2nd edition. Chichester, UK, Wiley-Blackwell, 2016, pp 160–163.

Refer to video PER-Q214.

214. C. Vertical vein.

No known normal structure courses between the inferior vena cava (IVC) and the abdominal aorta. When one is present, the likelihood of the structure being a vertical vein in the presence of infradiaphragmatic total anomalous pulmonary venous connection (TAPVC) is high. In order to help diagnose this form of TAPVC, a sweep between the IVC and aorta should be performed with two-dimensional (2D) imaging and then with color flow Doppler to identify venous flow draining away from the heart via a vertical vein draining into the portal vein, inferior vena cava, or hepatic veins.

▸ Allen HD, Driscoll DJ, Shaddy RE, et al: *Moss and Adams' Heart Disease in Infants, Children, and Adolescents: Including the Fetus and Young Adult*, 8th edition. Philadelphia, Lippincott Williams & Wilkins, 2013, p 826.

▸ Lai WW, Mertens LL, Cohen MS, et al (eds): *Echocardiography in Pediatric and Congenital Heart Disease: From Fetus to Adult*, 2nd edition. Chichester, UK, Wiley-Blackwell, 2016, pp 173, 182–187.

▸ Zwiebel WJ, Pellerito JS: *Introduction to Vascular Ultrasonography*, 5th edition. Philadelphia, Saunders, 2005, p 591.

Refer to video PER-Q215.

215. B. Intracardiac total anomalous pulmonary venous drainage.

Video PER-Q215 demonstrates leftward malalignment of the atrial septum, leaving all of the pulmonary veins returning to the right of the atrial septum. This is considered total anomalous pulmonary venous drainage of the cardiac type. The term "drainage" is used instead of "connection" in this scenario because the common pulmonary vein connected and then incorporated itself into the posterior aspect of the left atrium, making the "connection" normal. However, the malalignment of the atrial septum results in the pulmonary veins draining abnormally into the right atrium.

▶ Allen HD, Driscoll DJ, Shaddy RE, et al: *Moss and Adams' Heart Disease in Infants, Children, and Adolescents: Including the Fetus and Young Adult*, 8th edition. Philadelphia, Lippincott Williams & Wilkins, 2013, pp 809–815.

216. B. Failure of the common pulmonary vein–left atrial connection.

Failure of the common pulmonary vein to connect and incorporate into the posterior aspect of the left atrium (which then enables pulmonary venous return to the left atrium) is the process that leads to total anomalous pulmonary venous connection (TAPVC).

▶ Allen HD, Driscoll DJ, Shaddy RE, et al: *Moss and Adams' Heart Disease in Infants, Children, and Adolescents: Including the Fetus and Young Adult*, 8th edition. Philadelphia, Lippincott Williams & Wilkins, 2013, pp 810–812.

217. D. Intracardiac TAPVC.

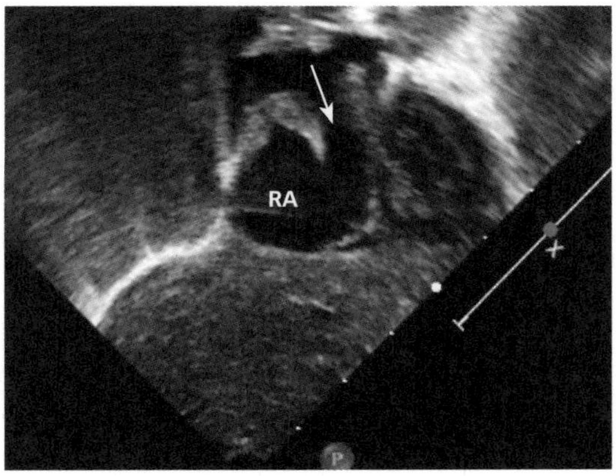

This image most accurately demonstrates TAPVC to the coronary sinus (arrow). The echocardiography community has described this view as having the appearance of a "whale's tale." Other reasons that a coronary sinus can be dilated include, but are not limited to, partial anomalous pulmonary

ANSWERS

venous connection, hepatic venous drainage to the coronary sinus, and left superior vena cava to the coronary sinus. RA = right atrium.

▶ Allen HD, Driscoll DJ, Shaddy RE, et al: *Moss and Adams' Heart Disease in Infants, Children, and Adolescents: Including the Fetus and Young Adult*, 8th edition. Philadelphia, Lippincott Williams & Wilkins, 2013, p 818.

▶ Lai WW, Mertens LL, Cohen MS, et al (eds): *Echocardiography in Pediatric and Congenital Heart Disease: From Fetus to Adult*, 2nd edition. Chichester, UK, Wiley-Blackwell, 2016, pp 172, 182–183, 190.

Refer to video PER-Q218.

218. C. Supracardiac total anomalous pulmonary venous connection.

Video PER-Q218 most accurately depicts supracardiac total anomalous pulmonary venous connection (TAPVC). Supracardiac TAPVC is the most common type of TAPVC, and it is seen with an atrial septal defect with right-to-left atrial shunting, which is essential to sustain life. Right heart dilatation, interventricular septal flattening, systemic arterial desaturation, and increased blood flow in the superior vena cava and innominate (brachiocephalic) vein are clues to the type of TAPVC, supracardiac. The subcostal and apical views are also important in the evaluation of this form of congenital heart disease.

▶ Allen HD, Driscoll DJ, Shaddy RE, et al: *Moss and Adams' Heart Disease in Infants, Children, and Adolescents: Including the Fetus and Young Adult*, 8th edition. Philadelphia, Lippincott Williams & Wilkins, 2013, p 825.

▶ Lai WW, Mertens LL, Cohen MS, et al (eds): *Echocardiography in Pediatric and Congenital Heart Disease: From Fetus to Adult*, 2nd edition. Chichester, UK, Wiley-Blackwell, 2016, pp 160–164.

219. A. Partial anomalous pulmonary venous connection.

Although dilatation and increased flow in the superior vena cava (SVC) can be signs of total anomalous pulmonary venous connection (TAPVC), a left-to-right atrial-level shunt excludes this abnormality. In TAPVC, shunting is from the morphologic right atrium to the morphologic left atrium. Left-to-right shunting and bidirectional shunting can be seen in a partial anomalous pulmonary venous connection (PAPVC). A left SVC shunting to the coronary sinus or a left SVC shunting directly to the left atrium does not generally cause dilatation of the right SVC.

▶ Allen HD, Driscoll DJ, Shaddy RE, et al: *Moss and Adams' Heart Disease in Infants, Children, and Adolescents: Including the Fetus and Young Adult*, 8th edition. Philadelphia, Lippincott Williams & Wilkins, 2013, p 827.

▶ Lai WW, Mertens LL, Cohen MS, et al (eds): *Echocardiography in Pediatric and Congenital Heart Disease: From Fetus to Adult*, 2nd edition. Chichester, UK, Wiley-Blackwell, 2016, pp 160, 182–183.

220. B. The vein is obstructed.

The likelihood that this vertical vein is obstructed is high and is due to compression from the passage of the vertical vein between the left pulmonary artery and the left mainstem bronchus. Careful sweeps using the parasternal short-axis views can help confirm this type of obstruction.

▶ Allen HD, Driscoll DJ, Shaddy RE, et al: *Moss and Adams' Heart Disease in Infants, Children, and Adolescents: Including the Fetus and Young Adult*, 8th edition. Philadelphia, Lippincott Williams & Wilkins, 2013, pp 825–829.

▶ Lai WW, Mertens LL, Cohen MS, et al (eds): *Echocardiography in Pediatric and Congenital Heart Disease: From Fetus to Adult*, 2nd edition. Chichester, UK, Wiley-Blackwell, 2016, p 160.

▶ Park MK: *Park's Pediatric Cardiology for Practitioners*, 6th edition. Philadelphia, Saunders, 2014, p 241.

ANSWERS

221. C. Left ventricular enlargement.

Care must be taken when answering this question. Partial anomalous pulmonary venous connection (PAPVC) can occur with and without an atrial septal defect. Right ventricular enlargement often occurs when the pulmonary veins drain to a systemic vein because the physiology is that of the left-to-right shunt, causing volume overload to the right heart. PAPVC would not be expected to cause left ventricular enlargement.

▶ Allen HD, Driscoll DJ, Shaddy RE, et al: *Moss and Adams' Heart Disease in Infants, Children, and Adolescents: Including the Fetus and Young Adult*, 8th edition. Philadelphia, Lippincott Williams & Wilkins, 2013, p 818.

▶ Park MK: *Park's Pediatric Cardiology for Practitioners*, 6th edition. Philadelphia, Saunders, 2014, pp 124–125.

222. D. Right lung hypoplasia.

The findings of heart dextroposition, no atrial-level shunting, right pulmonary veins to the inferior vena cava, and a small right pulmonary artery are consistent with Scimitar syndrome, in which there is associated right lung hypoplasia. The shift in the heart mass to the right, with the apex still pointing leftward, is caused by the hypoplastic right lung.

▶ Allen HD, Driscoll DJ, Shaddy RE, et al: *Moss and Adams' Heart Disease in Infants, Children, and Adolescents: Including the Fetus and Young Adult*, 8th edition. Philadelphia, Lippincott Williams & Wilkins, 2013, pp 817–821.

223. D. Diminished phasic flow.

See Color Plate 9 on page xxiii.

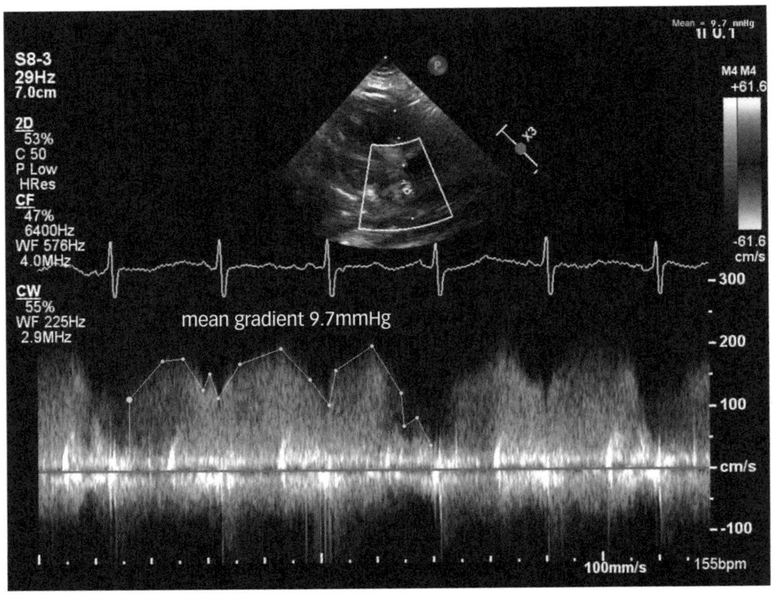

The spectral Doppler waveform demonstrates pulmonary vein stenosis. Upon inspection of the Doppler tracing, a few things stand out: loss of normal phasic laminar pulmonary vein flow, an essentially nonexistent retrograde A wave, and an increase in the mean pressure gradient.

▶ Lai WW, Mertens LL, Cohen MS, et al (eds): *Echocardiography in Pediatric and Congenital Heart Disease: From Fetus to Adult*, 2nd edition. Chichester, UK, Wiley-Blackwell, 2016, pp 164–165.

224. A. Biatrial enlargement.

Right atrial, right ventricular, and main pulmonary artery enlargement can be signs of pulmonary vein stenosis due to pulmonary hypertension. Left atrial enlargement is not normally associated with pulmonary vein stenosis because the obstruction is proximal to the left atrium. Left atrial enlargement is more likely to be seen with mitral valve regurgitation and/or mitral valve stenosis. Of the options given, biatrial enlargement is least likely to be associated with pulmonary vein stenosis.

▶ Lai WW, Mertens LL, Cohen MS, et al (eds): *Echocardiography in Pediatric and Congenital Heart Disease: From Fetus to Adult*, 2nd edition. Chichester, UK, Wiley-Blackwell, 2016, pp 165, 243–255.

▶ Park MK: *Park's Pediatric Cardiology for Practitioners*, 6th edition. Philadelphia, Saunders, 2014, pp 376–380.

225. C. Left ventricular anterolateral papillary muscle.

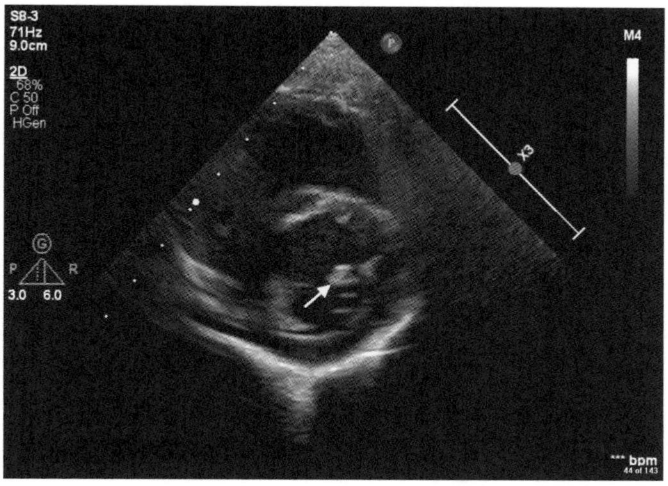

This parasternal short-axis image demonstrates the anterolateral papillary muscle (arrow) located at approximately 3 o'clock. The posteromedial papillary muscle is located at approximately 7 o'clock in this image.

▸ Lai WW, Mertens LL, Cohen MS, et al (eds): *Echocardiography in Pediatric and Congenital Heart Disease: From Fetus to Adult*, 2nd edition. Chichester, UK, Wiley-Blackwell, 2016, p 52.

226. C. Parachute mitral valve.

The findings are consistent with parachute mitral valve and can be visualized in your subcostal short-axis, parasternal short-axis, apical two-chamber, and apical four-chamber views. In Ebstein anomaly of the tricuspid valve, the posterior and septal leaflets of the tricuspid valve do not delaminate and the orifice of the valve is displaced apically. A double orifice mitral valve is characterized by two mitral valve openings, and a straddling mitral valve is seen in association with a ventricular septal defect, generally with mitral chordae tendineae crossing into the right ventricle.

▸ Allen HD, Driscoll DJ, Shaddy RE, et al: *Moss and Adams' Heart Disease in Infants, Children, and Adolescents: Including the Fetus and Young Adult*, 8th edition. Philadelphia, Lippincott Williams & Wilkins, 2013, pp 1010–1011.

▸ Lai WW, Mertens LL, Cohen MS, et al (eds): *Echocardiography in Pediatric and Congenital Heart Disease: From Fetus to Adult*, 2nd edition. Chichester, UK, Wiley-Blackwell, 2016, pp 66–68.

227. A. Chordae tendineae tethering.

The findings of chordae tendineae tethering are consistent with parachute mitral valve. Choices B (infundibulum) and D (chordal attachments of the atrioventricular valve to the interventricular septum) are associated with a morphologic right ventricle, not a morphologic left ventricle.

▶ Allen HD, Driscoll DJ, Shaddy RE, et al: *Moss and Adams' Heart Disease in Infants, Children, and Adolescents: Including the Fetus and Young Adult*, 8th edition. Philadelphia, Lippincott Williams & Wilkins, 2013, pp 1006–1010.

▶ Lai WW, Mertens LL, Cohen MS, et al (eds): *Echocardiography in Pediatric and Congenital Heart Disease: From Fetus to Adult*, 2nd edition. Chichester, UK, Wiley-Blackwell, 2016, pp 37–38, 246–247.

228. B. Mitral valve with redundant leaflets and a thickened appearance.

The myxomatous appearance of a mitral valve leaflet is usually characterized by leaflet rolling, thickened mitral valve leaflets, and a degree of incompetence. The histologic findings of a myxomatous mitral valve are different from those of normal mitral valve tissue, making choices A and C incorrect.

▶ Allen HD, Driscoll DJ, Shaddy RE, et al: *Moss and Adams' Heart Disease in Infants, Children, and Adolescents: Including the Fetus and Young Adult*, 8th edition. Philadelphia, Lippincott Williams & Wilkins, 2013, p 1017.

▶ Lai WW, Mertens LL, Cohen MS, et al (eds): *Echocardiography in Pediatric and Congenital Heart Disease: From Fetus to Adult*, 2nd edition. Chichester, UK, Wiley-Blackwell, 2016, p 243.

▶ Park MK: *Park's Pediatric Cardiology for Practitioners*, 6th edition. Philadelphia, Saunders, 2014, pp 383–385.

229. D. A possible finding with no other cardiac defects.

An isolated mitral valve cleft is a potential finding, especially when the location is in the anterior mitral valve leaflet. It can occur in the absence of an ostium primum defect and inlet ventricular septal defect. Although cleft mitral valves may exhibit incompetence (regurgitation), they can also be completely competent. Color flow Doppler is helpful in evaluating for regurgitation.

▶ Allen HD, Driscoll DJ, Shaddy RE, et al: *Moss and Adams' Heart Disease in Infants, Children, and Adolescents: Including the Fetus and Young Adult*, 8th edition. Philadelphia, Lippincott Williams & Wilkins, 2013, pp 1009–1011.

▶ Lai WW, Mertens LL, Cohen MS, et al (eds): *Echocardiography in Pediatric and Congenital Heart Disease: From Fetus to Adult*, 2nd edition. Chichester, UK, Wiley-Blackwell, 2016, p 245.

230. B. A ridge of tissue subdividing the left atrium that is located above the left atrial appendage.

Cor triatriatum is caused by incomplete incorporation of the common pulmonary vein into the left atrium, resulting in a ridge of tissue (with one or more openings) that separates the pulmonary vein segment of the left atrium from the embryonic left atrium (the left atrial appendage). Cor triatriatum is different from a supramitral valve ring (a membrane superior to the mitral valve) in regard to the position of the left atrial appendage in relation to the ridge of tissue: In cor triatriatum, the ridge of tissue lies above the appendage, while in supramitral ring the membrane lies below the appendage.

- Allen HD, Driscoll DJ, Shaddy RE, et al: *Moss and Adams' Heart Disease in Infants, Children, and Adolescents: Including the Fetus and Young Adult*, 8th edition. Philadelphia, Lippincott Williams & Wilkins, 2013, pp 833–836, 1008.
- Lai WW, Mertens LL, Cohen MS, et al (eds): *Echocardiography in Pediatric and Congenital Heart Disease: From Fetus to Adult*, 2nd edition. Chichester, UK, Wiley-Blackwell, 2016, p 250.

231. A. Ventricular septal defect.

A ventricular septal defect (VSD) is needed for a mitral valve to straddle. Straddling mitral valves can be seen with conotruncal abnormalities like double-outlet right ventricle and transposition of the great arteries (d-TGA) with a VSD.

- Lai WW, Mertens LL, Cohen MS, et al (eds): *Echocardiography in Pediatric and Congenital Heart Disease: From Fetus to Adult*, 2nd edition. Chichester, UK, Wiley-Blackwell, 2016, pp 245–246, 468.

232. C. Increased pulmonary vascular resistance and a PDA.

In the setting described in the question, the severity of pulmonary stenosis does not accurately correlate with the velocity. A pulmonary valve velocity of 1.8 m/sec is at the upper limit of normal and, taken by itself, would not suggest a significant pressure gradient across the pulmonary valve that would indicate valvular stenosis. However, the low transvalvular Doppler velocity can be misleading in a setting of elevated main pulmonary artery pressure, which can be produced by a moderate-sized patent ductus arteriosus (PDA) and/or elevated pulmonary vascular resistance. In the current question, a unicuspid, hypoplastic pulmonary valve is usually associated with stenosis, but in the presence of increased pulmonary vascular resistance (i.e., the newborn setting) and a PDA, the severity of stenosis can be underestimated by spectral Doppler.

▶ Lai WW, Mertens LL, Cohen MS, et al (eds): *Echocardiography in Pediatric and Congenital Heart Disease: From Fetus to Adult*, 2nd edition. Chichester, UK, Wiley-Blackwell, 2016, pp 281–287.

▶ Park MK: *Park's Pediatric Cardiology for Practitioners*, 6th edition. Philadelphia, Saunders, 2014, pp 119–123, 184–187.

Refer to video PER-Q233.

233. B. Anteriorly malaligned VSD.

Video PER-Q233 is of a patient with tetralogy of Fallot with an anteriorly malaligned ventricular septal defect (VSD), which is most often associated with some degree of pulmonary stenosis. Note that a posteriorly malaligned VSD (choice A) in normally related great vessels is usually associated with aortic obstruction. Mid-muscular VSDs (choice C) and apical VSDs (choice D) are not typically associated with the pulmonary valve stenosis seen in this video clip.

▶ Lai WW, Mertens LL, Cohen MS, et al (eds): *Echocardiography in Pediatric and Congenital Heart Disease: From Fetus to Adult*, 2nd edition. Chichester, UK, Wiley-Blackwell, 2016, pp 337–338, 408–409.

234. D. Depressed right ventricular systolic function.

A reduction in right ventricular function can depress the pulmonary gradient, leading to an underestimation of pulmonary stenosis severity and explaining why the gradient is only 15 mmHg.

▶ Lai WW, Mertens LL, Cohen MS, et al (eds): *Echocardiography in Pediatric and Congenital Heart Disease: From Fetus to Adult*, 2nd edition. Chichester, UK, Wiley-Blackwell, 2016, p 285.

▶ Park MK: *Park's Pediatric Cardiology for Practitioners*, 6th edition. Philadelphia, Saunders, 2014, pp 119–123, 186.

Refer to video PER-Q235.

235. A. Dome-shaped PV.

Video PER-Q235 demonstrates doming of the pulmonary valve leaflets. Note the shape of the leaflets during systole as they reach to the sinotubular junction but do not open fully, producing the domed appearance. The number of leaflets cannot be seen in this clip, so choices B (bicuspid pulmonary valve), C (normal pulmonary valve), and D (trileaflet pulmonary valve) are incorrect. Note that a normal pulmonary valve typically has three leaflets.

▶ Lai WW, Mertens LL, Cohen MS, et al (eds): *Echocardiography in Pediatric and Congenital Heart Disease: From Fetus to Adult*, 2nd edition. Chichester, UK, Wiley-Blackwell, 2016, pp 281–282.

236. C. Severe pulmonary valve insufficiency.

Flow reversal in the branch pulmonary arteries is a marker for severe pulmonary regurgitation, not stenosis. Tetralogy of Fallot repairs and tetralogy of Fallot with absent pulmonary valve syndrome are examples of situations in which one might encounter flow reversal in the branch pulmonary arteries in the setting of severe pulmonary regurgitation.

▶ Lai WW, Mertens LL, Cohen MS, et al (eds): *Echocardiography in Pediatric and Congenital Heart Disease: From Fetus to Adult*, 2nd edition. Chichester, UK, Wiley-Blackwell, 2016, pp 286, 422, 425.

Refer to video PER-Q237.

237. D. Tetralogy of Fallot with absent pulmonary valve syndrome.

Video PER-Q237 reveals the underdeveloped and "nubbin-like" appearance of the pulmonary valve in tetralogy of Fallot with absent pulmonary valve syndrome. Note the almost unguarded pulmonary valve orifice. The clip demonstrates significant pulmonary regurgitation that leads to right ventricular enlargement.

▶ Allen HD, Driscoll DJ, Shaddy RE, et al: *Moss and Adams' Heart Disease in Infants, Children, and Adolescents: Including the Fetus and Young Adult*, 8th edition. Philadelphia, Lippincott Williams & Wilkins, 2013, pp 974–976.

▶ Lai WW, Mertens LL, Cohen MS, et al (eds): *Echocardiography in Pediatric and Congenital Heart Disease: From Fetus to Adult*, 2nd edition. Chichester, UK, Wiley-Blackwell, 2016, p 425.

238. C. Absorption of the subaortic conus.

Anteriorly malaligned ventricular septal defect (VSD), double-chambered right ventricle (DCRV), and perimembranous VSD can be associated with subpulmonic stenosis. Anteriorly malaligned VSD can cause subpulmonary stenosis, as seen in tetralogy of Fallot. A perimembranous VSD is often associated with DCRV, which is a type of subpulmonary stenosis. Incomplete incorporation of the bulbus cordis into the right ventricle is considered to be the mechanism that causes DCRV. Absorption of the subaortic conus is a normal process in heart development and does not contribute to subpulmonary stenosis.

▶ Allen HD, Driscoll DJ, Shaddy RE, et al: *Moss and Adams' Heart Disease in Infants, Children, and Adolescents: Including the Fetus and Young Adult*, 8th edition. Philadelphia, Lippincott Williams & Wilkins, 2013, pp 150–152, 925–926.

▶ Lai WW, Mertens LL, Cohen MS, et al (eds): *Echocardiography in Pediatric and Congenital Heart Disease: From Fetus to Adult*, 2nd edition. Chichester, UK, Wiley-Blackwell, 2016, pp 38, 287–288, 337, 641–643.

239. D. Subcostal short-axis with angulation toward the right ventricular outflow tract/pulmonary valve.

The subpulmonic region is not well visualized using the parasternal long-axis and short-axis views at the levels indicated in choices A and C. Using the apical four-chamber view with superior and anterior angulation toward the pulmonary valve (choice B), the area immediately below the pulmonary valve is visualized and discrete membranes can be evaluated, but the infundibulum is not seen throughout its course to evaluate the anomalous muscle bundles that can cause the type of subpulmonic stenosis found in double-chambered right ventricle (DCRV). DCRV is best visualized with the subcostal short-axis view with angulation toward the right ventricular outflow tract. Another echocardiographic view to evaluate the subpulmonic region is the subcostal long axis with focus on the infundibulum (or conus arteriosus).

▶ Lai WW, Mertens LL, Cohen MS, et al (eds): *Echocardiography in Pediatric and Congenital Heart Disease: From Fetus to Adult*, 2nd edition. Chichester, UK, Wiley-Blackwell, 2016, pp 46–48, 287–289.

240. C. Between the sinus and infundibulum segments of the right ventricle.

Double-chambered right ventricle (DCRV) is division of the sinus and infundibular portions of the right ventricle. Note that the terms "conus arteriosus" and "infundibulum" are used interchangeably.

▶ Lai WW, Mertens LL, Cohen MS, et al (eds): *Echocardiography in Pediatric and Congenital Heart Disease: From Fetus to Adult*, 2nd edition. Chichester, UK, Wiley-Blackwell, 2016, pp 37–38, 287–288.

241. A. Right ventricular sinus.

The higher-pressure chamber in double-chambered right ventricle (DCRV) is the right ventricular sinus and the infundibulum (or conus arteriosus) is the lower-pressure chamber. The main pulmonary artery is continuous with the infundibular portion of the right ventricle and should have similar systolic pressure.

▶ Lai WW, Mertens LL, Cohen MS, et al (eds): *Echocardiography in Pediatric and Congenital Heart Disease: From Fetus to Adult*, 2nd edition. Chichester, UK, Wiley-Blackwell, 2016, pp 37, 288.

242. C. Perimembranous VSD.

Although double-chambered right ventricle (DCRV) has associations with both muscular and malalignment ventricular septal defects (VSDs), DCRV is most often seen with the perimembranous type of VSD.

- Allen HD, Driscoll DJ, Shaddy RE, et al: *Moss and Adams' Heart Disease in Infants, Children, and Adolescents: Including the Fetus and Young Adult*, 8th edition. Philadelphia, Lippincott Williams & Wilkins, 2013, pp 925–926.
- Lai WW, Mertens LL, Cohen MS, et al (eds): *Echocardiography in Pediatric and Congenital Heart Disease: From Fetus to Adult*, 2nd edition. Chichester, UK, Wiley-Blackwell, 2016, pp 217, 288.

243. B. Supravalvular pulmonary stenosis.

Alagille, Williams, and congenital rubella syndromes have all been associated with supravalvular pulmonary stenosis. Atrioventricular septal defects (AVSDs, also known as atrioventricular canal defects or AVCDs) are associated with trisomy 21 (Down syndrome), rhabdomyomas with tuberous sclerosis, and type B interrupted aortic arch (IAA) with DiGeorge syndrome.

- Allen HD, Driscoll DJ, Shaddy RE, et al: *Moss and Adams' Heart Disease in Infants, Children, and Adolescents: Including the Fetus and Young Adult*, 8th edition. Philadelphia, Lippincott Williams & Wilkins, 2013, pp 617–637.
- Lai WW, Mertens LL, Cohen MS, et al (eds): *Echocardiography in Pediatric and Congenital Heart Disease: From Fetus to Adult*, 2nd edition. Chichester, UK, Wiley-Blackwell, 2016, pp 292, 394, 625, 642.

244. A. Infants.

Peripheral branch pulmonary artery stenosis is a normal physiologic condition found in infants; it lessens over time and eventually resolves. The typical branch pulmonary artery velocities are generally less than 2 m/sec. Physiologic peripheral branch pulmonary artery stenosis is not generally encountered in teens, young adults, or middle-aged adults.

- Lai WW, Mertens LL, Cohen MS, et al (eds): *Echocardiography in Pediatric and Congenital Heart Disease: From Fetus to Adult*. Chichester, UK, Wiley-Blackwell, 2009, p 291.
- Park MK: *Park's Pediatric Cardiology for Practitioners*, 6th edition. Philadelphia, Saunders, 2014, p 114.

245. B. Aneurysmal branch pulmonary arteries.

In tetralogy of Fallot (TOF) with absent pulmonary valve syndrome, both branch pulmonary arteries are present and generally aneurysmal; the aneurysmally dilated pulmonary arteries cause compression of the bronchi. A ductus arteriosus is usually not present in TOF with absent pulmonary valve syndrome.

▶ Allen HD, Driscoll DJ, Shaddy RE, et al: *Moss and Adams' Heart Disease in Infants, Children, and Adolescents: Including the Fetus and Young Adult*, 8th edition. Philadelphia, Lippincott Williams & Wilkins, 2013, p 975.

▶ Lai WW, Mertens LL, Cohen MS, et al (eds): *Echocardiography in Pediatric and Congenital Heart Disease: From Fetus to Adult*, 2nd edition. Chichester, UK, Wiley-Blackwell, 2016, p 415.

246. D. Noonan syndrome.

Of the four syndromes listed, Noonan syndrome has a known association with pulmonary valve stenosis. Atrial and ventricular septal defects are associated with Holt-Oram syndrome. Turner syndrome usually involves congenital heart anomalies of the left side, such as coarctation of the aorta and bicuspid aortic valve. Trisomy 21 (Down syndrome) has a well-known association with atrioventricular septal defects as well as atrial septal and ventricular septal defects.

▶ Allen HD, Driscoll DJ, Shaddy RE, et al: *Moss and Adams' Heart Disease in Infants, Children, and Adolescents: Including the Fetus and Young Adult*, 8th edition. Philadelphia, Lippincott Williams & Wilkins, 2013, pp 618–634.

247. B. Coronary artery obstruction.

In pulmonary atresia with intact ventricular septum (PA/IVS), there can be fistulous connections (also called coronary sinusoids) directly between the right ventricle and one or more coronary arteries. When there are multiple stenoses in these connections, the areas of myocardium supplied by the coronary artery or arteries connected to the right ventricle (before the level of stenosis) will be dependent upon the antegrade flow from the right ventricle through the fistula(e) and into these coronaries. This is called right ventricle–dependent coronary circulation (RVDCC). While the presence of fistulous coronary connections can be suggested by echocardiography, the diagnosis of RVDCC cannot be made by echocardiography and instead must be established by cardiac catheterization and angiography. This is an important evaluation that is crucial in determining whether a two-ventricle repair can be performed in these patients; if RVDCC is present, a two-ventricle repair is contraindicated.

▶ Allen HD, Driscoll DJ, Shaddy RE, et al: *Moss and Adams' Heart Disease in Infants, Children, and Adolescents: Including the Fetus and Young Adult*, 8th edition. Philadelphia, Lippincott Williams & Wilkins, 2013, pp 959–967.

▶ Lai WW, Mertens LL, Cohen MS, et al (eds): *Echocardiography in Pediatric and Congenital Heart Disease: From Fetus to Adult*, 2nd edition. Chichester, UK, Wiley-Blackwell, 2016, pp 281–312.

▶ Park MK: *Park's Pediatric Cardiology for Practitioners*, 6th edition. Philadelphia, Saunders, 2014, pp 252–258.

Refer to video PER-Q248.

248. C. Coronary-cameral fistula.

Video PER-Q248 demonstrates a giant coronary-cameral fistula to the right atrium. Notice that the first clue that this is a coronary-cameral fistula is the abnormally large size of the right coronary artery. The echocardiographer used both the parasternal short-axis view at the level of the great vessels and then the parasternal long-axis right ventricular inflow tract (RVOT) view to identify the terminal end (arrow) of the coronary-cameral fistula into the right atrium.

▶ Lai WW, Mertens LL, Cohen MS, et al (eds): *Echocardiography in Pediatric and Congenital Heart Disease: From Fetus to Adult*, 2nd edition. Chichester, UK, Wiley-Blackwell, 2016, pp 602–603.

249. A. Right ventricle.

The right heart (right ventricle, right atrium, and pulmonary artery) is the most likely termination site for a coronary-cameral fistula; the left heart structures are less likely. A major clue in identifying a coronary-cameral fistula is the dilatation of the coronary artery that the fistula is connected to. However, it is important to remember that smaller fistulae might not be associated with dilated coronary arteries. Color Doppler sweeps demonstrating diastolic flow into a heart chamber are helpful in identifying the terminal end of a coronary-cameral fistula.

▶ Lai WW, Mertens LL, Cohen MS, et al (eds): *Echocardiography in Pediatric and Congenital Heart Disease: From Fetus to Adult*, 2nd edition. Chichester, UK, Wiley-Blackwell, 2016, pp 602–603.

250. D. Pulmonary atresia with intact ventricular septum.

Atrioventricular septal defect (choice A), tetralogy of Fallot with pulmonary stenosis (choice B), and common atrioventricular canal (choice C) have no known associations with coronary-cameral fistulae. In pulmonary atresia with intact ventricular septum, there can be fistulous connections (also called coronary sinusoids) directly between the right ventricle and one or more coronary arteries. When there are multiple stenoses in these connections, the areas of myocardium supplied by the coronary artery or arteries connected to the right ventricle (before the level of stenosis) will be dependent upon the antegrade flow from the right ventricle through the fistula(e) and into these coronaries. This is known as right ventricle–dependent coronary circulation (RVDCC).

▸ Allen HD, Driscoll DJ, Shaddy RE, et al: *Moss and Adams' Heart Disease in Infants, Children, and Adolescents: Including the Fetus and Young Adult*, 8th edition. Philadelphia, Lippincott Williams & Wilkins, 2013, pp 691–711, 930–940, 974.

▸ Lai WW, Mertens LL, Cohen MS, et al (eds): *Echocardiography in Pediatric and Congenital Heart Disease: From Fetus to Adult*, 2nd edition. Chichester, UK, Wiley-Blackwell, 2016, pp 602, 630.

251. B. Right ventricle–dependent coronary circulation.

In pulmonary atresia with intact ventricular septum (PA/IVS), there can be fistulous connections (also called coronary sinusoids) directly between the right ventricle and one or more coronary arteries. When there are multiple stenoses in these connections, the areas of myocardium supplied by the coronary artery or arteries connected to the right ventricle (before the level of stenosis) will be dependent upon the antegrade flow from the right ventricle through the fistula(e) and into these coronaries. This is known as right ventricle–dependent coronary circulation (RVDCC) and signifies dependence upon a high right ventricular pressure to maintain adequate coronary perfusion to either the right or left ventricle. In this setting, if a pulmonary valve perforation/dilatation (by cardiac catheterization) or surgical pulmonary valvotomy is performed, the right ventricle will be decompressed, right ventricular pressure will fall, and right ventricle–dependent coronary artery perfusion will be significantly compromised, potentially leading to infarction of the affected myocardial regions.

▸ Allen HD, Driscoll DJ, Shaddy RE, et al: *Moss and Adams' Heart Disease in Infants, Children, and Adolescents: Including the Fetus and Young Adult*, 8th edition. Philadelphia, Lippincott Williams & Wilkins, 2013, p 940.

▸ Park MK: *Park's Pediatric Cardiology for Practitioners*, 6th edition. Philadelphia, Saunders, 2014, pp 252–258.

252. C. Bicuspid.

The most common type of pulmonary valve morphology in tetralogy of Fallot is bicuspid.

▸ Allen HD, Driscoll DJ, Shaddy RE, et al: *Moss and Adams' Heart Disease in Infants, Children, and Adolescents: Including the Fetus and Young Adult*, 8th edition. Philadelphia, Lippincott Williams & Wilkins, 2013, p 974.

253. C. Tricuspid valve annulus diameter.

In a patient with pulmonary atresia with intact ventricular septum (PA/IVS), several studies (cited below) have shown that the diameter of the tricuspid valve annulus best correlates with right ventricular size.

- Bull C, de Leval MR, Mercanti C, et al: Pulmonary atresia and intact ventricular septum: a revised classification. Circulation 66:266–272, 1982.
- Lai WW, Mertens LL, Cohen MS, et al (eds): *Echocardiography in Pediatric and Congenital Heart Disease: From Fetus to Adult*, 2nd edition. Chichester, UK, Wiley-Blackwell, 2016, pp 63–70, 298.
- Zuberbuhler JR, Anderson RH: Morphological variations in pulmonary atresia with intact ventricular septum. Br Heart J 41:281–288, 1979.

254. B. Right-to-left atrial-level shunting.

A newborn with pulmonary atresia with intact ventricular septum (PA/IVS) is reliant upon an unobstructed right-to-left atrial-level shunt, as well as a patent ductus arteriosus (PDA), for survival. The subcostal long- and short-axis views are important echocardiographic windows for evaluating atrial-level shunting with color flow imaging and spectral Doppler. A mean gradient obtained with spectral Doppler of the atrial-level shunt is important to determine whether restrictive right-to-left atrial-level shunting is present.

- Allen HD, Driscoll DJ, Shaddy RE, et al: *Moss and Adams' Heart Disease in Infants, Children, and Adolescents: Including the Fetus and Young Adult*, 8th edition. Philadelphia, Lippincott Williams & Wilkins, 2013, p 946.
- Lai WW, Mertens LL, Cohen MS, et al (eds): *Echocardiography in Pediatric and Congenital Heart Disease: From Fetus to Adult*, 2nd edition. Chichester, UK, Wiley-Blackwell, 2016, pp 46–48, 304–305.

255. B. Acquire a ductal view to visualize the patency of the ductus arteriosus.

This clinical scenario is an example of critical pulmonary valve stenosis. When the patent ductus arteriosus (PDA) closes, it becomes apparent that the right ventricle cannot pump enough blood across the very stenotic pulmonary valve to provide adequate blood flow to the lungs; blood flow then returns to the left atrium via the pulmonary veins. Instead, a significant amount of systemic venous (deoxygenated) blood returning to the right atrium shunts across the atrial septum into the left atrium, mixing with the small amount of oxygenated blood returning from the pulmonary veins. This results in significant systemic arterial hypoxemia—in this case the oxygen saturations are in the low 60s. When pulmonary valve stenosis is severe enough that an acceptable systemic arterial oxygen saturation is dependent on the presence of a PDA, the patient is diagnosed as having critical pulmonary valve stenosis. Therefore, in this scenario, the echocardiographic exam should first begin with the most immediate questions that must be answered—the patency and size of the PDA.

- Lai WW, Mertens LL, Cohen MS, et al (eds): *Echocardiography in Pediatric and Congenital Heart Disease: From Fetus to Adult*, 2nd edition. Chichester, UK, Wiley-Blackwell, 2016, pp 281–282.
- Park MK: *Park's Pediatric Cardiology for Practitioners*, 6th edition. Philadelphia, Saunders, 2014, pp 483–494.

256. C. A morphologic right atrial to morphologic left atrial shunt.

Atrial-level shunting in this scenario will be morphologic right atrium to morphologic left atrium. Given the presence of tricuspid atresia, this shunting is vital for the patient's survival. Hence, an intact atrial septum would not be compatible with survival, and if atrial-level shunting is deemed to be restrictive, a balloon atrial septostomy (or surgical atrial septectomy) might be indicated.

- Lai WW, Mertens LL, Cohen MS, et al (eds): *Echocardiography in Pediatric and Congenital Heart Disease: From Fetus to Adult*, 2nd edition. Chichester, UK, Wiley-Blackwell, 2016, pp 446–460, 520–526.
- Park MK: *Park's Pediatric Cardiology for Practitioners*, 6th edition. Philadelphia, Saunders, 2014, pp 446–460.

257. D. Left-sided juxtaposition of the atrial appendages.

Left-sided juxtaposition of the atrial appendages can be seen in tricuspid valve anomalies like tricuspid atresia. Stella Van Praagh et al. reported that the incidence of left-sided juxtaposition of the atrial appendages is high if patients have right ventricular hypoplasia and abnormally related great arteries, such as transposition of the great arteries (d-TGA) or double-outlet right ventricle. Bilateral left atrial appendages (left atrial isomerism, choice A) and bilateral right atrial appendages (right atrial isomerism, choice C) are excluded because (as noted in the question) visceroatrial situs is solitus; therefore the atrial situs is normal and there is no isomerism. Choice B, right-sided juxtaposition of the atrial appendages, is very rare and is generally not associated with tricuspid atresia. Of note: While scanning a heart with juxtaposition of the atrial appendages, care must be taken not to confuse the juxtaposed appendages for a large atrial septal defect or dilated coronary sinus.

- Lai WW, Mertens LL, Cohen MS, et al (eds): *Echocardiography in Pediatric and Congenital Heart Disease: From Fetus to Adult*, 2nd edition. Chichester, UK, Wiley-Blackwell, 2016, pp 520–526, 563–566.
- Van Praagh S, O'Sullivan J, Brili S, et al: Juxtaposition of the morphologically right atrial appendage in situs solitus and inversus atria: a study of 35 postmortem cases. Am Heart J 132:382–390, 1996.

Refer to video PER-Q258.

258. A. Abdominal visceral situs inversus.

Video PER-Q258 demonstrates visceral situs inversus. The clip shows a left-sided liver, left-sided inferior vena cava, right-sided abdominal aorta, and right-sided stomach.

- Lai WW, Mertens LL, Cohen MS, et al (eds): *Echocardiography in Pediatric and Congenital Heart Disease: From Fetus to Adult*, 2nd edition. Chichester, UK, Wiley-Blackwell, 2016, pp 31–37.

Refer to video PER-Q259.

259. B. Muscular tricuspid atresia.

Video PER-Q259 represents tricuspid atresia of the muscular type with an interventricular septal defect. The floor of the right atrium in this clip is muscular, with no visible tricuspid valve. The right ventricle is hypoplastic. An unbalanced common atrioventricular canal (choice A) is incorrect because the patient does not have a common atrioventricular valve. Hypoplastic left heart syndrome (HLHS, choice C) is incorrect because there is a good-sized mitral valve and left ventricle, ruling out HLHS. Pulmonary atresia with intact ventricular septum (choice D) is also incorrect; although the right ventricle may also be hypoplastic in patients with this condition, the interventricular septal defect seen in the video clip excludes this choice.

- Lai WW, Mertens LL, Cohen MS, et al (eds): *Echocardiography in Pediatric and Congenital Heart Disease: From Fetus to Adult*, 2nd edition. Chichester, UK, Wiley-Blackwell, 2016, pp 259–264, 357–366, 520–526.

260. B. Restrictive atrial-level shunting.

Patients with tricuspid atresia require a widely patent atrial communication so that systemic venous blood can return unobstructed to the left atrium and ventricle. In this setting, a restrictive atrial septal defect will in turn lead to elevated right atrial and inferior/superior vena caval pressures. These elevated systemic venous pressures will in turn produce hepatomegaly. None of the other choices for this question would be expected to produce hepatomegaly.

- Allen HD, Driscoll DJ, Shaddy RE, et al: *Moss and Adams' Heart Disease in Infants, Children, and Adolescents: Including the Fetus and Young Adult*, 8th edition. Philadelphia, Lippincott Williams & Wilkins, 2013, pp 877–879.

261. D. Right aortic arch.

A right aortic arch (RAA) is seen in approximately 25% of patients with tetralogy of Fallot (TOF). Persistence of the fifth aortic arch (choice A) and a double aortic arch (choice C) can be seen with TOF, but not with the same increased frequency as RAA. No relevant statistical information is found for choice B, left aortic arch with aberrant right subclavian artery.

- Allen HD, Driscoll DJ, Shaddy RE, et al: *Moss and Adams' Heart Disease in Infants, Children, and Adolescents: Including the Fetus and Young Adult*, 8th edition. Philadelphia, Lippincott Williams & Wilkins, 2013, pp 758–786.
- Lai WW, Mertens LL, Cohen MS, et al (eds): *Echocardiography in Pediatric and Congenital Heart Disease: From Fetus to Adult*, 2nd edition. Chichester, UK, Wiley-Blackwell, 2016, pp 414–415.

262. C. The pulmonary arteries are discontinuous.

This scenario describes tetralogy of Fallot (TOF) in which there is a right aortic arch and the pulmonary arteries are discontinuous, with the right pulmonary artery arising from the main pulmonary artery and the left pulmonary artery supplied completely by a patent ductus arteriosus (PDA) originating from the base of the left innominate (brachiocephalic) artery. Maintaining patency of this left-sided PDA with prostaglandin E1 (PGE1) might be necessary to provide continued perfusion to the left pulmonary artery. Of note, when there is TOF with a right aortic arch with mirror-image branching and a PDA, it is common for the ductus arteriosus to arise from the left innominate artery instead of its usual origin from the undersurface of the aortic arch.

- Allen HD, Driscoll DJ, Shaddy RE, et al: *Moss and Adams' Heart Disease in Infants, Children, and Adolescents: Including the Fetus and Young Adult*, 8th edition. Philadelphia, Lippincott Williams & Wilkins, 2013, pp 758–786, 974.
- Knight L, Edwards JE: Right aortic arch: types and associated cardiac anomalies. Circulation 50:1047–1051, 1974.
- Lai WW, Mertens LL, Cohen MS, et al (eds): *Echocardiography in Pediatric and Congenital Heart Disease: From Fetus to Adult*, 2nd edition. Chichester, UK, Wiley-Blackwell, 2016, pp 407–418.

Refer to video PER-Q263.

263. C. Hemitruncus.

Video PER-Q263 demonstrates a right pulmonary artery originating from the ascending aorta, which historically has been called "hemitruncus." Hemitruncus is not considered to be in the category of truncus arteriosus because it is an abnormality of great artery (not outflow tract) development. Unlike truncus arteriosus, hemitruncus is associated with a fully developed pulmonary artery and aorta, and two separate semilunar valves.

▸ Lai WW, Mertens LL, Cohen MS, et al (eds): *Echocardiography in Pediatric and Congenital Heart Disease: From Fetus to Adult*, 2nd edition. Chichester, UK, Wiley-Blackwell, 2016, p 327.

Refer to video PER-Q264.

264. D. High left parasternal, ductal view.

Video PER-Q264 was obtained in a high left parasternal view with the index marker pointing to approximately 12 o'clock. Notice that in this view one can visualize the main pulmonary artery, the descending aorta, and the shunting pattern of the patent ductus arteriosus (PDA). This view is helpful when evaluating a PDA that shunts from right to left, and it is useful in distinguishing the PDA from the left pulmonary artery. A PDA that shunts from right to left indicates an elevated main pulmonary artery pressure, which can be seen in various clinical settings that produce pulmonary hypertension, including total anomalous pulmonary venous connection (TAPVC) and congenital diaphragmatic hernia. Right-to-left PDA shunting can also be found in certain types of congenital heart disease characterized by left-sided obstructive lesions accompanied by some degree of aortic hypoplasia/obstruction; these include hypoplastic left heart syndrome, interrupted aortic arch, severe coarctation, and critical aortic valve stenosis.

▸ Lai WW, Mertens LL, Cohen MS, et al (eds): *Echocardiography in Pediatric and Congenital Heart Disease: From Fetus to Adult*, 2nd edition. Chichester, UK, Wiley-Blackwell, 2016, pp 54, 317–329, 382–402.

▸ Park MK: *Park's Pediatric Cardiology for Practitioners*, 6th edition. Philadelphia, Saunders, 2014, pp 204, 258–259, 483–490.

ANSWERS

See Color Plate 10 on page xxiv.

265. B. Normal pulmonary vascular resistance (PVR).

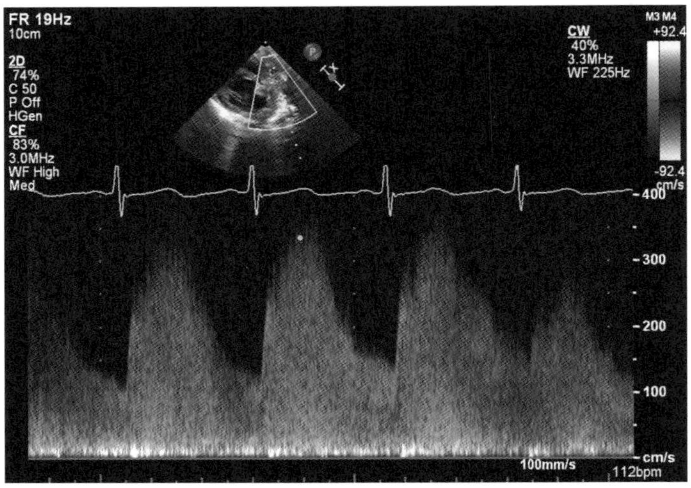

This spectral Doppler image is of a small restrictive patent ductus arteriosus (PDA). The spectral tracing displays continuous left-to-right flow with a peak systolic velocity (PSV) of approximately 3.4 m/sec, which indicates a high systemic to pulmonary artery gradient and therefore a low pulmonary artery pressure and likely normal pulmonary vascular resistance (PVR). In the setting of pulmonary hypertension, there will be a low systolic gradient between the aorta and the pulmonary artery, resulting in a low-systolic-velocity left-to-right shunt across the PDA. A large PDA will generally result in elevated pulmonary artery pressure and a low- (not high-) velocity left-to-right PDA shunt. Interrupted aortic arch (IAA) anomalies will have obligate right-to-left systolic shunting at the level of the PDA.

▸ Lai WW, Mertens LL, Cohen MS, et al (eds): *Echocardiography in Pediatric and Congenital Heart Disease: From Fetus to Adult*, 2nd edition. Chichester, UK, Wiley-Blackwell, 2016, pp 317–329.

Refer to video PER-Q266.

266. A. Mesocardia.

Video PER-Q266 demonstrates a midline heart, also termed mesocardia. In this clip, the apex points inferiorly. However, it is important to realize that with mesocardia the cardiac mass is located in the midline but the apex of the heart can point in any direction. Scimitar syndrome and absent right pulmonary artery are conditions in which mesocardia occurs. The hypoplasia of the right lung in Scimitar syndrome can cause a rightward shift in the ventricular mass, so that the heart is situated in the midline.

▸ Allen HD, Driscoll DJ, Shaddy RE, et al: *Moss and Adams' Heart Disease in Infants, Children, and Adolescents: Including the Fetus and Young Adult*, 8th edition. Philadelphia, Lippincott Williams & Wilkins, 2013, pp 817–821.

ANSWERS

▸ Lai WW, Mertens LL, Cohen MS, et al (eds): *Echocardiography in Pediatric and Congenital Heart Disease: From Fetus to Adult*, 2nd edition. Chichester, UK, Wiley-Blackwell, 2016, pp 34, 160, 166–167.

Refer to video PER-Q267.

267. B. Anomalous left coronary artery from the pulmonary artery.

Refer to video PER-Q267. This parasternal short-axis clip demonstrates anomalous left coronary artery from the pulmonary artery (ALCAPA). The most frequent origin of ALCAPA is the left or posterior segment of the main pulmonary artery, but it can also arise closer to the right pulmonary artery.

▸ Lai WW, Mertens LL, Cohen MS, et al (eds): *Echocardiography in Pediatric and Congenital Heart Disease: From Fetus to Adult*, 2nd edition. Chichester, UK, Wiley-Blackwell, 2016, pp 44–59, 591–594.

268. B. Coronary artery steal.

Several phases describe the physiology of anomalous left coronary artery from the pulmonary artery (ALCAPA), but the cause of myocardial ischemia is the coronary arterial "steal" that occurs when left coronary artery blood—which normally fills antegrade to perfuse the left ventricular myocardium—instead drains retrograde into the main pulmonary artery. As a result, there is significant coronary hypoperfusion of the left ventricle, leading to myocardial ischemia and (in some instances) infarction.

▸ Lai WW, Mertens LL, Cohen MS, et al (eds): *Echocardiography in Pediatric and Congenital Heart Disease: From Fetus to Adult*, 2nd edition. Chichester, UK, Wiley-Blackwell, 2016, pp 591–594.

Refer to video PER-Q269.

269. B. Anomalous right coronary artery from the pulmonary artery.

Video PER-Q269 demonstrates anomalous right coronary artery from the pulmonary artery (ARCAPA). With this condition, coronary artery "steal" physiology can lead to myocardial ischemia. With color Doppler imaging, this abnormal steal phenomenon can be visualized as retrograde flow into the main pulmonary artery. Unlike anomalous left coronary artery from the pulmonary artery (ALCAPA), ARCAPA has a peak age of diagnosis beyond infancy. Angina, congestive heart failure, and dyspnea can be symptoms of ARCAPA, with sudden death being the worst outcome. However, the natural history of ARCAPA is much more variable than that of ALCAPA; some patients have little to no symptomatology and a more benign course.

- Gupta R, Marwah A, Shrivastva S: Anomalous origin of right coronary artery from pulmonary artery. Ann Pediatr Cardiol 5:95–96, 2012.
- Lai WW, Mertens LL, Cohen MS, et al (eds): *Echocardiography in Pediatric and Congenital Heart Disease: From Fetus to Adult*, 2nd edition. Chichester, UK, Wiley-Blackwell, 2016, pp 595–596.
- Thomas Collins R, Davis E, Stephens P: Asymptomatic anomalous right coronary artery from the pulmonary trunk. Cardiol Young 19:391–392, 2009.
- Williams IA, Gersony WM, Hellenbrand WE: Anomalous right coronary artery arising from the pulmonary artery: a report of 7 cases and a review of the literature. Am Heart J 152:1004.e9–.e17, 2006.

270. A. The LMCA courses between the two great vessels, partially within the walls of the aorta.

An intramural course of the left main coronary artery (LMCA) is a potentially life-threatening congenital coronary abnormality that can lead to syncope and/or sudden death. Careful examination of the coronary artery origins should be performed with 2D imaging as well as color flow Doppler. An intramural LMCA arises from the right coronary sinus of the aorta and courses to the left between the two great arteries, with a portion of the LMCA traveling within the wall of the aorta (hence the term "intramural"). The use of color flow Doppler is helpful in demonstrating the coronary artery within the luminal wall of the aorta and thus in diagnosing the anomaly. A parasternal short-axis view is essential for making this diagnosis. Other helpful echocardiographic techniques include sweeps from an apical four-chamber to five-chamber view and the parasternal long-axis view.

- Allen HD, Driscoll DJ, Shaddy RE, et al: *Moss and Adams' Heart Disease in Infants, Children, and Adolescents: Including the Fetus and Young Adult*, 8th edition. Philadelphia, Lippincott Williams & Wilkins, 2013, p 748.
- Lai WW, Mertens LL, Cohen MS, et al (eds): *Echocardiography in Pediatric and Congenital Heart Disease: From Fetus to Adult*, 2nd edition. Chichester, UK, Wiley-Blackwell, 2016, pp 597–598.

271. A. Descending aorta.

Aortopulmonary collateral vessels (APCs) are mostly likely to originate from the descending aorta, innominate (brachiocephalic) artery, or abdominal aorta. A color Doppler sweep from the subcostal short-axis view with emphasis on the aorta is helpful in identifying APCs. Other helpful views include the suprasternal long- and short-axis views, emphasizing the thoracic aorta and head and neck vessels, with color flow Doppler.

▶ Lai WW, Mertens LL, Cohen MS, et al (eds): *Echocardiography in Pediatric and Congenital Heart Disease: From Fetus to Adult*, 2nd edition. Chichester, UK, Wiley-Blackwell, 2016, pp 47, 53–54.

▶ Nichols DG, Ungerleider RM, Spevak PJ, et al: *Critical Heart Disease in infants and Children*, 2nd edition. Philadelphia, Mosby Elsevier, 2006, p 450.

272. B. Tetralogy of Fallot with pulmonary atresia.

Aortopulmonary collateral vessels (APCs) are most likely to be seen in tetralogy of Fallot (TOF) with pulmonary atresia. When performing a study, the echocardiographer must pay particular attention to the head and neck arteries, descending thoracic aorta, and abdominal aorta to rule out APCs. These APCs appear as small, tortuous arteries with continuous flow, are often difficult to follow completely, and have an uncertain point of drainage (due to the fact that they usually empty into sites deep within the lungs). Severe aortic coarctation, Van Praagh type A1 truncus arteriosus, and hypoplastic left heart syndrome with mitral atresia and aortic atresia are not typically associated with APCs.

▶ Nichols DG, Ungerleider RM, Spevak PJ, et al: *Critical Heart Disease in infants and Children*, 2nd edition. Philadelphia, Mosby Elsevier, 2006, pp 755–766.

273. B. Color flow Doppler.

Aortopulmonary collateral vessels (APCs) are generally difficult to visualize by 2D imaging only, and most of the time color Doppler flow imaging is required to aid in their identification. After the aortopulmonary collateral flow is identified by color Doppler, a spectral Doppler pulsed wave can be used to identify their arterial flow pattern. M-mode imaging and speckle tracking echocardiography are not useful for evaluation of aortopulmonary collaterals.

▶ Lai WW, Mertens LL, Cohen MS, et al (eds): *Echocardiography in Pediatric and Congenital Heart Disease: From Fetus to Adult*, 2nd edition. Chichester, UK, Wiley-Blackwell, 2016, pp 317–322, 416.

274. C. Williams-Beuren syndrome.

Supravalvular aortic stenosis and supravalvular pulmonary stenosis are typically associated with Williams-Beuren (also known simply as Williams) syndrome. Note that supravalvular pulmonary stenosis (branch pulmonary arteries) in patients with Williams-Beuren syndrome may improve over time. In contrast, supravalvular aortic stenosis in patients with Williams-Beuren progresses over time. When performing echocardiography on a patient with Williams syndrome, you must take care to rule out supravalvular aortic stenosis using appropriate echocardiographic views such as the parasternal long-axis and suprasternal views of the ascending aorta, as well as the apical five-chamber view in some cases. Color flow acceleration, starting at the sinotubular junction and continuing into the ascending aorta, serves as a clue for supravalvular aortic stenosis. Down syndrome (trisomy 21), Holt-Oram syndrome, and Char syndrome are not associated with supravalvular aortic stenosis.

- Allen HD, Driscoll DJ, Shaddy RE, et al: *Moss and Adams' Heart Disease in Infants, Children, and Adolescents: Including the Fetus and Young Adult*, 8th edition. Philadelphia, Lippincott Williams & Wilkins, 2013, pp 617–637.
- Lai WW, Mertens LL, Cohen MS, et al (eds): *Echocardiography in Pediatric and Congenital Heart Disease: From Fetus to Adult*, 2nd edition. Chichester, UK, Wiley-Blackwell, 2016, pp 51–54, 326, 336.

275. B. Sinotubular junction.

The sinotubular junction is the most common site for supravalvular aortic stenosis, but hypoplasia of the aortic arch can also occur within the same patient. Sliding the transducer medially (toward the patient's sternum) in a parasternal long-axis sweep enables the echocardiographer to visualize the ascending aorta and interrogate it for supravalvular aortic stenosis. Color Doppler often demonstrates a discrete increase in velocity at the site of narrowing.

- Lai WW, Mertens LL, Cohen MS, et al (eds): *Echocardiography in Pediatric and Congenital Heart Disease: From Fetus to Adult*, 2nd edition. Chichester, UK, Wiley-Blackwell, 2016, pp 345–347.

276. D. Coronary ostial stenosis.

Stenoses of the coronary artery origins can be seen with supravalvular aortic stenosis, and these can be extremely problematic. These stenoses can be difficult to visualize by echocardiography but should be suspected when the origins of the coronary arteries lie close to the area of supravalvular narrowing.

- Allen HD, Driscoll DJ, Shaddy RE, et al: *Moss and Adams' Heart Disease in Infants, Children, and Adolescents: Including the Fetus and Young Adult*, 8th edition. Philadelphia, Lippincott Williams & Wilkins, 2013, p 1038.
- Lai WW, Mertens LL, Cohen MS, et al (eds): *Echocardiography in Pediatric and Congenital Heart Disease: From Fetus to Adult*, 2nd edition. Chichester, UK, Wiley-Blackwell, 2016, p 345.

277. C. C.

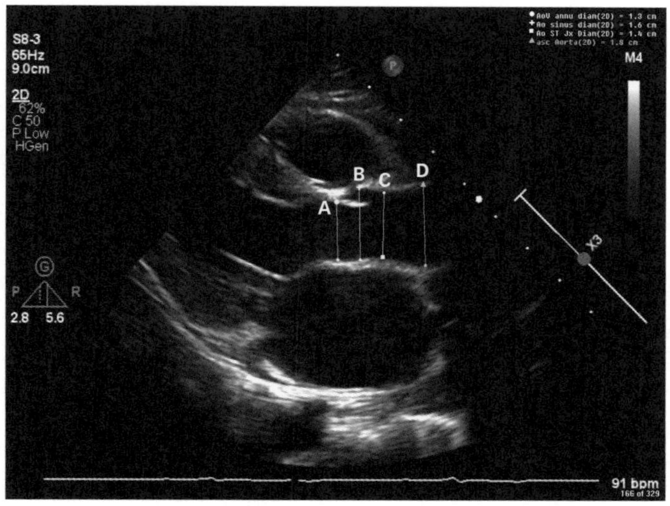

In this image the letter C identifies the aortic sinotubular junction, which is the most common site of supravalvular aortic stenosis. The letter A identifies the aortic valve annulus, B the aortic sinuses of Valsalva, and D the ascending aorta.

- Lai WW, Mertens LL, Cohen MS, et al (eds): *Echocardiography in Pediatric and Congenital Heart Disease: From Fetus to Adult*, 2nd edition. Chichester, UK, Wiley-Blackwell, 2016, pp 345–346.
- Lopez L, Colan SD, Frommelt PC, et al: Recommendations for quantification methods during the performance of a pediatric echocardiogram: a report from the Pediatric Measurements Writing Group of the American Society of Echocardiography Pediatric and Congenital Heart Disease Council. J Am Soc Echocardiogr 23:465–495, 2010.

278. A. Right anterior cardinal vein.

The primitive embryologic cardinal veins form the superior systemic venous system. The right anterior cardinal vein becomes the right-sided superior vena cava (SVC). The left cardinal system usually involutes or, if it persists, becomes a left-sided SVC. The splanchnic system forms the pulmonary veins. The right vitelline vein becomes the inferior vena cava (IVC).

- Lai WW, Mertens LL, Cohen MS, et al (eds): *Echocardiography in Pediatric and Congenital Heart Disease: From Fetus to Adult*, 2nd edition. Chichester, UK, Wiley-Blackwell, 2016, p 181.

279. D. It contains the limbus of the fossa ovalis.

The morphologic right atrium always contains the limbus of the fossa ovalis. Although the right atrium usually receives the systemic veins, this is not always the case—as when the left superior vena cava drains directly to the left atrium, or in the case of heterotaxy syndrome, where the inferior vena cava may drain to the left atrium. The tricuspid valve is almost always associated with the right ventricle (not the right atrium).

▶ Lai WW, Mertens LL, Cohen MS, et al (eds): *Echocardiography in Pediatric and Congenital Heart Disease: From Fetus to Adult*, 2nd edition. Chichester, UK, Wiley-Blackwell, 2016, p 36.

280. A. Dilated azygos vein.

When the inferior vena cava (IVC) is interrupted, the venous blood from the lower portion of the body usually drains via an azygos vein that then drains to the superior vena cava (SVC) below the insertion of the innominate (brachiocephalic) vein. The innominate vein is thus not involved. The azygos does not drain to a left-sided SVC. The pulmonary veins are not involved.

▶ Lai WW, Mertens LL, Cohen MS, et al (eds): *Echocardiography in Pediatric and Congenital Heart Disease: From Fetus to Adult*, 2nd edition. Chichester, UK, Wiley-Blackwell, 2016, p 187.

281. B. Rhabdomyomas.

The natural history of rhabdomyomas is that they tend to be multiple and tend to regress over time. The other masses—fibromas, teratomas, and myxomas—do not have that characteristic. Fibromas usually occur as singular masses, myxomas tend to be located in the atria, and teratomas tend to be pericardial.

▶ Lai WW, Mertens LL, Cohen MS, et al (eds): *Echocardiography in Pediatric and Congenital Heart Disease: From Fetus to Adult*, 2nd edition. Chichester, UK, Wiley-Blackwell, 2016, pp 641–648.

282. A. Tuberous sclerosis.

Rhabdomyomas are highly associated with tuberous sclerosis and are not associated with Down, Turner, or DiGeorge syndrome.

▶ Lai WW, Mertens LL, Cohen MS, et al (eds): *Echocardiography in Pediatric and Congenital Heart Disease: From Fetus to Adult*, 2nd edition. Chichester, UK, Wiley-Blackwell, 2016, pp 641–648.

Refer to video PER-Q283.

283. D. Myxoma.

Video PER-Q283 shows a mass with the typical appearance and location of a myxoma—pedunculated with a stalk and adherent to the atrial septum. Fibromas and rhabdomyomas tend to be located in the ventricles. Teratomas tend to be pericardial.

▶ Lai WW, Mertens LL, Cohen MS, et al (eds): *Echocardiography in Pediatric and Congenital Heart Disease: From Fetus to Adult*, 2nd edition. Chichester, UK, Wiley-Blackwell, 2016, pp 646–647.

284. C. Total anomalous pulmonary venous connection.

The individual pulmonary veins arise from the splanchnic system and then join the common pulmonary vein. The common pulmonary vein is then incorporated into the left atrium. Partial incorporation results in cor triatriatum. Complete lack of incorporation results in total anomalous pulmonary venous connection without any pulmonary venous drainage to the left atrium. Instead, the pulmonary veins drain to one or more systemic veins or to the right atrium. Partial anomalous pulmonary venous connection occurs when one or more pulmonary veins do not connect to the left atrium and instead drain to a systemic vein or the right atrium. However, at least one or more pulmonary veins will still return to the left atrium. Supravalvular mitral ring is not an abnormality of the common pulmonary vein.

▶ Lai WW, Mertens LL, Cohen MS, et al (eds): *Echocardiography in Pediatric and Congenital Heart Disease: From Fetus to Adult*, 2nd edition. Chichester, UK, Wiley-Blackwell, 2016, p 160.

285. A. Cor triatriatum.

See the answer to question 284.

▶ Lai WW, Mertens LL, Cohen MS, et al (eds): *Echocardiography in Pediatric and Congenital Heart Disease: From Fetus to Adult*, 2nd edition. Chichester, UK, Wiley-Blackwell, 2016, p 159.

286. B. Left anterior cardinal system.

The primitive embryologic cardinal veins form the systemic venous system. The inferior vena cava (IVC) and superior vena cava (SVC) are remnants of the horns of the sinus venosus, which are right-sided. The left cardinal system usually involutes or, if it persists, becomes a left-sided SVC. The splanchnic system forms the pulmonary veins. The umbilicovitelline system develops into portions of the IVC and the hepatic veins.

▶ Lai WW, Mertens LL, Cohen MS, et al (eds): *Echocardiography in Pediatric and Congenital Heart Disease: From Fetus to Adult*, 2nd edition. Chichester, UK, Wiley-Blackwell, 2016, p 181.

287. A. Left atrial appendage.

The relationship of the membrane you are evaluating to the left atrial appendage will help you determine whether it is most likely cor triatriatum or a supravalvular mitral ring. With the partial incorporation of the common pulmonary vein that results in cor triatriatum, the membrane in the left atrium is

ANSWERS

located superior to the left atrial appendage. A supravalvular mitral ring is an abnormality more inherent in the mitral valve structure, and the membrane is located inferior to the left atrial appendage, just above the mitral valve annulus. Neither of these structures has a direct relationship to the right-sided pulmonary veins, fossa ovalis, or coronary sinus.

▸ Lai WW, Mertens LL, Cohen MS, et al (eds): *Echocardiography in Pediatric and Congenital Heart Disease: From Fetus to Adult*, 2nd edition. Chichester, UK, Wiley-Blackwell, 2016, pp 165–166.

Refer to video PER-Q288.

288. C. Extension of Wilms tumor.

Video PER-Q288 presents an example of a Wilms tumor—not a primary cardiac tumor—infiltrating up the inferior vena cava (IVC) from the kidneys. Fibromas and rhabdomyomas tend to be located in the ventricles. Myxomas are primary cardiac tumors that are commonly located in the atria and usually attached to the atrial septum.

▸ Lai WW, Mertens LL, Cohen MS, et al (eds): *Echocardiography in Pediatric and Congenital Heart Disease: From Fetus to Adult*, 2nd edition. Chichester, UK, Wiley-Blackwell, 2016, p 647.

289. A. Common pulmonary vein.

Partial incorporation of the common pulmonary vein into the left atrium results in cor triatriatum. The systemic venous system, such as the cardinal system and azygos veins, is not involved. The crista terminalis—the ridge between the true right atrium and horns of the sinus venosus—is a hallmark of the morphologic right atrium.

▸ Lai WW, Mertens LL, Cohen MS, et al (eds): *Echocardiography in Pediatric and Congenital Heart Disease: From Fetus to Adult*, 2nd edition. Chichester, UK, Wiley-Blackwell, 2016, p 159.

Refer to video PER-Q290.

290. C. Retroaortic innominate vein.

Video PER-Q290 is an example of an innominate (brachiocephalic) vein passing beneath the aortic arch, known as a retroaortic innominate vein. Neither an azygos nor a pulmonary vein will cross underneath the aortic arch. An interrupted inferior vena cava is usually manifested by a dilated azygos vein.

▸ Lai WW, Mertens LL, Cohen MS, et al (eds): *Echocardiography in Pediatric and Congenital Heart Disease: From Fetus to Adult*, 2nd edition. Chichester, UK, Wiley-Blackwell, 2016, p 192.

291. B. Coronary sinus.

A left-sided superior vena cava is a remnant of the left cardinal system and most commonly drains to the coronary sinus. On rare occasions, it may drain directly to the left atrium, but that is far less common. There is no connection to the pulmonary veins or coronary arteries.

▶ Lai WW, Mertens LL, Cohen MS, et al (eds): *Echocardiography in Pediatric and Congenital Heart Disease: From Fetus to Adult*, 2nd edition. Chichester, UK, Wiley-Blackwell, 2016, p 182.

292. D. Dilated coronary sinus.

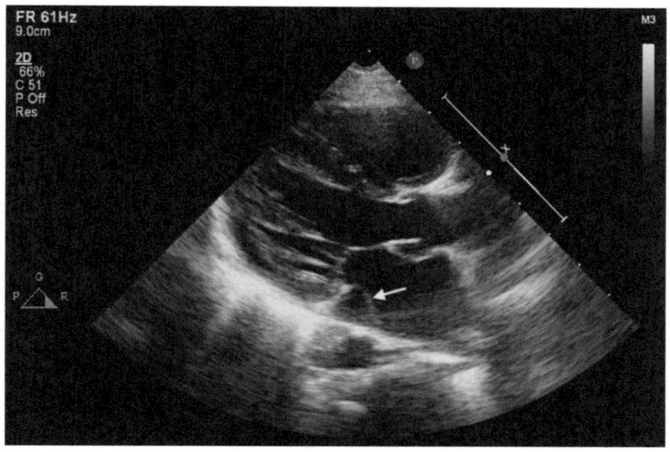

This image shows a dilated coronary sinus (arrow) as it runs in the left-sided atrioventricular (AV) groove. The descending aorta is usually more posterior and not nestled in the AV groove. This structure is distinct from the left atrium and is not associated with an abnormality of the mitral valve.

▶ Lai WW, Mertens LL, Cohen MS, et al (eds): *Echocardiography in Pediatric and Congenital Heart Disease: From Fetus to Adult*, 2nd edition. Chichester, UK, Wiley-Blackwell, 2016, p 190.

293. A. Left-sided superior vena cava.

A left-sided superior vena cava (SVC) is a remnant of the left cardinal system and most commonly drains to the coronary sinus. This is not an inherent abnormality of the mitral valve. An interrupted inferior vena cava (IVC) is associated with a dilated azygos vein, which drains into the right-sided SVC and does not involve the coronary sinus. Supracardiac total anomalous pulmonary venous connection (TAPVC) would not result in a dilated coronary sinus.

▶ Lai WW, Mertens LL, Cohen MS, et al (eds): *Echocardiography in Pediatric and Congenital Heart Disease: From Fetus to Adult*, 2nd edition. Chichester, UK, Wiley-Blackwell, 2016, p 182.

294. C. Teratoma.

Teratomas are often pericardial and associated with an effusion. Myxomas, rhabdomyomas, and fibromas are usually located within the cardiac structures and less likely associated with a primary effusion.

▶ Lai WW, Mertens LL, Cohen MS, et al (eds): *Echocardiography in Pediatric and Congenital Heart Disease: From Fetus to Adult*, 2nd edition. Chichester, UK, Wiley-Blackwell, 2016, p 645.

295. B. Dextroposition.

Dextroposition occurs when the apex of the heart is normally pointed leftward but the heart itself has been shifted rightward due to external factors. This often happens if a left-sided mass or other abnormality shifts the heart rightward or when there is a loss of volume on the right, which then also shifts the heart rightward. Dextrocardia occurs when the heart is on the right side of the thoracic cavity and the apex is pointed rightward. Dextroversion is rare and occurs when the atria are in normal position and the heart has been flipped on its vertical axis such that the apex is toward the right. Dextromethorphan is a cough suppressant.

▶ Lai WW, Mertens LL, Cohen MS, et al (eds): *Echocardiography in Pediatric and Congenital Heart Disease: From Fetus to Adult*, 2nd edition. Chichester, UK, Wiley-Blackwell, 2016, p 558.

296. C. Dextrocardia.

Patients with Kartagener syndrome have mirror-image dextrocardia with the cardiac apex pointing rightward. Levocardia is the normal leftward positioning of the heart. Dextroposition involves levocardia with the heart shifted rightward. Dextroversion is rare and occurs when the atria are in normal position and the heart has been flipped on its vertical axis so that the apex is toward the right.

▶ Allen HD, Shaddy RE, Penny DJ, et al: *Moss and Adams' Heart Disease in Infants, Children, and Adolescents, Including the Fetus and Young Adult*, 9th edition. Philadelphia, Wolters Kluwer, 2016, p 1254.

297. A. Situs inversus.

Patients with Kartagener syndrome have situs inversus totalis so that everything is mirror-image flipped. Thus the morphologic right atrium is on the left and the morphologic left atrium is on the right. Situs solitus is normally positioned atria. Situs ambiguus is more common, with heterotaxy where the situs cannot be determined. Bronchus suis is an anatomic variation of the tracheobronchial tree.

▶ Lai WW, Mertens LL, Cohen MS, et al (eds): *Echocardiography in Pediatric and Congenital Heart Disease: From Fetus to Adult*, 2nd edition. Chichester, UK, Wiley-Blackwell, 2016, p 32.

298. B. Anomalous pulmonary vein.

A left-sided superior vena cava (SVC) would be draining down toward the heart, not up into the innominate (brachiocephalic) vein. An azygos vein drains into the SVC directly. An arteriovenous malformation does not have a low-velocity phasic pattern; rather, it has more of a continuous flow pattern. An isolated left-sided pulmonary vein can drain anomalously into the innominate vein and is a common form of partial anomalous pulmonary venous connection.

▶ Lai WW, Mertens LL, Cohen MS, et al (eds): *Echocardiography in Pediatric and Congenital Heart Disease: From Fetus to Adult*, 2nd edition. Chichester, UK, Wiley-Blackwell, 2016, pp 66–67.

Refer to video PER-Q299.

299. C. Bilateral bidirectional Glenn.

Video PER-Q299 shows flow from both right- and left-sided superior venae cavae (SVCs) to the branch pulmonary arteries, which is a hallmark of bilateral bidirectional Glenn surgery. Fontan completion is anastomosis of the inferior vena cava to the branch pulmonary artery. LeCompte involves bringing the branch pulmonary arteries anterior to the ascending aorta, usually in the setting of an arterial switch procedure. A Norwood procedure with a Sano conduit involves creation of a neoaorta and placement of a right ventricle–to–pulmonary artery nonvalved conduit.

▶ Lai WW, Mertens LL, Cohen MS, et al (eds): *Echocardiography in Pediatric and Congenital Heart Disease: From Fetus to Adult*, 2nd edition. Chichester, UK, Wiley-Blackwell, 2016, pp 376–377.

300. D. Total anomalous pulmonary venous drainage.

The volume load to the right side from total anomalous pulmonary venous connection (TAPVC) results in dilatation of the right ventricle and is not related to a drop in pulmonary vascular resistance. A patent foramen ovale does not cause

ANSWERS

chamber dilatation. A patent ductus arteriosus can cause left-sided chamber dilatation. Tricuspid atresia is associated with a small right ventricle.

▶ Lai WW, Mertens LL, Cohen MS, et al (eds): *Echocardiography in Pediatric and Congenital Heart Disease: From Fetus to Adult*, 2nd edition. Chichester, UK, Wiley-Blackwell, 2016, p 168.

301. B. Vertical vein with supracardiac total anomalous pulmonary venous connection.

The vertical vein with supracardiac total anomalous pulmonary venous connection (TAVPC) will drain superiorly toward the innominate (brachiocephalic) vein or superior vena cava (SVC). A vertical vein with infracardiac TAPVC will not be seen from the high parasternal view and would be draining inferiorly. A left-sided SVC would drain inferiorly toward the heart. A retroaortic innominate vein is located just underneath the aortic arch and drains slightly inferiorly to the right-sided SVC.

▶ Lai WW, Mertens LL, Cohen MS, et al (eds): *Echocardiography in Pediatric and Congenital Heart Disease: From Fetus to Adult*, 2nd edition. Chichester, UK, Wiley-Blackwell, 2016, pp 168–173.

302. B. Cor triatriatum dextrum.

This is an example of cor triatriatum dextrum, which is an embryologic remnant of the horns of the sinus venosus and has a typical wind-sock appearance in the right atrium. Cor triatriatum sinister is the more common form of cor triatriatum and results from incomplete incorporation of the common pulmonary vein into the left atrium. An atrial myxoma does not have a membranous appearance and resembles a solid tumor. Ebstein anomaly involves incomplete delamination of the septal leaflet of the tricuspid valve, with inferior displacement of the hinge point of the septal leaflet.

▶ Lai WW, Mertens LL, Cohen MS, et al (eds): *Echocardiography in Pediatric and Congenital Heart Disease: From Fetus to Adult*, 2nd edition. Chichester, UK, Wiley-Blackwell, 2016, p 240.

303. A. Dilated superior vena cava.

Patients with interrupted inferior vena cava (IVC) have drainage via a large azygos vein draining to the superior vena cava (SVC), which causes dilatation of the SVC. None of the other structures are involved and thus they are not dilated.

▶ Lai WW, Mertens LL, Cohen MS, et al (eds): *Echocardiography in Pediatric and Congenital Heart Disease: From Fetus to Adult*, 2nd edition. Chichester, UK, Wiley-Blackwell, 2016, p 187.

304. C. Maintain normal positioning of the transducer and do nothing different.

When imaging a patient with dextrocardia from the apical or subcostal view, always maintain normal positioning of the transducer or else the reader will not be able to determine whether the patient has dextrocardia. Having the patient lie on the left side only makes imaging of the right-sided heart more challenging.

▶ Lai WW, Mertens LL, Cohen MS, et al (eds): *Echocardiography in Pediatric and Congenital Heart Disease: From Fetus to Adult*, 2nd edition. Chichester, UK, Wiley-Blackwell, 2016, pp 560–561.

305. D. The IVC and hepatic veins can have various connections.

In heterotaxy patients, vascular connections are quite varied and thus there is no standard rule for where the inferior vena cava and hepatic veins may drain.

▶ Lai WW, Mertens LL, Cohen MS, et al (eds): *Echocardiography in Pediatric and Congenital Heart Disease: From Fetus to Adult*, 2nd edition. Chichester, UK, Wiley-Blackwell, 2016, p 566.

306. B. Interrupted inferior vena cava.

The patient has an interrupted inferior vena cava (IVC), and the structure you see is a prominent azygos vein, which is positioned posteriorly alongside the aorta and is draining up to the superior vena cava (SVC). Infracardiac total anomalous pulmonary venous connection (TAPVC) would have a vertical vein positioned anterior to the descending aorta, closer to the liver and draining inferiorly. A Fontan completion involves anastomosis of the IVC to the branch pulmonary artery, and no extra vessel is noted below the diaphragm. Hepatic arteriovenous malformations (AVMs) are abnormal vascular connections contained within the liver.

▶ Lai WW, Mertens LL, Cohen MS, et al (eds): *Echocardiography in Pediatric and Congenital Heart Disease: From Fetus to Adult*, 2nd edition. Chichester, UK, Wiley-Blackwell, 2016, pp 187–188.

307. C. Hypoplastic left heart syndrome.

Turner syndrome has a known association with hypoplastic left heart syndrome (HLHS). When HLHS is encountered, chromosomal analysis can be performed to evaluate for this genetic anomaly, in which one female X chromosome is absent (45,XO) or structurally altered in all cells in the patient's body.

ANSWERS

Some Turner syndrome patients will have this chromosomal abnormality in only some (not all) of their cells; this is known as mosaicism. With HLHS, a patent ductus arteriosus (PDA) is essential for survival in order to allow the dominant right heart to provide blood supply to the body as well as to the coronary arteries. In addition, a good-sized atrial communication (such as an atrial septal defect) is necessary to allow egress of left atrial blood to the right side of the heart. Other congenital cardiac defects that have a well-known association with Turner syndrome include coarctation of the aorta, bicuspid aortic valve, and partial anomalous pulmonary venous connection.

- Allen HD, Shaddy RE, Penny DJ, et al: *Moss and Adams' Heart Disease in Infants, Children, and Adolescents, Including the Fetus and Young Adult*, 9th edition. Philadelphia, Wolters Kluwer, 2016, p 626.
- Lai WW, Mertens LL, Cohen MS, et al (eds): *Echocardiography in Pediatric and Congenital Heart Disease: From Fetus to Adult*, 2nd edition. Chichester, UK, Wiley-Blackwell, 2016, pp 357–382.
- Park MK: *Park's Pediatric Cardiology for Practitioners*, 6th edition. Philadelphia, Saunders, 2014, p 14.

308. D. Left to right.

The most likely atrial-level shunting pattern seen in a 1-week-old patient with HLHS is left to right. This left-to-right atrial shunt is essential for survival, allowing oxygenated blood (returning from the pulmonary veins) to cross to the right side of the heart, where it can mix with deoxygenated blood returning from the systemic veins. The right ventricle then ejects this mixture of oxygenated and deoxygenated blood though a patent ductus arteriosus (PDA) to provide necessary perfusion of the organs and coronary arteries. Rarely, an intact atrial septum can be found with HLHS; these patients are usually very sick at birth and require emergency care. In cases with HLHS and intact atrial septum, there can be an alternate egress of blood from the left atrium by way of a levoatrial cardinal vein. This vein connects the left atrium or pulmonary veins directly to the innominate (brachiocephalic) vein, enabling blood to bypass the intact atrial septum.

- Rudolph AM: *Congenital Diseases of the Heart: Clinical-Physiological Considerations*, 3rd edition. Chichester, UK, Wiley Blackwell, 2009, pp 258, 277.

309. A. Retrograde from the patent ductus arteriosus.

Coronary and cerebral perfusion in hypoplastic left heart syndrome (HLHS) with aortic atresia (AA) and mitral atresia (MA) is accomplished via a patent ductus arteriosus (PDA), by way of retrograde perfusion through the aortic arch, delivering blood to the head and neck vessels and ascending aorta. This means that a PDA is essential for the patient's survival (a condition known as ductal dependence). Note that atrial-level shunting in HLHS with MA/AA should be left to right, and no forward flow will be seen across the aortic valve and ascending aorta. A levoatrial cardinal artery does not appear in the congenital heart disease literature.

▶ Rudolph AM: *Congenital Diseases of the Heart: Clinical-Physiological Considerations*, 3rd edition. Chichester, UK, Wiley Blackwell, 2009, p 258.

Refer to video PER-Q310.

310. B. Hypoplastic left heart syndrome.

Video PER-Q310 demonstrates hypoplastic left heart syndrome (HLHS) with a very small (but present) mitral valve, which eliminates an unguarded mitral valve orifice (choice A). The septal leaflet of the tricuspid valve is not inferiorly displaced; therefore, this patient does not have Ebstein anomaly of the tricuspid valve (choice C).

▶ Lai WW, Mertens LL, Cohen MS, et al (eds): *Echocardiography in Pediatric and Congenital Heart Disease: From Fetus to Adult*, 2nd edition. Chichester, UK, Wiley-Blackwell, 2016, pp 357–358.

Refer to video PER-Q311.

311. C. Atrial-level shunting appears restrictive (left-to-right shunt), but further investigation is needed.

Video PER-Q311 demonstrates an atrial septal defect that looks small and possibly restrictive by 2D imaging and color Doppler; however, further echocardiographic investigation is needed to confirm this suspicion. The use of an additional view, such as the subcostal short-axis view at the level of the atrial septum, can be helpful in further evaluating the atrial-level shunt with color flow and spectral Doppler. The use of spectral Doppler to record a mean gradient can be useful, as a waveform that does not return to the spectral Doppler baseline—which demonstrates a maintained increased flow velocity—can be a sign of restriction. Notice the color flow aliasing that is occurring with a relatively high Nyquist limit of 92.4 cm/sec; this implies an increased shunt velocity, which also suggests a restrictive atrial defect.

▶ Lai WW, Mertens LL, Cohen MS, et al (eds): *Echocardiography in Pediatric and Congenital Heart Disease: From Fetus to Adult*, 2nd edition. Chichester, UK, Wiley-Blackwell, 2016, p 364.

Refer to video PER-Q312.

312. B. Morphologic right-to-left atrial shunt.

Video PER-Q312 demonstrates a secundum atrial septal defect versus a patent foramen ovale with right-to-left atrial shunting. This is an obligatory right-to-left atrial shunt because of the atretic pulmonary valve. From this subcostal long-axis view the area where a superior sinus venous defect would exist looks intact.

▶ Lai WW, Mertens LL, Cohen MS, et al (eds): *Echocardiography in Pediatric and Congenital Heart Disease: From Fetus to Adult*, 2nd edition. Chichester, UK, Wiley-Blackwell, 2016, p 198.

Refer to video PER-Q313.

313. A. Aortic valve atresia in the setting of hypoplastic left heart syndrome.

Video PER-Q313 demonstrates an extremely small aorta with aortic valve atresia. Because the aortic valve is atretic, flow to the head and neck arteries and coronary arteries must be supplied in retrograde fashion from a patent ductus arteriosus; this is shown by the red (retrograde) flow seen in the aortic arch. When scanning an aorta of this size, the echocardiographer should use the highest-frequency transducer that allows good visualization. The superior vena cava is not visualized in this video clip. Total anomalous pulmonary venous connection and double aortic arch do not cause reversal of flow in the aortic arch. When scanning and sweeping from the suprasternal window, care must be taken not to accidentally miss the markedly small ascending aorta.

▶ Lai WW, Mertens LL, Cohen MS, et al (eds): *Echocardiography in Pediatric and Congenital Heart Disease: From Fetus to Adult*, 2nd edition. Chichester, UK, Wiley-Blackwell, 2016, pp 98, 359.

Refer to video PER-Q314.

314. C. Ebstein anomaly of the tricuspid valve.

Video PER-Q314 demonstrates Ebstein anomaly of the tricuspid valve. Notice the apical (inferior) displacement of the tricuspid valve septal leaflet and the atrialized portion of the right ventricle.

▶ Lai WW, Mertens LL, Cohen MS, et al (eds): *Echocardiography in Pediatric and Congenital Heart Disease: From Fetus to Adult*, 2nd edition. Chichester, UK, Wiley-Blackwell, 2016, pp 231–233.

PART 4

Postoperative Anatomy

315. B. The patient will need a pulmonary valve replacement, most likely before 18 years of age, to address progressive pulmonary valve insufficiency with right heart dilatation.

In patients with tetralogy of Fallot (TOF), the main pulmonary artery and pulmonary valve are often very small. Most patients undergo the placement of a transannular patch to widen the pulmonary annulus and pulmonary artery, in addition to closure of the ventricular septal defect and removal of right ventricular outflow tract muscle bundles. The surgical treatment allows for a widely patent right ventricular outflow tract but also disturbs the integrity of the pulmonary valve. This results in incompetency of the pulmonary valve, leading to progressive pulmonary insufficiency, which in turn can lead to progressive right ventricular dilatation over time. The increasing right ventricular dilatation in postoperative TOF patients is associated with ventricular arrhythmias, right ventricular dysfunction, and right heart failure accompanied by left ventricular dysfunction. To prevent these complications, pulmonary valve replacement is generally required, often before 18 years of age. The integrity of the aortic valve is not affected by surgery. A vascular ring is not generally associated with TOF, and if not initially present it will not develop over time.

- Geva T: Indications for pulmonary valve replacement in repaired tetralogy of Fallot: the quest continues. Circulation 128:1855–1857, 2013.
- Lai WW, Mertens LL, Cohen MS, et al (eds): *Echocardiography in Pediatric and Congenital Heart Disease: From Fetus to Adult*, 2nd edition. Chichester, UK, Wiley-Blackwell, 2016, pp 420–423.
- Lewin MB, Stout K (eds): *Echocardiography in Congenital Heart Disease*. Philadelphia, Elsevier Saunders, 2012, pp 89–92.

316. A. Residual shunting across the ventricular septal defect.

Pulmonary valve insufficiency and pulmonary stenosis are all associated with tetralogy of Fallot (TOF). The left ventricular outflow tract is not affected in TOF. After surgery, no significant residual ventricular shunting should be seen, although occasionally a small residual ventricular septal defect can be found post repair.

- Geva T: Indications for pulmonary valve replacement in repaired tetralogy of Fallot: the quest continues. Circulation 128:1855–1857, 2013.
- Lewin MB, Stout K (eds): *Echocardiography in Congenital Heart Disease*. Philadelphia, Elsevier Saunders, 2012, pp 89–92.

ANSWERS

317. D. The pulmonary artery pressure cannot be determined.

Pulmonary artery systolic pressure can be estimated using the tricuspid regurgitant jet peak velocity. However, this can be done only in the absence of pulmonary valve or pulmonary artery obstruction. In this case there is pulmonary valve stenosis as well as some degree of branch pulmonary artery stenosis. A noninvasive estimation of right and left pulmonary artery pressures, and therefore a determination of whether pulmonary hypertension is present, cannot be made accurately.

- Lai WW, Mertens LL, Cohen MS, et al (eds): *Echocardiography in Pediatric and Congenital Heart Disease: From Fetus to Adult*, 2nd edition. Chichester, UK, Wiley-Blackwell, 2016, pp 420–423.
- Lewin MB, Stout K (eds): *Echocardiography in Congenital Heart Disease*. Philadelphia, Elsevier Saunders, 2012, pp 89–92.

318. D. Severe.

This patient has a history of tetralogy of Fallot status post repair. Tetralogy of Fallot is associated with DiGeorge syndrome. Pulmonary valve insufficiency is a known complication of tetralogy of Fallot repair. Right ventricular dilatation occurs secondary to pulmonary insufficiency. Significant dilatation of the ventricle can cause an upward "tilt" or displacement of the tricuspid valve, resulting in an abnormal tricuspid annular plane systolic excursion (TAPSE). The description of the echo findings is most consistent with severe pulmonary insufficiency.

- Lai WW, Mertens LL, Cohen MS, et al (eds): *Echocardiography in Pediatric and Congenital Heart Disease: From Fetus to Adult*, 2nd edition. Chichester, UK, Wiley-Blackwell, 2016, pp 420–423.
- Lewin MB, Stout K (eds): *Echocardiography in Congenital Heart Disease*. Philadelphia, Elsevier Saunders, 2012, pp 89–92.

319. C. The finding is common and expected post TOF repair.

This finding is expected for a postoperative patient with TOF. The echobright portion of the septum represents a patch placed in the septum by the surgeon to close the ventricular septal defect associated with tetralogy of Fallot (TOF). Such patches are made of Dacron, Gore-Tex, or another material that appears echobright on the echocardiogram. This portion of the septum has poor mobility and may appear flat or hypokinetic, but that finding alone does not suggest pulmonary hypertension in this patient. Ligation of a conal branch from the right coronary artery at the time of surgery is not uncommon, as conal branches often cross the right ventricular outflow tract in the region where the surgeon places the transannular patch. However, if ligation of the conal branch occurred, it would cause wall motion abnormality of the right ventricular outflow tract (not the base of the interventricular septum).

▶ Lai WW, Mertens LL, Cohen MS, et al (eds): *Echocardiography in Pediatric and Congenital Heart Disease: From Fetus to Adult*, 2nd edition. Chichester, UK, Wiley-Blackwell, 2016, pp 345, 420–423.

▶ Lewin MB, Stout K (eds): *Echocardiography in Congenital Heart Disease*. Philadelphia, Elsevier Saunders, 2012, pp 89–92.

320. B. Left upper pulmonary vein diameter.

Postoperatively, patients with tetralogy of Fallot can develop pulmonary artery or pulmonary valve stenosis. While it is important to perform a complete echocardiographic exam whenever possible, the pulmonary veins are generally not affected in tetralogy of Fallot, and surgical repair of this condition does not involve any type of repair or manipulation of the pulmonary veins.

▶ Lai WW, Mertens LL, Cohen MS, et al (eds): *Echocardiography in Pediatric and Congenital Heart Disease: From Fetus to Adult*, 2nd edition. Chichester, UK, Wiley-Blackwell, 2016, pp 416–423.

▶ Lewin MB, Stout K (eds): *Echocardiography in Congenital Heart Disease*. Philadelphia, Elsevier Saunders, 2012, pp 89–92.

321. D. Right ventricular dilatation.

Right ventricular dilatation secondary to significant pulmonary insufficiency results in displacement or tilting of the tricuspid valve annulus superiorly. In some instances, the right ventricle can dilate so severely that it can displace the left ventricle; the right ventricle thereby becomes the apex-forming ventricle.

▶ Lai WW, Mertens LL, Cohen MS, et al (eds): *Echocardiography in Pediatric and Congenital Heart Disease: From Fetus to Adult*, 2nd edition. Chichester, UK, Wiley-Blackwell, 2016, pp 416–423.

▶ Lewin MB, Stout K (eds): *Echocardiography in Congenital Heart Disease*. Philadelphia, Elsevier Saunders, 2012, pp 89–92.

322. D. Right ventricle to pulmonary artery.

A conduit is a tube that generally connects the right ventricle to the pulmonary artery. It typically has a bioprosthetic valve placed inside it. This bioprosthetic valve usually wears out over time and needs to be replaced periodically.

▶ Lai WW, Mertens LL, Cohen MS, et al (eds): *Echocardiography in Pediatric and Congenital Heart Disease: From Fetus to Adult*, 2nd edition. Chichester, UK, Wiley-Blackwell, 2016, pp 420–421.

▸ Lewin MB, Stout K (eds): *Echocardiography in Congenital Heart Disease*. Philadelphia, Elsevier Saunders, 2012, pp 89–92.

323. A. Typical findings post transannular patch repair.

These findings are typical for a child with tetralogy of Fallot status post transannular patch repair. There is mild right ventricular dilatation secondary to the pulmonary insufficiency. Septal flattening is typically seen in the septum in the region of the patch. A small, restrictive residual ventricular septal defect (VSD) can sometimes be found after repair. It is important to note any residual VSDs for endocarditis prophylaxis recommendations, although most will not be of any hemodynamic significance, nor will the majority require reintervention.

▸ Lai WW, Mertens LL, Cohen MS, et al (eds): *Echocardiography in Pediatric and Congenital Heart Disease: From Fetus to Adult*, 2nd edition. Chichester, UK, Wiley-Blackwell, 2016, pp 420–423.

▸ Lewin MB, Stout K (eds): *Echocardiography in Congenital Heart Disease*. Philadelphia, Elsevier Saunders, 2012, pp 89–92.

324. D. All of the above.

A complete echocardiographic evaluation of a patient with a history of aortic coarctation includes evaluation of the aortic valve. This is because a bicuspid aortic valve is associated with coarctation of the aorta in 50%–85% of patients. Doppler evaluation of the abdominal aorta can suggest the presence of a residual coarctation, particularly if flow continuation is seen in diastole. It is also important to evaluate the isthmus and descending aorta to ensure that there are no areas of residual aortic arch hypoplasia or narrowing.

▸ Lai WW, Mertens LL, Cohen MS, et al (eds): *Echocardiography in Pediatric and Congenital Heart Disease: From Fetus to Adult*, 2nd edition. Chichester, UK, Wiley-Blackwell, 2016, pp 339–348.

▸ Lewin MB, Stout K (eds): *Echocardiography in Congenital Heart Disease*. Philadelphia, Elsevier Saunders, 2012, pp 176–179.

325. D. More information is needed to make this calculation.

The velocity suggests that there is a residual coarctation. However, in the setting of proximal stenosis, the simplified Bernoulli equation, $\Delta P = 4V^2$, cannot be used, as this equation assumes a normal proximal velocity that is negligible in the calculation. In the setting of aortic or supravalvular aortic stenosis, the proximal velocity in the ascending aorta might be *increased, in which case it is no longer negligible and needs to be used in the expanded (modified) Bernoulli equation*

$$\Delta P = 4\ (V_2^2 - V_1^2)$$

to calculate an accurate gradient. Failure to do so can cause an overestimation of the gradient.

- Lai WW, Mertens LL, Cohen MS, et al (eds): *Echocardiography in Pediatric and Congenital Heart Disease: From Fetus to Adult*, 2nd edition. Chichester, UK, Wiley-Blackwell, 2016, pp 339–348.
- Lewin MB, Stout K (eds): *Echocardiography in Congenital Heart Disease*. Philadelphia, Elsevier Saunders, 2012, pp 176–179.

326. C. Balloon aortoplasty for coarctation of the aorta.

In infants, the preferred method for repair of most patients with a coarctation is a surgical approach. After infancy, balloon angioplasty can often be used for relief of a coarctation. Stent placement is generally not used for infants and small children due to their small aortic size. Stent placement is generally reserved for older children, because a larger stent can be deployed and can be expanded to accommodate the child's growth (often to adult size). Robotic surgery for coarctation repair does not exist. Direct dilatation with an aortic dilator would require surgery and is generally not used.

- Lai WW, Mertens LL, Cohen MS, et al (eds): *Echocardiography in Pediatric and Congenital Heart Disease: From Fetus to Adult*, 2nd edition. Chichester, UK, Wiley-Blackwell, 2016, pp 348–349.
- Lewin MB, Stout K (eds): *Echocardiography in Congenital Heart Disease*. Philadelphia, Elsevier Saunders, 2012, pp 176–179.

327. D. V_1 represents the velocity in the ascending aorta and V_2 the velocity in the descending aorta.

V_1 represents the velocity proximal to the coarctation, and V_2 represents the velocity distal to the coarctation. It is important to use both velocities in the modified Bernoulli equation when evaluating a patient with a history of coarctation who has any proximal aortic obstruction, such as valvular or supravalvular aortic stenosis. The other choices can be dismissed as incorrect because none of the other velocities mentioned is obtained from the portion of the aorta immediately proximal to the coarctation.

- Lai WW, Mertens LL, Cohen MS, et al (eds): *Echocardiography in Pediatric and Congenital Heart Disease: From Fetus to Adult*, 2nd edition. Chichester, UK, Wiley-Blackwell, 2016, pp 339–348.
- Lewin MB, Stout K (eds): *Echocardiography in Congenital Heart Disease*. Philadelphia, Elsevier Saunders, 2012, pp 176–179.

328. A. Bicuspid aortic valve and ventricular septal defect.

During evaluation of a patient with coarctation of the aorta (CoA), it is important to ensure there are no other cardiac lesions present. CoA can be associated with many lesions, the most common being bicuspid aortic valve and ventricular septal defect.

▶ Lai WW, Mertens LL, Cohen MS, et al (eds): *Echocardiography in Pediatric and Congenital Heart Disease: From Fetus to Adult*, 2nd edition. Chichester, UK, Wiley-Blackwell, 2016, pp 339–340.

▶ Lewin MB, Stout K (eds): *Echocardiography in Congenital Heart Disease*. Philadelphia, Elsevier Saunders, 2012, pp 176–179.

329. C. Subcostal views.

Subcostal views will allow for imaging of the abdominal aorta. Doppler of the abdominal aorta demonstrating blunted upstroke and diastolic flow continuation suggests a residual coarctation.

▶ Lai WW, Mertens LL, Cohen MS, et al (eds): *Echocardiography in Pediatric and Congenital Heart Disease: From Fetus to Adult*, 2nd edition. Chichester, UK, Wiley-Blackwell, 2016, pp 341–345.

▶ Lewin MB, Stout K (eds): *Echocardiography in Congenital Heart Disease*. Philadelphia, Elsevier Saunders, 2012, pp 176–179.

330. B. Double envelope Doppler waveform.

A double envelope Doppler waveform indicates a difference in the proximal and distal velocities. This is a classic finding with coarctation of the aorta. A dagger-shaped Doppler waveform may indicate dynamic obstruction.

▶ Lewin MB, Stout K (eds): *Echocardiography in Congenital Heart Disease*. Philadelphia, Elsevier Saunders, 2012, pp 176–178.

331. D. The cursor is not well aligned and there is peripheral branch pulmonary stenosis.

In this patient, the cursor is most likely not well aligned. The normal pulsed-wave Doppler at the site of coarctation repair indicates that there is no significant re-coarctation. Continuous-wave Doppler is characterized by range ambiguity; hence peripheral branch pulmonary stenosis could be sampled along the line of the Doppler cursor. In the setting of a re-coarctation, the abdominal aorta, on color Doppler and pulsed-wave Doppler, could also be expected to have increased velocities; the question stipulates a normal velocity by pulsed-wave Doppler in the region of repair, so re-coarctation is excluded. After surgical coarctation repair, the ductus arteriosus would have been ligated.

- Lai WW, Mertens LL, Cohen MS, et al (eds): *Echocardiography in Pediatric and Congenital Heart Disease: From Fetus to Adult*, 2nd edition. Chichester, UK, Wiley-Blackwell, 2016, pp 339–345.
- Lewin MB, Stout K (eds): *Echocardiography in Congenital Heart Disease*. Philadelphia, Elsevier Saunders, 2012, pp 176–179.

332. A. Widening of the distance between the left subclavian and left carotid arteries.

Coarctation of the aorta (CoA) is associated with an increased distance between the left subclavian artery and the left carotid artery. CoA can also be associated with a posterior shelf near the isthmus as well as a bicuspid aortic valve and a ventricular septal defect. Diastolic flow continuation would be seen in patients with residual coarctation. A bovine arch and aberrant right subclavian artery can be found in association with CoA, but these findings are not typically seen with coarctation and furthermore can be difficult to diagnose if attention is not paid to the branching pattern of the head and neck vessels.

- Kantoch M, Pieroni D, Roland JM, et al: Association of distal displacement of the left subclavian artery and coarctation of the aorta. Pediatr Cardiol 13:164–169, 1992.
- Lai WW, Mertens LL, Cohen MS, et al (eds): *Echocardiography in Pediatric and Congenital Heart Disease: From Fetus to Adult*, 2nd edition. Chichester, UK, Wiley-Blackwell, 2016, pp 339–345.

333. C. An absent left subclavian artery because it was used for a subclavian flap coarctation repair.

An older surgical technique used for coarctation repair, known as a Waldhausen repair, involves sacrificing the left subclavian artery. This technique is performed by creating a flap out of the left subclavian artery to widen the narrowed region of the aorta. Because this surgery utilizes native tissue, it has the advantage of enabling the repaired area to grow with the patient. However, patients who underwent this form of CoA repair were noted to have shorter arms on the left and absent left arm pulses, even though collateral vessels had developed to provide flow to the arm. Contrary to the myths about this surgery, there was no risk of the arm "falling off." Techniques have since evolved, and more popular surgical approaches now include an end-to-end anastomosis, in which the narrowed region is removed and the aorta is brought back together. If extra patch material is required to augment the arch (generally a homograft is used), it does not encircle the aorta, allowing the aorta to grow with the patient.

- Adams EE, Davidson WR, Swallow NA, et al: Long-term results of the subclavian flap repair for coarctation of the aorta in infants. World J Pediatr Congenit Heart Surg 4:13–18, 2013.
- Brown ML, Burkhart HM, Connolly HM, et al: Coarctation of the aorta: lifelong surveillance is mandatory following surgical repair. J Am Coll Cardiol 62:1020–1025, 2013.

334. B. Pulmonary valve.

Patients with left-sided cardiac lesions can have multiple abnormalities on the left side of the heart. It is important to perform a complete evaluation with special attention to all left-sided cardiac lesions, including the left ventricle (which may be small or hypertrophied), the aortic arch (which may be hypoplastic or have a coarctation/interrupted aortic arch), and the mitral valve (which may also be abnormal). It is very uncommon to have both right-sided and left-sided valvular lesions, such as aortic and pulmonary stenoses, so the pulmonary valve is not usually affected in patients with left-sided obstructive lesions.

- Lai WW, Mertens LL, Cohen MS, et al (eds): *Echocardiography in Pediatric and Congenital Heart Disease: From Fetus to Adult*, 2nd edition. Chichester, UK, Wiley-Blackwell, 2016, pp 340–343.
- Lewin MB, Stout K (eds): *Echocardiography in Congenital Heart Disease*. Philadelphia, Elsevier Saunders, 2012, pp 170–176.

335. A. There may be significant residual aortic stenosis in the setting of poor cardiac output.

The degree of aortic stenosis can be underestimated in the setting of poor cardiac output. Valve thickness, leaflet excursion, and other factors can and should be used to give an indication of the potential for significant aortic stenosis, as the degree of stenosis can be underestimated based on the Doppler velocity when poor ventricular systolic function is present.

- Lai WW, Mertens LL, Cohen MS, et al (eds): *Echocardiography in Pediatric and Congenital Heart Disease: From Fetus to Adult*, 2nd edition. Chichester, UK, Wiley-Blackwell, 2016, pp 340–344.
- Lewin MB, Stout K (eds): *Echocardiography in Congenital Heart Disease*. Philadelphia, Elsevier Saunders, 2012, pp 170–176.

336. B. Shone syndrome.

The findings described are consistent with Shone syndrome. Shone syndrome (also known as Shone complex) consists of multiple left-sided lesions including coarctation of the aorta, a mitral valve abnormality (typically a supravalvular mitral ring and parachute mitral valve), and subaortic stenosis. The left ventricle is often small. Patau syndrome (trisomy 13) can be associated with many cardiac lesions, including ventricular septal defects, atrial septal defects, and patent ductus arteriosus. DiGeorge syndrome is often associated with cardiac lesions such as tetralogy of Fallot, pulmonary atresia, and interrupted aortic arch. Down syndrome (trisomy 21) is also associated with cardiac lesions, including endocardial cushion defects, ventricular septal defects, and tetralogy of Fallot.

▸ Lai WW, Mertens LL, Cohen MS, et al (eds): *Echocardiography in Pediatric and Congenital Heart Disease: From Fetus to Adult*, 2nd edition. Chichester, UK, Wiley-Blackwell, 2016, pp 340–343, 383.

▸ Lewin MB, Stout K (eds): *Echocardiography in Congenital Heart Disease*. Philadelphia, Elsevier Saunders, 2012, pp 170–176.

ANSWERS

337. C. A mean gradient consistent with moderate stenosis.

Mitral gradients are assessed using mean mitral valve inflow gradients from Doppler tracings. A mean inflow gradient between 5 and 10 mmHg is considered moderate mitral stenosis.

▸ Baumgartner H, Hung J, Bermejo J, et al: Echocardiographic assessment of valve stenosis: EAE/ASE recommendations for clinical practice. J Am Soc Echocardi 22:1–23, 2009.

▸ Lewin MB, Stout K (eds): *Echocardiography in Congenital Heart Disease*. Philadelphia, Elsevier Saunders, 2012, p 172.

338. A. AS cannot be determined without knowing the baseline gradient obtained early after valve implantation.

When assessing mechanical valves, one must be aware that there is an increase in the baseline velocity that can vary depending upon the manufacturer and type of valve. Published charts can provide the expected baseline measurement for most valves, but it is also important to trend measurements within the same patient to grade the degree of stenosis.

▸ Nishimura RA, Otto CM, Bonow RO, et al: 2014 AHA/ACC guideline for the management of patients with valvular heart disease: a report of the American College of Cardiology/American Heart Association Task Force on Practice Guidelines. Circulation 129:2440–2492, 2014.

339. D. Both A and B.

Following balloon pulmonary valvuloplasty, most children will have a mild degree of pulmonary stenosis and pulmonary insufficiency. Cardiologists are willing to accept the tradeoff between correcting pulmonary stenosis and risking pulmonary insufficiency. The more aggressive the valvuloplasty, the more successful the improvement in pulmonary stenosis—but the higher the risk for pulmonary insufficiency. Moderate pulmonary insufficiency may be seen after valvuloplasty, but in the hands of a skilled pediatric interventionist most children will, at worst, have only mild insufficiency.

▶ Lai WW, Mertens LL, Cohen MS, et al (eds): *Echocardiography in Pediatric and Congenital Heart Disease: From Fetus to Adult*, 2nd edition. Chichester, UK, Wiley-Blackwell, 2016, pp 281–287.

▶ Lewin MB, Stout K (eds): *Echocardiography in Congenital Heart Disease*. Philadelphia, Elsevier Saunders, 2012, pp 156–162.

340. A. Closing the tricuspid valve with a fenestrated patch, thereby excluding the right ventricle.

The Starnes procedure is a surgical approach to extend the lives of patients with severe Ebstein anomaly as well as other severe tricuspid valve anomalies. The Starnes procedure consists of closing the tricuspid valve and excluding the right ventricle (i.e., surgically creating tricuspid atresia). This method is mainly limited to patients with severe Ebstein anomaly; left untreated, many such patients would otherwise not survive.

▶ Reemsten BL, Starnes VA: Fenestrated right ventricular exclusion (Starnes' procedure) for severe neonatal Ebstein's anomaly. Oper Tech Thorac Cardiovasc Surg 13:91–100, 2008.

341. C. Moderate to severe.

Flow reversal in the descending aorta indicates at least moderate aortic valve insufficiency. Doppler evaluation of the abdominal aorta is an important factor in assessing the degree of aortic regurgitation.

▶ Lai WW, Mertens LL, Cohen MS, et al (eds): *Echocardiography in Pediatric and Congenital Heart Disease: From Fetus to Adult*, 2nd edition. Chichester, UK, Wiley-Blackwell, 2016, p 83.

▶ Lewin MB, Stout K (eds): *Echocardiography in Congenital Heart Disease*. Philadelphia, Elsevier Saunders, 2012, pp 61–65.

342. B. Moderate pulmonary stenosis only.

There is an increased velocity across the pulmonary valve, indicating moderate pulmonary stenosis with a peak velocity of 49 mmHg. The tricuspid regurgitant (TR) jet may be used only to estimate pulmonary artery systolic pressure in the absence of distal obstruction. Thus, in the setting of pulmonary stenosis, the TR jet estimates right ventricular systolic pressure (secondary to the presence of pulmonary stenosis) but cannot estimate pulmonary artery systolic pressures distal to the site of pulmonary stenosis. Nonetheless, given the elevated gradient across the pulmonary valve and the nearly equivalent TR and pulmonary valve velocities, it seems very unlikely that distal pulmonary artery pressures are elevated—that is, it is highly unlikely that this patient has pulmonary hypertension.

- Lai WW, Mertens LL, Cohen MS, et al (eds): *Echocardiography in Pediatric and Congenital Heart Disease: From Fetus to Adult*, 2nd edition. Chichester, UK, Wiley-Blackwell, 2016, pp 79–82.

343. D. Mild to moderate pulmonary valve insufficiency.

A Ross procedure places a patient's native pulmonary valve in the aortic position. It is used for treatment of aortic valve pathology (aortic valve stenosis and/or regurgitation). A conduit or tissue pulmonary valve is generally used to replace the native pulmonary valve. The new pulmonary valve is thoroughly interrogated to ensure that there is no evidence of valvular insufficiency or stenosis prior to placement. The pulmonary valve must also be approximately the same size as the native aortic valve. However, because a tissue valve (or often a valved conduit) is used in the pulmonary position, these valves often deteriorate and become insufficient over time, resulting in worsening pulmonary insufficiency. Nevertheless, the Ross procedure is useful in younger patients because the neoaortic valve (the former pulmonary valve) is composed of living tissue, which can theoretically grow in proportion to the patient's somatic growth. Also, it allows patients to avoid using anticoagulation medications such as warfarin (Coumadin); this is particularly important for patients who want to remain active in sports (since severe bleeding due to a sports injury becomes less of a concern) or in young women who might get pregnant in the future (since warfarin has known teratogenic effects on the fetus).

- Bowdish ME, Kumar SR, Starnes VA: The Ross procedure: an excellent option in the right hands. Ann Transl Med 4:471, 2016.
- Lai WW, Mertens LL, Cohen MS, et al (eds): *Echocardiography in Pediatric and Congenital Heart Disease: From Fetus to Adult*, 2nd edition. Chichester, UK, Wiley-Blackwell, 2016, p 339.

344. B. Patency of Norwood anastomosis.

The infant in this scenario has reduced systolic function. Obstruction of the Norwood anastomosis will have two negative effects. First, it will impose an increased afterload on the single right ventricle, and this can be detrimental to ventricular systolic function. Second, if there is no antegrade aortic root flow, the coronaries will be fed solely in retrograde fashion through the native ascending aorta that arises from the Norwood anastomosis. If the obstruction is proximal to the takeoff of the native ascending aorta, coronary perfusion could be compromised. Therefore, evaluation of the patency of the Norwood connection is imperative, as stenosis may require additional surgical intervention. Atrial septal and pulmonary blood flow patency is important to evaluate in the setting of excessive cyanosis post Norwood. Tricuspid valve dysfunction (in particular, tricuspid valve regurgitation) is important to recognize because it can occur as a result of reduced ventricular systolic function, but a treatable cause of ventricular systolic function (such as obstruction of the Norwood anastomosis) should still be sought.

▸ Bartram U, Grünenfelder J, Van Praagh R: Causes of death after the modified Norwood procedure: a study of 122 postmortem cases. Ann Thorac Surg 64:1795–1802, 1997.

▸ Lai WW, Mertens LL, Cohen MS, et al (eds): *Echocardiography in Pediatric and Congenital Heart Disease: From Fetus to Adult*, 2nd edition. Chichester, UK, Wiley-Blackwell, 2016, pp 370–378.

345. C. Assessment of the atrial septum.

As part of the Norwood procedure, some type of systemic–to–pulmonary artery connection must be established to enable enough blood to be oxygenated via the pulmonary arteries to maintain an adequate systemic arterial saturation. This generally occurs via a systemic–to–pulmonary artery shunt (e.g., a Blalock-Taussig shunt) or a right ventricle–to–pulmonary artery (Sano) conduit. In either type of systemic–to–pulmonary artery connection, a high-velocity Doppler signal (usually greater than 2.5–3 m/sec) should be obtained. This particular infant has what appears to be a patent Sano conduit, although there is unexpectedly low velocity noted across the conduit. Etiologies could include pulmonary vascular disease or restriction in the egress of pulmonary blood flow back to the heart. This obstruction can occur at the level of the pulmonary veins or at the level of the atrial septum. Despite atrial septectomy at the time of Norwood, the atrial septum may grow back. The patency of the atrial communication should be assessed during all echocardiographic evaluations.

▸ Bartram U, Grünenfelder J, Van Praagh R: Causes of death after the modified Norwood procedure: a study of 122 postmortem cases. Ann Thorac Surg 64:1795–1802, 1997.

▸ Lai WW, Mertens LL, Cohen MS, et al (eds): *Echocardiography in Pediatric and Congenital Heart Disease: From Fetus to Adult*, 2nd edition. Chichester, UK, Wiley-Blackwell, 2016, pp 370–378.

346. A. Modified Blalock-Taussig shunt.

See Color Plate 11 on page xxiv.

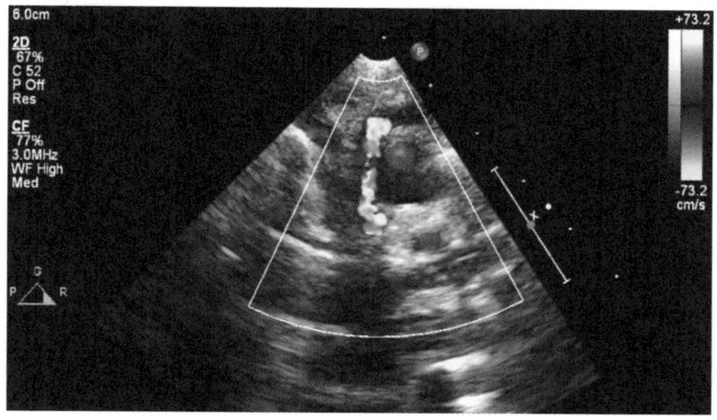

This image, obtained using a suprasternal coronal window, demonstrates the modified Blalock-Taussig shunt descending from the innominate (brachiocephalic) artery into the right pulmonary artery. Note the aliasing color Doppler with the Nyquist set in the 70s, suggesting high-velocity flow.

▸ Lai WW, Mertens LL, Cohen MS, et al (eds): *Echocardiography in Pediatric and Congenital Heart Disease: From Fetus to Adult*, 2nd edition. Chichester, UK, Wiley-Blackwell, 2016, pp 370–378.

347. B. Normal for Norwood, with Blalock-Taussig (systemic-to-pulmonary artery) shunt.

See Color Plate 12 on page xxv.

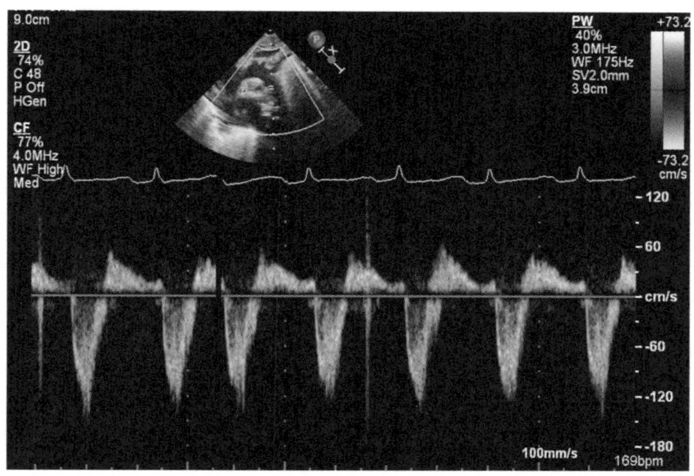

This pattern represents the normal unobstructed flow down the descending aorta, with retrograde diastolic flow seen into the modified Blalock-Taussig shunt. A Sano shunt does not produce retrograde flow in the descending aorta. The systolic Doppler pattern is not blunted, as would be expected with a coarctation. Severe tricuspid insufficiency does not produce retrograde diastolic flow in the descending aorta.

▸ Lai WW, Mertens LL, Cohen MS, et al (eds): *Echocardiography in Pediatric and Congenital Heart Disease: From Fetus to Adult*, 2nd edition. Chichester, UK, Wiley-Blackwell, 2016, pp 370–378.

348. C. Pulmonary artery.

An example of a case where a Blalock-Taussig shunt (BTS) is used to stabilize pulmonary blood flow is in a patient with hypoplastic left heart syndrome (HLHS). A Norwood procedure is the first-stage palliative procedure in patients with HLHS. The Norwood procedure consists of an atrial septectomy, aortic reconstruction to a neoaorta (using the patient's own pulmonary artery), patent ductus arteriosus ligation, and establishment of a BTS or Sano conduit. A BTS is sewn onto the innominate (brachiocephalic) artery and then the central pulmonary artery. A Sano conduit is sewn onto the right ventricle and then the central pulmonary artery. A BTS or Sano conduit would not be sewn to the inferior vena cava or the left ventricle.

- Allen HD, Driscoll DJ, Shaddy RE, et al: *Moss and Adams' Heart Disease in Infants, Children, and Adolescents: Including the Fetus and Young Adult*, 8th edition. Philadelphia, Lippincott Williams & Wilkins, 2013, pp 1074–1080.
- Lai WW, Mertens LL, Cohen MS, et al (eds): *Echocardiography in Pediatric and Congenital Heart Disease: From Fetus to Adult*, 2nd edition. Chichester, UK, Wiley-Blackwell, 2016, pp 361–366.

349. D. Coronary sinus.

Among the options given, the only vein that drains desaturated blood that continues to drain to the heart after a nonfenestrated Fontan palliation is the coronary sinus; the Thebesian veins (not given as an option) also do so. The other options—the hepatic veins, the hemiazygos vein, and the azygos vein—drain passively to the pulmonary arteries through either the Glenn or Fontan pathway.

- Lai WW, Mertens LL, Cohen MS, et al (eds): *Echocardiography in Pediatric and Congenital Heart Disease: From Fetus to Adult*, 2nd edition. Chichester, UK, Wiley-Blackwell, 2016, pp 370–378.

350. D. Patent right-sided SVC to right pulmonary artery and patent left-sided SVC to left-sided pulmonary artery connections.

A bidirectional Glenn surgery consists of anastomosis of the right-sided superior vena cava (SVC) to the right pulmonary artery (RPA). Bilateral bidirectional Glenn consists of right-sided SVC to RPA and left-sided SVC to LPA. An inferior vena cava (IVC) to pulmonary artery connection is a Fontan completion. An aortopulmonary connection is usually a Blalock-Taussig or central shunt.

- Lai WW, Mertens LL, Cohen MS, et al (eds): *Echocardiography in Pediatric and Congenital Heart Disease: From Fetus to Adult*, 2nd edition. Chichester, UK, Wiley-Blackwell, 2016, pp 376–377.

351. C. Inferior vena cava.

The inferior vena cava, with its desaturated blood flow, is sewn to an extracardiac Fontan conduit. Therefore, choices A, B, and D are incorrect.

▶ Lai WW, Mertens LL, Cohen MS, et al (eds): *Echocardiography in Pediatric and Congenital Heart Disease: From Fetus to Adult*, 2nd edition. Chichester, UK, Wiley-Blackwell, 2016, p 545.

352. D. Flow through a right ventricle–to–pulmonary artery conduit.

See Color Plate 13 on page xxv.

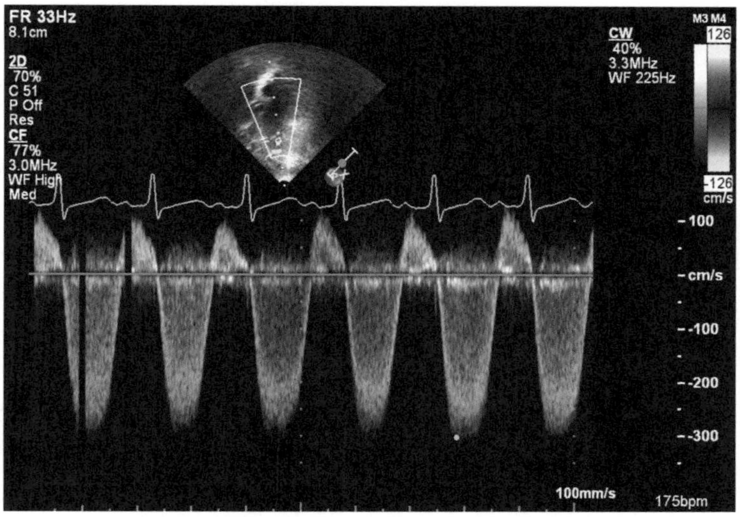

The to-and-fro pattern observed here is classic for the non-valved right ventricle–to–pulmonary artery (Sano) conduit used as palliation in hypoplastic left heart syndrome. Flow through a modified Blalock-Taussig shunt would be expected to demonstrate a continuously antegrade pattern throughout the cardiac cycle. The Doppler flow pattern across a pulmonary artery is systolic, generally high-velocity, and without a diastolic component (assuming the absence of pulmonary valve regurgitation). Flow through the tricuspid valve is diastolic and low-velocity.

▶ Lai WW, Mertens LL, Cohen MS, et al (eds): *Echocardiography in Pediatric and Congenital Heart Disease: From Fetus to Adult*, 2nd edition. Chichester, UK, Wiley-Blackwell, 2016, pp 370–378.

353. B. Superior vena cava.

In a right-sided bidirectional Glenn procedure, the right superior vena cava (SVC) is divided and then is sewn (anastomosed) to the right pulmonary artery. In a left-sided bidirectional Glenn procedure, a left SVC is divided and then anastomosed to the left pulmonary artery. In a bidirectional Glenn shunt, desaturated venous blood flows from the SVC to the branch pulmonary artery, making choices A, C, and D incorrect.

▶ Lai WW, Mertens LL, Cohen MS, et al (eds): *Echocardiography in Pediatric and Congenital Heart Disease: From Fetus to Adult*, 2nd edition. Chichester, UK, Wiley-Blackwell, 2016, pp 183, 376, 545.

Refer to video PER-Q354.

354. B. Obstructed modified Blalock-Taussig shunt.

Video PER-Q354 demonstrates a nearly completely occluded modified Blalock-Taussig shunt, which is the reason for cyanosis in this patient. Branch pulmonary artery stenosis could be a contributing factor but is not seen in the video. The flow pattern is not typical of the low-velocity continuous flow seen through a bidirectional Glenn anastomosis. Excessive pulmonary blood flow should not result in significant cyanosis; if anything, oxygen saturations could be higher than usual.

▶ Lai WW, Mertens LL, Cohen MS, et al (eds): *Echocardiography in Pediatric and Congenital Heart Disease: From Fetus to Adult*, 2nd edition. Chichester, UK, Wiley-Blackwell, 2016, pp 370–378.

355. B. There is diastolic runoff through the shunt.

Diastolic runoff through a modified Blalock-Taussig shunt can minimize the antegrade diastolic flow across an arch obstruction; the blood flow through the shunt, instead of the coarctation, is following the path of least resistance. The resultant decreased flow through the coarctation can result in a lower than expected flow velocity across the aortic arch. Patients with gradually noted aortic arch obstruction can often have an initial increase in oxygen saturations, followed by a drop as overall cardiac output decreases.

▶ Lai WW, Mertens LL, Cohen MS, et al (eds): *Echocardiography in Pediatric and Congenital Heart Disease: From Fetus to Adult*, 2nd edition. Chichester, UK, Wiley-Blackwell, 2016, pp 370–378.

356. A. Bidirectional Glenn anastomosis.

See Color Plate 14 on page xxvi.

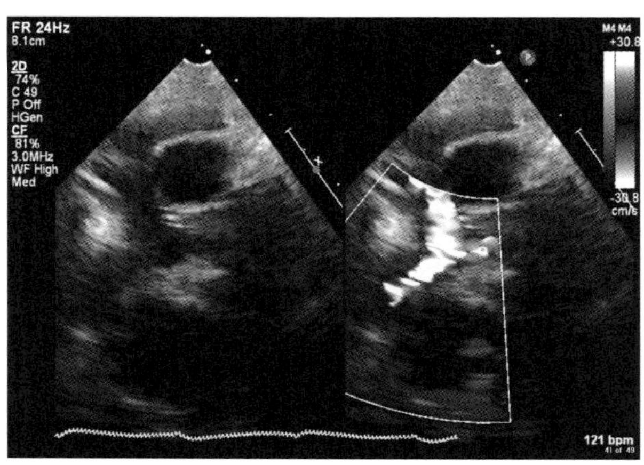

This is a bidirectional Glenn anastomosis as seen from a suprasternal coronal view. Note the low Nyquist limit and low-velocity flow from the superior vena cava into the right pulmonary artery, with color Doppler flow seen going into the distal right and central portion of the pulmonary arteries. Variations of the subsequent Fontan procedure will connect the inferior vena cava and/or hepatic veins directly to the branch pulmonary arteries.

▸ Lai WW, Mertens LL, Cohen MS, et al (eds): *Echocardiography in Pediatric and Congenital Heart Disease: From Fetus to Adult*, 2nd edition. Chichester, UK, Wiley-Blackwell, 2016, pp 370–378.

357. C. Interrupted inferior vena cava (IVC) with azygos or hemiazygos continuation to the SVC.

A Kawashima Glenn is most often performed in the setting of heterotaxy/polysplenia (left isomerism) with an interrupted IVC and azygos or hemiazygos continuation to the superior vena cava (SVC). This type of Glenn palliation incorporates the upper-body and most of the lower-body venous flow. The hepatic veins and coronary sinus are typically the only systemic veins returning directly to the heart. The hepatic veins are subsequently incorporated into a Fontan type of pathway that redirects hepatic vein flow directly to the pulmonary arteries.

▸ Lai WW, Mertens LL, Cohen MS, et al (eds): *Echocardiography in Pediatric and Congenital Heart Disease: From Fetus to Adult*, 2nd edition. Chichester, UK, Wiley-Blackwell, 2016, pp 370–378.

358. D. Suprasternal coronal view.

Because of the LeCompte maneuver, the pulmonary artery branches are moved anteriorly and straddle the ascending aorta. It can be very difficult to visualize these branches with a standard parasternal short-axis view. The suprasternal coronal window offers the best view to evaluate the anteriorly positioned left and right pulmonary arteries.

▸ Lai WW, Mertens LL, Cohen MS, et al (eds): *Echocardiography in Pediatric and Congenital Heart Disease: From Fetus to Adult*, 2nd edition. Chichester, UK, Wiley-Blackwell, 2016, p 460.

359. A. Supravalvular neopulmonary stenosis.

Following an arterial switch operation, the most common early complication is supravalvular pulmonary stenosis, which relates to tension at the pulmonary artery anastomosis if the branch pulmonary arteries are not sufficiently mobilized.

This can create tension on the main pulmonary artery. In addition, there can be circumferential narrowing at the suture line and/or bowstringing of one branch pulmonary artery over the aorta (LeCompte position). Coronary artery obstruction can be an early complication, especially in the setting of more complicated coronary artery patterns.

▶ Allen HD, Shaddy RE, Penny DJ, et al: *Moss and Adams' Heart Disease in Infants, Children, and Adolescents, Including the Fetus and Young Adult*, 9th edition. Philadelphia, Wolters Kluwer, 2016, pp 1122–1142.

360. A. Superior vena cava pathway obstruction.

The most common complication after an atrial switch operation (Mustard or Senning procedure) to correct transposition of the great arteries (d-TGA) is superior vena cava (SVC) pathway obstruction below the true SVC/RA junction, which occurs in 5%–10% of cases. Obstruction of the inferior vena cava (IVC) is rare but has been observed in approximately 1% of cases. Supravalvular pulmonary stenosis is seen after an arterial switch procedure but not typically after an atrial switch operation. Moderate to severe tricuspid insufficiency is also a complication noted after an atrial switch operation (1%–2% of cases) and is more frequently seen in patients who also have a ventricular septal defect (5%–10% of cases). Subaortic obstruction is rarely if ever seen following an atrial switch operation for d-TGA.

▶ Allen HD, Shaddy RE, Penny DJ, et al: *Moss and Adams' Heart Disease in Infants, Children, and Adolescents, Including the Fetus and Young Adult*, 9th edition. Philadelphia, Wolters Kluwer, 2016, pp 1122–1142.

361. C. Transposition of the great arteries (d-TGA) following an arterial switch operation.

See Color Plate 15 on page xxvi.

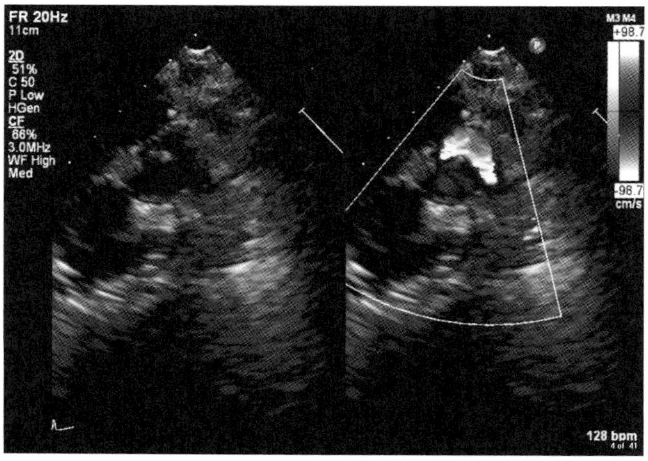

The image represents a parasternal short-axis view with the branch pulmonary arteries (blue) more anterior and wrapped around the ascending aorta (red), in the LeCompte position. The LeCompte maneuver typically places the pulmonary arteries anterior to the ascending aorta so that they "straddle" the ascending aorta.

▶ Lai WW, Mertens LL, Cohen MS, et al (eds): *Echocardiography in Pediatric and Congenital Heart Disease: From Fetus to Adult*, 2nd edition. Chichester, UK, Wiley-Blackwell, 2016, pp 459–463.

Refer to video PER-Q362.

362. B. Fontan thrombus.

In video PER-Q362, echogenic material is seen inside the extracardiac Fontan conduit, most likely representing thrombus.

▶ Lai WW, Mertens LL, Cohen MS, et al (eds): *Echocardiography in Pediatric and Congenital Heart Disease: From Fetus to Adult*, 2nd edition. Chichester, UK, Wiley-Blackwell, 2016, pp 377–378.

Refer to video PER-Q363.

363. D. Hybrid palliation.

Video PER-Q363 represents the hybrid palliation for hypoplastic left heart syndrome (HLHS). Hybrid palliation emerged in the early 2000s as an alternative to the conventional Norwood procedure to address stage 1 palliation of HLHS. It involves bilateral pulmonary artery banding and placement of a ductal stent but does not address the hypoplastic aortic arch, which is still perfused primarily or exclusively via retrograde flow from the stented ductus arteriosus. This leaves the ascending aorta/transverse arch vulnerable to possible obstruction from the ductal stent (also known as "jailing"). The video demonstrates retrograde filling of the aortic arch during systole. Of the answer choices, hybrid palliation for HLHS is the only one that fits the retrograde filling of the entire aortic arch seen in this clip during systole.

▶ Lai WW, Mertens LL, Cohen MS, et al (eds): *Echocardiography in Pediatric and Congenital Heart Disease: From Fetus to Adult*, 2nd edition. Chichester, UK, Wiley-Blackwell, 2016, pp 370–379.

364. C. Antegrade systolic pulmonary artery flow and retrograde diastolic flow via a ductal stent.

Hybrid palliation for hypoplastic left heart syndrome includes an atrial septostomy, ductal stent, and bilateral branch pulmonary artery bands. A continuous antegrade flow pattern is seen in the branch pulmonary arteries because they receive blood supply from both systolic antegrade flow through the main pulmonary artery and retrograde diastolic flow back through the ductal stent. A modified Blalock-Taussig shunt and a right ventricle–to–pulmonary artery (Sano) conduit are not usually a standard part of the hybrid palliation.

- Fenstermaker B, Berger GE, Rowland DG, et al: Interstage echocardiographic changes in patients undergoing hybrid stage I palliation for hypoplastic left heart syndrome. J Am Soc Echocardiogr 21:1222–1228, 2008.
- Lai WW, Mertens LL, Cohen MS, et al (eds): *Echocardiography in Pediatric and Congenital Heart Disease: From Fetus to Adult*, 2nd edition. Chichester, UK, Wiley-Blackwell, 2016, pp 370–379.

365. D. Normal systemic venous return.

Intravenous (IV) line location is critical in the contrast assessment of cyanosis following a bidirectional Glenn procedure. Two possible causes of post-Glenn cyanosis include venovenous collaterals and pulmonary arteriovenous malformations. To assess for these, the IV must be placed in an extremity that returns venous flow to the Glenn anastomosis—in other words, in an IV located in one of the upper (not lower) extremities. With this patient a lower extremity IV line will only demonstrate normal return of contrast to the right heart.

- Allen HD, Shaddy RE, Penny DJ, et al: *Moss and Adams' Heart Disease in Infants, Children, and Adolescents, Including the Fetus and Young Adult*, 9th edition. Philadelphia, Wolters Kluwer, 2016, pp 1080–1082.

366. A. Venovenous collaterals.

Venovenous collaterals may form due to distal obstruction in the venous circuit. The presence of a gradient at the site of the Glenn anastomosis suggests Glenn obstruction, which is a stimulus for the formation of venovenous collaterals. It should be noted that, even in the presence of obstruction, a gradient across the Glenn anastomosis might not be present (or might not be high) when there are venovenous collaterals, due to decompression ("popoff") of the superior vena cava (SVC) or innominate (brachiocephalic) vein blood through the collaterals, thereby bypassing the Glenn anastomosis.

- Allen HD, Shaddy RE, Penny DJ, et al: *Moss and Adams' Heart Disease in Infants, Children, and Adolescents, Including the Fetus and Young Adult*, 9th edition. Philadelphia, Wolters Kluwer, 2016, pp 1080–1082.

367. A. Atria.

The assessment of post Glenn procedure cyanosis with contrast should focus on the atria. This focus will demonstrate the location of contrast return to the heart and ideally will reveal the source of the cyanosis. If return to the left atrium comes quickly (<3 beats), cyanosis is most likely due to pulmonary arteriovenous malformations. Return via the inferior vena cava (IVC) into the right atrium suggests venovenous collateral flow, with the collateral vessels returning below the diaphragm. Return into the right or left atrium could suggest a residual left superior vena cava (SVC) draining to the coronary sinus or directly back to the atrium. Venovenous flow into the coronary sinus and pulmonary veins can also be seen but is less common. While assessment of the SVC and distal branch pulmonary arteries can confirm successful injection, it does not evaluate cyanosis effectively. Assessment of the aorta (for appearance of contrast) is not useful in this setting.

▸ Allen HD, Shaddy RE, Penny DJ, et al: *Moss and Adams' Heart Disease in Infants, Children, and Adolescents, Including the Fetus and Young Adult*, 9th edition. Philadelphia, Wolters Kluwer, 2016, pp 1080–1082.

368. C. Reduction in pulmonary vascular resistance.

Increased modified Blalock-Taussig (BT) shunt velocity is a common finding after palliation of single-ventricle anatomy and should be measured in the clinical context. In this setting, the lower BT shunt velocity was likely due to marginal postoperative clinical status with associated high pulmonary vascular resistance, which in turn produced a lower BT shunt velocity and lower systemic oxygen saturation. Several weeks later, following clinical improvement, the increased oxygen saturation likely represents a reduction in pulmonary vascular resistance, allowing for increased pulmonary blood flow and the higher Doppler velocity obtained (and correlating with the higher oxygen saturations). BT shunt obstruction may result in a higher velocity across the shunt, but generally this will produce lower systemic oxygen saturation. Aortopulmonary (AP) collateral flow should not affect the velocity across the BT shunt. Coarctation of the distal Norwood anastomosis might result in higher pressures in the aortic arch, resulting in a higher (not lower) velocity across the BT shunt.

▸ Allen HD, Shaddy RE, Penny DJ, et al: *Moss and Adams' Heart Disease in Infants, Children, and Adolescents, Including the Fetus and Young Adult*, 9th edition. Philadelphia, Wolters Kluwer, 2016, pp 1074–1080.

ANSWERS

369. B. He has had a fenestrated Fontan procedure with right-to-left shunting.

A

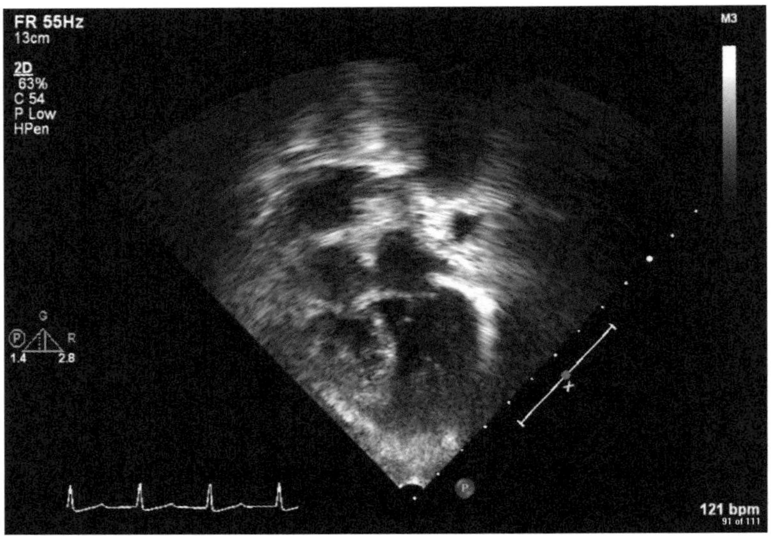

B

See Color Plate 16 on page xxvii.

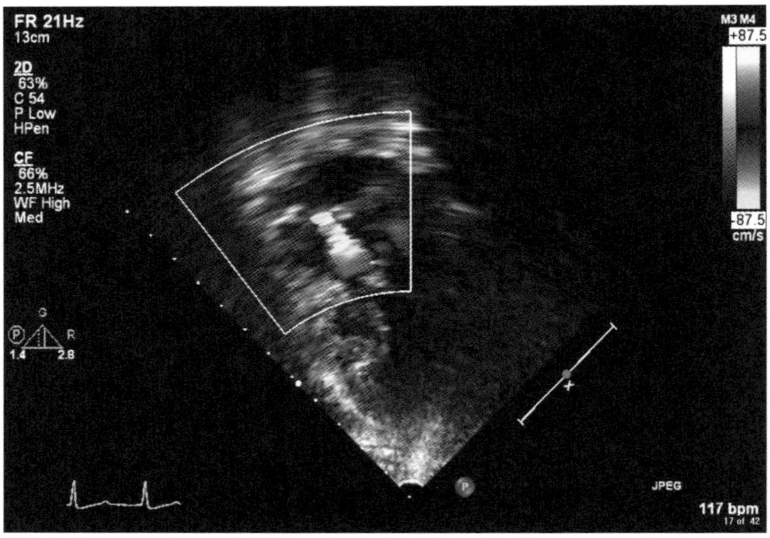

The images represent an apical view of his anatomy: pulmonary atresia with intact ventricular septum. The extracardiac Fontan conduit is noted posterior to the right atrium. The color Doppler image demonstrates color flow from the Fontan conduit (containing systemic venous blood) into his right atrium (now in continuity with the left atrium and pulmonary veins), thereby representing a physiologic right-to-left shunt. The combined systemic/pulmonary venous blood (with a lower than normal oxygen saturation) then empties into the left ventricle and is ejected into his systemic arterial system.

▸ Lai WW, Mertens LL, Cohen MS, et al (eds): *Echocardiography in Pediatric and Congenital Heart Disease: From Fetus to Adult*, 2nd edition. Chichester, UK, Wiley-Blackwell, 2016, pp 546–555.

370. D. Occlusion of an isolated left anterior descending coronary artery.

Segmental wall motion abnormalities in children with transposition of the great arteries (d-TGA) status post arterial switch operation should prompt evaluation for coronary hypoperfusion. The left anterior descending artery is the only vessel clearly affected in this case and arises independently in 10%–15% of patients. The fact that the wall motion abnormalities are segmental (confined to the ventricular septum and the left ventricular apex) rules out kinking of the entire left main coronary artery system. The pulmonary artery position would be remote from this coronary artery, and any geometrical distortion would be expected in the immediate postoperative period. Dilatation of the mitral valve annulus is unlikely to cause the wall motion abnormalities seen in this patient.

▶ Allen HD, Shaddy RE, Penny DJ, et al: *Moss and Adams' Heart Disease in Infants, Children, and Adolescents, Including the Fetus and Young Adult*, 9th edition. Philadelphia, Wolters Kluwer, 2016, pp 1132–1138.

▶ Lai WW, Mertens LL, Cohen MS, et al (eds): *Echocardiography in Pediatric and Congenital Heart Disease: From Fetus to Adult*, 2nd edition. Chichester, UK, Wiley-Blackwell, 2016, p 450.

371. A. Spontaneous complete heart block.

The conduction system in congenitally corrected transposition of the great arteries (ccTGA) is abnormally positioned and known to be unstable. Of the options listed, the most likely etiology of a regular bradycardia in this patient would be spontaneous complete heart block or complete atrioventricular (AV) dissociation. Sinus node dysfunction is possible given the atrial switch procedure but is not listed as an option. Atrial fibrillation is unlikely in this patient, and she would most likely manifest a rapid ventricular response at this age. Complete heart block related to VSD closure or hypoperfusion of the AV node would be expected to manifest much sooner after cardiac surgery.

▶ Allen HD, Shaddy RE, Penny DJ, et al: *Moss and Adams' Heart Disease in Infants, Children, and Adolescents, Including the Fetus and Young Adult*, 9th edition. Philadelphia, Wolters Kluwer, 2016, p 1149.

372. C. Pulmonary atresia with intact ventricular septum (PA/IVS) and mild tricuspid valve/right ventricular hypoplasia.

In those patients with pulmonary atresia with intact ventricular septum (PA/IVS) who also have a reasonable tricuspid valve annulus and membranous atresia of the pulmonary valve, radiofrequency perforation and balloon pulmonary

ANSWERS

valvuloplasty can be performed to establish antegrade pulmonary blood flow. In such cases, the right ventricular volume can increase to the point that a biventricular circulation might be possible. If ventricular volumes are insufficient for a full cardiac output, additional sources of pulmonary blood flow may be necessary (using a ductal stent or modified Blalock-Taussig shunt in the short term and bidirectional Glenn anastomosis for the long term). The remaining three choices in this question—hypoplastic left heart syndrome with mitral atresia, double-outlet right ventricle with mitral atresia, and tricuspid atresia with non-restrictive ventricular septal defect and normally related great arteries—all have atresia of one of the atrioventricular (AV) valves. In such cases a biventricular circulation would not be possible because atretic AV valves cannot be made to function successfully in a biventricular repair.

▸ Allen HD, Shaddy RE, Penny DJ, et al: *Moss and Adams' Heart Disease in Infants, Children, and Adolescents, Including the Fetus and Young Adult*, 9th edition. Philadelphia, Wolters Kluwer, 2016, pp 954–955.

373. D. Significant preoperative cyanosis.

Fenestrations have been shown to improve initial postoperative morbidity and shorten the length of hospital stays. Patients in whom fenestration appears to show the most predictable benefit include those who are undergoing important concomitant procedures or single-lung Fontan palliation, patients with an elevated pulmonary vascular resistance or transpulmonary gradient, patients with significant atrioventricular (AV) valve regurgitation, and patients with poor ventricular function. Since the fenestration results in right-to-left shunting and reduced postoperative systemic oxygen saturations, significant preoperative cyanosis would not be an indication for fenestration—and in fact might well be a contraindication.

▸ Lemler MS, Scott WA, Leonard SR, et al: Fenestration improves clinical outcome of the Fontan procedure: a prospective, randomized study. Circulation 105:207–212, 2002.

▸ Salazar JD, Zafar F, Siddiqui K, et al: Fenestration during Fontan palliation: now the exception instead of the rule. Journal Thorac Cardiovasc Surg 140:129–136, 2010.

374. D. Patients with double-outlet right ventricle, a subpulmonary VSD, and right ventricular outflow tract obstruction.

Double-outlet right ventricle (DORV) with a subpulmonary ventricular septal defect (VSD) and side-by-side great arteries is also known as Taussig-Bing anomaly. This anomaly has a physiology similar to that of transposition of the great arteries (d-TGA). However, Taussig-Bing anomaly can also be associated with right ventricular outflow tract (RVOT) obstruction (subaortic) and potential aortic arch obstruction. In general, single-stage repair of Taussig-Bing anomaly requires an arterial switch operation, VSD closure, relief of the RVOT obstruction (the pulmonary outflow tract following the arterial switch), and repair of aortic arch obstruction, as well as ligation/division of the ductus arteriosus. For multiple reasons, repair of Taussig-Bing anomaly can be very complex. Therefore, compared to the other options in this question, single-stage repair of Taussig-Bing anomaly is associated with a considerably higher risk of mortality. Important complicating factors include RVOT obstruction, potential aortic arch obstruction, and unusual coronary artery variations that are commonly found with Taussig-Bing anomaly. Certain coronary variations can significantly increase the difficulty of the arterial switch operation (due to difficulties in coronary translocation), and they can also limit potential relief of the RVOT obstruction. In some instances of RVOT narrowing, a right ventricle–to–pulmonary artery conduit might be necessary to bypass the obstruction, but its position could lie in close proximity to a coronary course, creating a risk of coronary compression.

▸ Allen HD, Shaddy RE, Penny DJ, et al: *Moss and Adams' Heart Disease in Infants, Children, and Adolescents, Including the Fetus and Young Adult*, 9th edition. Philadelphia, Wolters Kluwer, 2016, pp 1138–1142.

375. C. D-TGA with VSD and left ventricular outflow tract (LVOT) obstruction.

The Rastelli procedure was originally described for transposition of the great arteries (d-TGA) with ventricular septal defect (VSD) and left ventricular outflow tract (LVOT) (subpulmonary) obstruction. The Rastelli operation involves suturing a large intraventricular baffle (basically a large VSD patch) into place in order to close the VSD and direct left ventricular outflow to the transposed aortic valve; the main pulmonary artery is ligated and a right ventricle–to–pulmonary artery conduit is placed.

▸ Lai WW, Mertens LL, Cohen MS, et al (eds): *Echocardiography in Pediatric and Congenital Heart Disease: From Fetus to Adult*, 2nd edition. Chichester, UK, Wiley-Blackwell, 2016, pp 458–462.

376. D. To evaluate for proximal coronary artery obstruction.

Echocardiography is generally sufficient for the assessment of most postoperative concerns following an arterial switch operation for transposition of the great arteries (d-TGA). However,

ANSWERS

following arterial switch, long-term follow-up studies have shown that there can be an increased risk of morbidity and mortality (up to 8%) related to coronary artery pathology. This pathology can be present even with normal cardiac function and no apparent resting wall motion abnormalities. In such patients, echocardiography is insufficient to evaluate potential coronary artery pathology. Cardiac magnetic resonance imaging (MRI) studies more accurately assess proximal coronary patency in a majority of patients at this age, as well as evaluating ventricular function and identifying any evidence of a myocardial scar. MRI studies can also evaluate for other vascular concerns, such as supravalvular pulmonary stenosis and aortic root dilatation. In this patient, a 15-year-old boy, routine evaluation of the coronaries by cardiac MRI is warranted.

▶ Cohen MS, Eidem BW, Cetta F, et al: Multimodality imaging guidelines of patients with transposition of the great arteries: a report from the American Society of Echocardiography developed in collaboration with the Society for Cardiovascular Magnetic Resonance and the Society of Cardiovascular Computed Tomography. J Am Soc Echocardiogr 29:571–621, 2016.

▶ Warnes CA, Williams RG, Bashore TM, et al: ACC/AHA 2008 guidelines for the management of adults with congenital heart disease: a report of the American College of Cardiology/American Heart Association Task Force on Practice Guidelines (writing committee to develop guidelines on the management of adults with congenital heart disease). Circulation 118:e714–e833, 2008.

377. B. Intramural left coronary artery.

An intramural coronary artery in a patient with transposition of the great arteries (d-TGA) has the highest risk of complications of surgery; studies have demonstrated a sixfold increase in mortality. However, while an intramural coronary pattern carries the highest risk following the arterial switch operation, other coronary artery patterns found in d-TGA can also affect outcomes. Those infants with d-TGA and single coronary artery variations have a threefold increase in mortality, likely owing to the greater impact of stretching or kinking of the only cardiac source of blood.

▶ Pasquali SK, Hasselblad V, Li JS, et al: Coronary artery pattern and outcome of arterial switch operation for transposition of the great arteries: a meta-analysis. Circulation 106:2575–2580, 2002.

378. A. Replacement of the aortic valve with the native pulmonary valve.

Aortic valve replacement with an artificial prosthesis is challenging in the pediatric population due to limited valve sizes, the patient's rapid somatic growth, and the need for ongoing anticoagulation post procedure. The Ross procedure was proposed as a surgical alternative to mechanical aortic valve replacement. The Ross procedure is an autograft surgery that moves the normal pulmonary valve to the aortic position to replace a diseased aortic valve. The pulmonary valve is replaced with an allograft from the right ventricle (RV) to the pulmonary artery (PA). This RV-to-PA conduit can be created from a donated human cadaveric pulmonary or aortic homograft, or it can be a xenograft (porcine or bovine vessel with valve). The coronary arteries must also be transferred as button grafts from the native aortic root to the transplanted pulmonary root. The diseased aortic valve is discarded.

▶ Kouchoukos NT, Dávila-Román VG, Spray TL, et al: Replacement of the aortic root with a pulmonary autograft in children and young adults with aortic-valve disease. N Engl J Med 330:1–6, 1994.

379. D. It is a surgery that replaces two valves instead of one.

One of the main disadvantages to the Ross procedure is that it is a double-valve surgery. This is because the native pulmonary valve is removed and placed in the aortic valve position, thus necessitating a pulmonary allograft be placed in the right ventricular outflow tract to pulmonary artery position. Although the new native aortic (neoaortic) valve will grow as the pediatric patient grows to adulthood, the pulmonary allograft will not grow with the patient and usually will develop valve dysfunction with age. Hence, depending on the age at which the Ross procedure is performed, one or more future surgeries will be necessary to replace the allograft from the right ventricle to the pulmonary artery. After the Ross procedure, patients don't need ongoing postoperative anticoagulation therapy.

▶ Otto CM, Bonow RO: *Valvular Heart Disease: A Companion to Braunwald's Heart Disease*, 4th edition. Philadelphia, Saunders Elsevier, 2014, pp 199–218.

380. B. Neoaortic valve insufficiency.

The most common post-Ross complication involving the neoaortic valve is development of neoaortic valve insufficiency. Obstruction of the right ventricle–to–pulmonary artery conduit (which does not involve the new aortic valve) is also a common postoperative complication. In approximately 25% of patients who have undergone the Ross procedure these sequelae may require reintervention by 8 years post procedure. While other left ventricular outflow tract complications are possible, none of the other answer choices—including neoaortic stenosis, supravalvular aortic stenosis, and subaortic stenosis—is as commonly seen following the Ross procedure.

▶ Pasquali SK, Shera D, Wernovsky G, et al: Midterm outcomes and predictors of reintervention after the Ross procedure in infants, children, and young adults. J Thorac Cardiovasc Surg 133:893–899, 2007.

381. C. Neoaortic root (pulmonary autograft).

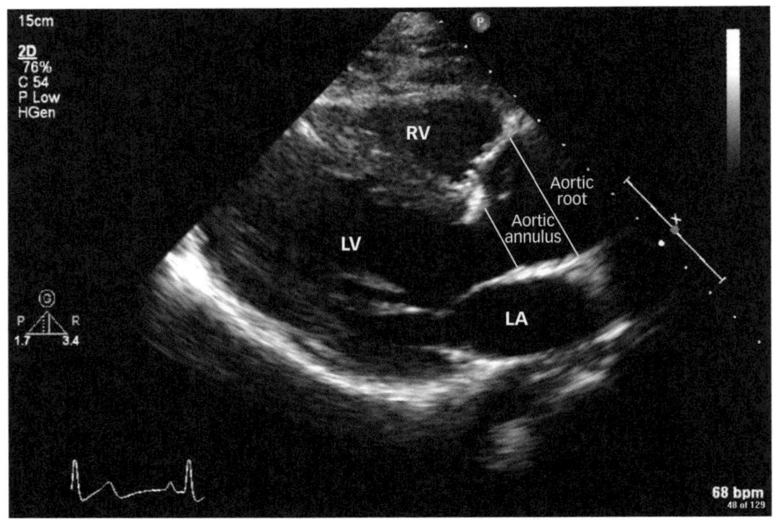

The neoaortic root (pulmonary autograft) is the vascular structure most at risk for dilatation following the Ross procedure. Nonetheless, the long-term outcomes of the Ross procedure in infants and toddlers are favorable despite moderate dilatation of the pulmonary autograft with age. Reintervention at the right ventricular outflow tract is also common. In a study of 34 patients who underwent pediatric Ross procedures, Elder et al. (2013) found that the freedom from autograft reintervention at 10 years post procedure was 95.5%, but follow-up echocardiograms did show significant enlargement of the autograft annulus, sinus, and sinotubular junction over that time period. Most patients (n = 17) maintained less than mild aortic insufficiency (AI), while one developed mild to moderate AI and one other developed moderate AI. None of the patients developed aortic stenosis. One patient required reoperation for AI and one patient required reoperation for subaortic stenosis. This image shows the correct technique for measuring the neoaortic root. LV = left ventricle, RV = right ventricle, LA = left atrium.

▶ Elder RW, Quaegebeur JM, Bacha EA, et al: Outcomes of the infant Ross procedure for congenital aortic stenosis followed into adolescence. J Thorac Cardiovasc Surg 145:1504–1511, 2013.

382. A. Right ventricle–to–pulmonary artery conduit.

Neoaortic valve insufficiency and right ventricle–to–pulmonary artery conduit obstruction are common postoperative sequelae that may require reintervention in up to 25% of patients by 8 years post procedure. Pasquali et al. (2007) reported that in a population of 121 pediatric patients who underwent a Ross procedure, freedom from right ventricular outflow tract (RVOT) reintervention at 8 years was 81%. Smaller homograft size was the strongest predictor of RVOT reintervention. Elder et al. (2013) reported on a population of 34 pediatric patients who underwent a Ross procedure for congenital aortic stenosis at a median age of 6 months. In this series the freedom from RVOT reintervention was 85% at 5 years and 64% at 10 years post procedure.

▸ Elder RW, Quaegebeur JM, Bacha EA, et al: Outcomes of the infant Ross procedure for congenital aortic stenosis followed into adolescence. J Thorac Cardiovasc Surg 145:1504–1511, 2013.

▸ Pasquali SK, Shera D, Wernovsky G, et al: Midterm outcomes and predictors of reintervention after the Ross procedure in infants, children, and young adults. J Thorac Cardiovasc Surg 133:893–899, 2007.

383. B. New or worsening neoaortic valve insufficiency.

Subaortic stenosis is an uncommon complication following the Ross procedure, but it has been described. When suspected prior to the Ross procedure, an additional surgical intervention, called a Konno procedure, can be performed. This involves resection of the subaortic area with a myotomy and myomectomy of the ventricular septum. Indications for reintervention in patients with subaortic stenosis include a Doppler-derived gradient of greater than 50 mmHg or the development of increasing aortic valve insufficiency.

▸ Elder RW, Quaegebeur JM, Bacha EA, et al: Outcomes of the infant Ross procedure for congenital aortic stenosis followed into adolescence. J Thorac Cardiovasc Surg 145:1504–1511, 2013.

▸ Pasquali SK, Shera D, Wernovsky G, et al: Midterm outcomes and predictors of reintervention after the Ross procedure in infants, children, and young adults. J Thorac Cardiovasc Surg 133:893–899, 2007.

384. A. Pulmonary hypertension.

Early postoperative instability after repair of total anomalous pulmonary venous connection (TAPVC) is usually caused by pulmonary hypertension in the patient secondary to increased pulmonary vascular resistance. The incidence of early mortality has been reported at approximately 15%, but the presence of obstructed TAPVC has been associated

ANSWERS

with higher rates of perioperative death. Diffuse pulmonary lymphangiectasia can also be found in some infants with TAPVC and is associated with higher mortality.

▶ Allen HD, Shaddy RE, Penny DJ, et al: *Moss and Adams' Heart Disease in Infants, Children, and Adolescents, Including the Fetus and Young Adult,* 9th edition. Philadelphia, Wolters Kluwer, 2016, p 903.

385. C. Pulmonary venous anastomosis obstruction.

See Color Plate 17 on page xxvii.

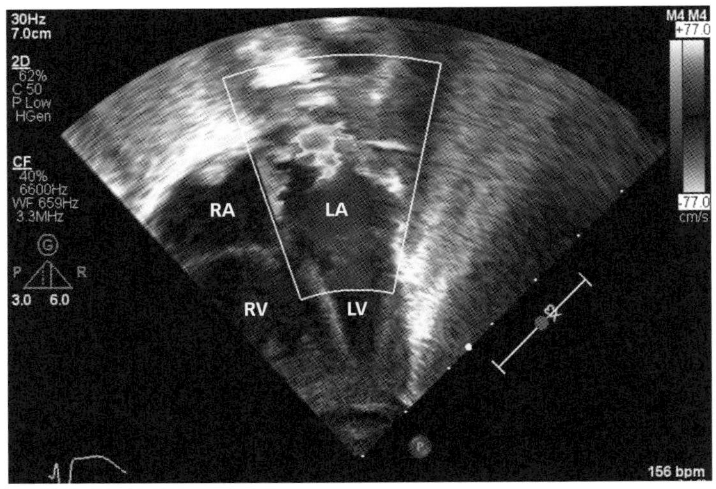

The development of postoperative pulmonary venous anastomosis obstruction can occur in up to 10%–15% of repaired cases of total anomalous pulmonary venous connection (TAPVC). The site of reobstruction is often at the left atrial–pulmonary venous anastomosis, but it can also be due to a diffuse fibrosis within the pulmonary veins themselves. This can occur months or even years after the initial repair and can present with severe respiratory failure, hypoxia, and pulmonary congestion. Surgical correction of this complication has a poor prognosis, as it has an increased rate of recurrence and a 30%–45% risk of mortality. This image demonstrates pulmonary venous anastomosis obstruction as shown by color Doppler.

▶ Allen HD, Driscoll DJ, Shaddy RE, et al: *Moss and Adams' Heart Disease in Infants, Children, and Adolescents: Including the Fetus and Young Adult,* 8th edition. Philadelphia, Lippincott Williams & Wilkins, 2013, p 903.

386. D. Pulmonary venous anastomosis.

The development of postoperative pulmonary venous anastomosis obstruction can occur in up to 10%–15% of repaired cases of total anomalous pulmonary venous connection (TAPVC). The site of reobstruction is often at the left atrial–pulmonary venous anastomosis, but it can also be due to a diffuse fibrosis within the pulmonary veins themselves. This can occur months or even years after the initial repair and can present with respiratory symptoms and exercise intolerance. Reobstruction in the pulmonary venous connection must be evaluated when there is evidence of pulmonary hypertension. In some cases, elevated estimates of either right ventricular or pulmonary artery pressure may be the first sign of pulmonary venous reobstruction. An attempt should be made to thoroughly investigate the left atrial–pulmonary venous anastomosis and pulmonary veins themselves using color Doppler and pulsed-wave Doppler. Surgical correction of this complication has a poor prognosis, as it has increased rate of recurrence and a 30%–45% risk for mortality.

- Allen HD, Driscoll DJ, Shaddy RE, et al: *Moss and Adams' Heart Disease in Infants, Children, and Adolescents: Including the Fetus and Young Adult*, 8th edition. Philadelphia, Lippincott Williams & Wilkins, 2013, p 903.
- Wong PC, Miller-Hance WC (eds): *Transesophageal Echocardiography for Congenital Heart Disease*, London, Springer-Verlag, 2014, pp 162–163.

387. C. SVC baffle stenosis.

A

See Color Plate 18 on page xxvii.

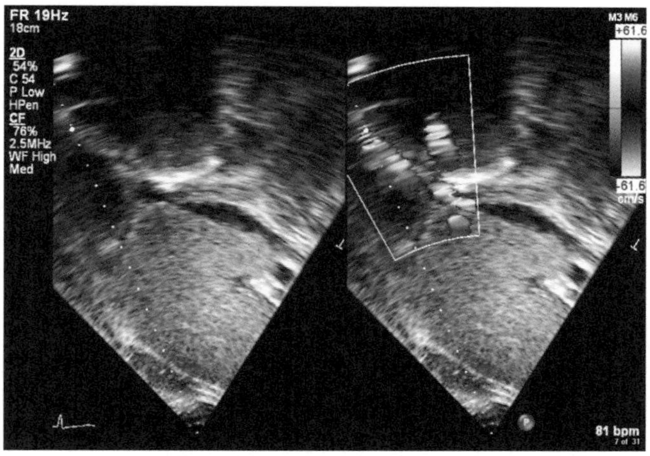

B

See Color Plate 19 on page xxviii.

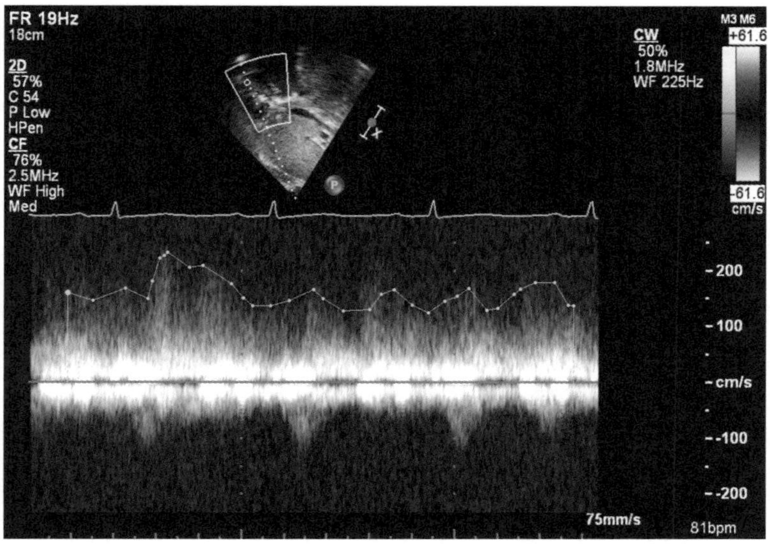

*These images show **A** a subcostal sagittal view of the superior vena cava (SVC) and **B** a spectral Doppler waveform of SVC flow. Normal flow in the SVC is characterized by biphasic forward flow in systole and early diastole with a brief halt to forward flow and reversed flow during atrial contraction. In children the systolic flow is greater than the diastolic flow and the atrial wave reversal is usually very low-velocity and brief. SVC anastomosis obstruction can occur as a postsurgical complication, particularly after repair of a sinus venosus atrial septal defect (ASD) with right-sided partial anomalous pulmonary venous connection (PAPVC) that involved baffling of an anomalous right upper pulmonary vein (RUPV) to the SVC–right atrial junction. Doppler findings in SVC obstruction include increased peak velocity, increased mean gradient, and loss of phase, as seen in image **B**. However, the absolute Doppler gradient can vary depending upon preload status of the patient at the time of the echocardiogram and also can be underestimated due to the capacitance of the venous bed proximal to the obstruction. Thus, assessment of the Doppler pattern is often more important than the Doppler gradient itself. In cases of venous obstruction, this pattern will primarily show loss of the normal biphasic flow pattern, along with an increased mean gradient as measured over several cardiac cycles.*

- Allen HD, Driscoll DJ, Shaddy RE, et al: *Moss and Adams' Heart Disease in Infants, Children, and Adolescents: Including the Fetus and Young Adult*, 8th edition. Philadelphia, Lippincott Williams & Wilkins, 2013, p 894.
- Wong PC, Miller-Hance WC (eds): *Transesophageal Echocardiography for Congenital Heart Disease*, London, Springer-Verlag, 2014, pp 164–165.

388. B. Pulmonary venous baffle obstruction.

See Color Plate 20 on page xxviii.

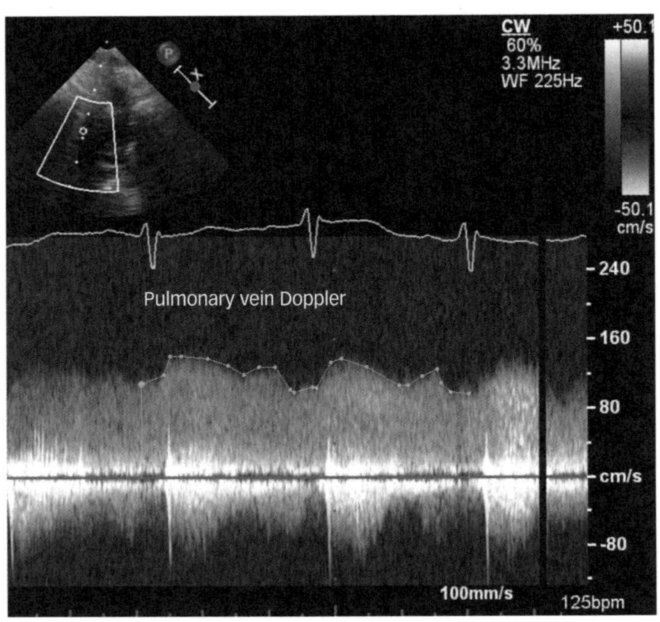

Normal pulmonary venous Doppler flow is characterized by a triphasic forward flow pattern in early systole (atrial relaxation), late systole (right ventricular contraction), and diastole (left ventricular relaxation and filling), with a brief halt to forward flow and reversed flow during atrial contraction (A wave). In children, a biphasic forward flow pattern is more common with a single systolic waveform. Pulmonary vein stenosis can occur as an isolated lesion or secondary to surgery or other interventions. Obstruction in the right pulmonary veins after surgical repair of partial anomalous pulmonary venous connection (PAPVC) to the superior vena cava (SVC) is a known complication. The evaluation of the right pulmonary veins by 2D, color Doppler flow, and pulsed-wave Doppler is critical to the diagnosis of obstruction. The peak velocity and peak systolic gradient might not accurately reflect the severity of obstruction due to flow redistribution away from the lung segment drained by the stenotic vein. Thus, it is important not only to assess the pulmonary venous Doppler gradients but also to evaluate the Doppler flow pattern. Stenosis is manifested primarily by loss of phasic flow pattern in the veins and can also be demonstrated by an elevated mean Doppler gradient assessed over several cardiac cycles, as opposed to a measurement of peak velocity at an isolated point in the cardiac cycle.

- Allen HD, Driscoll DJ, Shaddy RE, et al: *Moss and Adams' Heart Disease in Infants, Children, and Adolescents: Including the Fetus and Young Adult*, 8th edition. Philadelphia, Lippincott Williams & Wilkins, 2013, p 894.
- Wong PC, Miller-Hance WC (eds): *Transesophageal Echocardiography for Congenital Heart Disease*, London, Springer-Verlag, 2014, pp 164–165.

389. B. Tetralogy of Fallot.

Pulmonary artery (PA) banding is performed by encircling the main PA with a ring of prosthetic material via either a median sternotomy or a left thoracotomy. The PA band works to effectively restrict pulmonary blood flow, increase systemic perfusion, and protect the pulmonary vasculature from prolonged exposure to pulmonary hypertension that could lead to progressive changes resulting in pulmonary vascular disease. The PA band can be done as a temporary measure or staging approach in cases where a more definitive cardiac repair or palliation cannot be performed safely in the current clinical setting. A PA band may also be useful in addressing heart defects in which excessive pulmonary blood flow needs to be prevented, and in which a definitive surgical option is not available. These may include single-ventricle lesions, multiple ventricular septal defects (VSDs), atrioventricular

ANSWERS

septal defects (AVSDs), and a double-outlet right or left ventricle (DORV or DOLV). In contrast, tetralogy of Fallot (TOF) typically involves obstruction of the right ventricular outflow tract due to subvalvular, valvular, or supravalvular pulmonary stenosis resulting in diminished pulmonary blood flow and associated with cyanosis. Thus, PA banding is not used in cases of TOF.

▶ Muller WH Jr, Danimann JF Jr: The treatment of certain congenital malformations of the heart by the creation of pulmonic stenosis to reduce pulmonary hypertension and excessive pulmonary blood flow: a preliminary report. Surg Gynecol Obstet 95:213–219, 1952.

▶ Pizarro C, Norwood WI: Pulmonary artery banding before Norwood procedure. Ann Thorac Surg 75:1008–1010, 2003.

390. A. Increasing LV wall thickness and LV mass.

Pulmonary artery (PA) banding can also be used for "training" the LV in neonates with transposition of the great arteries (d-TGA) that was not repaired in the neonatal period. In patients with d-TGA without a ventricular septal defect (VSD), the LV is pumping blood to the main PA and is not exposed to systemic pressures. In this situation, the LV only pumps against the lower pulmonary resistance, which, over time, leads to "deconditioning" of the LV. The wall of the LV can thicken only when exposed to systemic pressures in the first few weeks after birth and will slowly start to lose its ability to generate systemic pressure by the second or third week after birth. If performed too late in life, an arterial switch operation will suddenly expose an unprepared LV to systemic pressure; unable to adapt to the sudden change in pressure, the unprepared LV will often fail. A solution to this is PA banding, which forces the LV to pump against an artificially created pulmonary artery obstruction, thus inducing LV wall thickening and increasing LV mass prior to the arterial switch operation.

▶ Corno AE, Hurni M, Payot M, et al: Adequate left ventricular preparation allows for arterial switch despite late referral. Cardiol Young 13:49–52, 2003.

▶ Naughton P, Mossad E: Retraining the left ventricle after arterial switch operation: emerging uses for the left ventricular assist device in pediatric cardiac surgery. J Cardiothorac Vasc Anesth 14:454–456, 2000.

▶ Norwood WI, Dobell AR, Freed MD, et al: Intermediate results of the arterial switch repair: a 20-institution study. J Thorac Cardiovasc Surg 96:854–863, 1988.

391. D. Compromised branch pulmonary artery flow.

The most common complications of pulmonary artery (PA) banding include dilatation of the proximal portion of the PA, pulmonary valve dysfunction, and branch PA compromise. If placed too close to the pulmonary valve, the band can cause pulmonary valve injury, resulting in pulmonary valve insufficiency, or compress the pulmonary valve, causing stenosis. If the band migrates distally, blood flow may be compromised through the branch PAs; the right PA in particular can be affected. If undetected this blood flow compromise can cause a true stenosis of the compressed branch pulmonary artery.

- Albus RA, Trusler GA, Izukawa T, et al: Pulmonary artery banding. J Thorac Cardiovasc Surg 88:645–653, 1984.
- Freedom RM, Mawson JB, Yoo SJ, et al: *Congenital Heart Disease: Textbook of Angiocardiography*. Armonk, NY, Futura, 1997, pp 473–478.
- Stark J, Berry CL, Silove ED: The evaluation of materials used for pulmonary artery banding: experimental study in piglets. Ann Thorac Surg 13:163–169, 1972.

392. D. PA band that is too tight.

In this clinical scenario the patient has had an interval increase of the peak Doppler gradient across the pulmonary artery (PA) band, with the corresponding clinical finding of cyanosis due to increased right-to-left shunting of blood across the ventricular septal defects (VSDs). The PA band has become too tight over time, probably due to somatic growth of the child, and now the patient has insufficient pulmonary blood flow to maintain adequate systemic arterial oxygenation, resulting in cyanosis. This patient does not have pulmonary hypertension, as that would cause the PA band gradient to decrease over time due to equalization of PA and right ventricular pressure. The PA band was noted to be in good position and not impinging on the branch PAs; if it had been compressing a branch PA, the resulting stenosis could also have caused the progressive cyanosis, but that was not the case in this patient. Pulmonary valve insufficiency would not cause cyanosis.

- Albus RA, Trusler GA, Izukawa T, et al: Pulmonary artery banding. J Thorac Cardiovasc Surg 88:645–653, 1984.
- Freedom RM, Mawson JB, Yoo SJ, et al: *Congenital Heart Disease: Textbook of Angiocardiography*. Armonk, NY, Futura, 1997, pp 473–478.

393. C. PA band is too loose.

In this clinical scenario the patient has a low peak Doppler gradient across the pulmonary artery (PA) band with corresponding clinical findings of congestive heart failure (CHF), which is due to excessive pulmonary blood flow from left-to-right shunting across the ventricular septal defects (VSDs). Pulmonary hypertension can also cause the PA band peak Doppler gradient to be lower than expected due to equalization of PA and right ventricular pressure. However, this patient does not have clinical findings suggestive of worsening pulmonary hypertension, such as worsening cyanosis and diminished pulmonary blood flow on chest x-ray. A PA band was noted to be in good position and not impinging on the branch PAs, but this could also cause a low PA gradient due to downstream obstruction. Thus, it is important to confirm that both branch PAs are widely patent with normal flow pattern. Furthermore, both pulmonary hypertension and distal branch PA stenosis would cause elevated RV pressure and thus right-to-left shunting at the level of the VSDs, which was not seen. Pulmonary valve insufficiency and PA dilatation would not cause signs of CHF.

▶ Albus RA, Trusler GA, Izukawa T, et al: Pulmonary artery banding. J Thorac Cardiovasc Surg 88:645–653, 1984.

▶ Freedom RM, Mawson JB, Yoo SJ, et al: *Congenital Heart Disease: Textbook of Angiocardiography*. Armonk, NY, Futura, 1997, pp 473–478.

394. A. PA band migration with compromised RPA flow.

In this clinical scenario, the patient has an increased peak Doppler gradient across the PA band with corresponding findings of increased left pulmonary artery (LPA) flow velocity and no visible right pulmonary artery (RPA) flow. The patient has the clinical finding of lower systemic oxygen saturations. This should raise concern for slippage or migration of the PA band onto the RPA as a cause of compromised RPA flow. The increased flow to the LPA is compensatory and should not be misinterpreted as LPA branch stenosis. A tight PA band would cause an increased PA band gradient but would also result in signs of decreased pulmonary blood flow (equally to both the RPA and the LPA) and potentially increased right-to-left shunting at the level of the ventricular septal defect (VSD), leading to significant cyanosis. A loose PA band would result in features of heart failure, including persistent difficulties feeding, increased work of breathing, and increased pulmonary vascular markings or pulmonary edema on chest x-ray. The PA band position was not well documented in this scenario. Thus, it is important to confirm that both branch pulmonary arteries are patent, with normal flow to each shown by color flow and pulsed-wave Doppler. Pulmonary valve insufficiency and PA dilatation, while common postoperative findings after PA banding, would not be expected to cause lower oxygen saturations in a patient.

▶ Albus RA, Trusler GA, Izukawa T, et al: Pulmonary artery banding. J Thorac Cardiovasc Surg 88:645–653, 1984.

▶ Freedom RM, Mawson JB, Yoo SJ, et al: *Congenital Heart Disease: Textbook of Angiocardiography*. Armonk, NY, Futura, 1997, pp 473–478

395. B. Rastelli.

In certain cases of transposition of the great arteries (d-TGA) with a ventricular septal defect (VSD) and obstruction of the left ventricular outflow tract (LVOT), it may be difficult to perform an arterial switch operation alone, as this can result in long-term issues with recurrent subaortic stenosis and/or neoaortic valve stenosis. In these patients, the arterial switch operation is not suitable. Initially, the repair in these patients involved an atrial switch/baffle, closure of the VSD, and repair of the LVOT obstruction—with either resection of the stenosis or placement of a conduit from the left ventricle to the pulmonary arteries. While this redirects blood flow to achieve a physiologic repair of d-TGA, the right ventricle remains the systemic pumping chamber at long-term risk of failure, and the risk for recurrent LVOT obstruction is considerable. The Rastelli operation was devised to address this situation by bypassing the LVOT obstruction altogether by closing off the LVOT, dividing the pulmonary artery (PA) just above the valve, and creating an intraventricular baffle with a patch that redirects blood flow from the left ventricle through the VSD and into the ascending aorta. A right ventricle–to–pulmonary artery connection is then created with an external conduit, typically a pulmonary allograft. This procedure corrects the abnormal blood flow pattern of d-TGA at the ventricular level and allows the left ventricle to continue functioning as the systemic pumping chamber. The Rastelli operation can also be performed in the setting of double-outlet right ventricle (DORV) with malposition of the great arteries, VSD, and severe pulmonary valve stenosis. However, in the case of DORV with transposed aorta and subpulmonary VSD (Taussig-Bing type) the surgery requires an arterial switch operation.

▶ McGoon DC, Rastelli GC, Ongley PA: An operation for the correction of truncus arteriosus. JAMA 205:69–73, 1968.

▶ Morell VO, Jacobs JP, Quintessenza JA: Surgical management of transposition with ventricular septal defect and obstruction to the left ventricular outflow tract. Cardiol Young 15 (suppl 1):102–105, 2005.

▶ Rastelli GC. A new approach to "anatomic" repair of transposition of the great arteries. Mayo Clin Proc 44:1–12, 1969.

396. A. Placement of an intraventricular baffle and an RV-to-PA conduit.

See the answer to question 395. The Rastelli repair involves placement of an intraventricular baffle to redirect blood flow from the left ventricle through the VSD to the native ascending aorta, and placement of a right ventricle to the pulmonary artery conduit.

▶ McGoon DC, Rastelli GC, Ongley PA: An operation for the correction of truncus arteriosus. JAMA 205:69–73, 1968.

▶ Morell VO, Jacobs JP, Quintessenza JA: Surgical management of transposition with ventricular septal defect and obstruction to the left ventricular outflow tract. Cardiol Young 15 (suppl 1):102–105, 2005.

▶ Rastelli GC. A new approach to "anatomic" repair of transposition of the great arteries. Mayo Clin Proc 44:1–12, 1969.

397. A. Right ventricle–to–pulmonary artery conduit stenosis.

The Rastelli procedure involves placement of an external right ventricle–to–pulmonary artery (RV-PA) conduit, typically a pulmonary allograft (homograft). These RV-PA homografts have a specific size and do not grow with the patient. Thus, they have a limited lifespan and eventually will need to be changed (upsized) due to gradual stenosis or hypoplasia that occurs from somatic growth of the child. Depending on the size of the conduit and the type of narrowing, it might be possible to perform catheter balloon angioplasty or stenting to delay the need for surgery. If catheter-based intervention is unsuccessful or the narrowing of the conduit extends through a long segment, then surgical replacement will be required. RV-PA conduit insufficiency is also common but requires intervention less often. While decreased systolic function can occur, that complication is generally treated with medical therapy. Developing atrioventricular valve regurgitation that requires intervention is less likely following a Rastelli repair.

▶ Kreutzer C, De Vive J, Oppido G, et al: Twenty-five-year experience with Rastelli repair for transposition of the great arteries. J Thorac Cardiovasc Surg 120:211–223, 2000.

398. D. Left ventricular outflow tract obstruction.

The Rastelli procedure was introduced for patients with transposition of the great arteries (d-TGA) with ventricular septal defect (VSD) and left ventricular outflow tract obstruction (LVOT), recognizing the difficulty of accessing and repairing left ventricular outflow tract obstruction (LVOTO). Despite the Rastelli repair bypassing the original left ventricular (subpulmonary) outflow tract, there is still a risk for developing stenosis across the intraventricular baffle that redirects blood from the left ventricle through the ventricular septal defect (VSD) and into the ascending aorta. The length of the baffle and degree of subaortic stenosis can sometimes lead to the development of LVOTO over years. Addressing LVOTO can be challenging and sometimes requires that the VSD be enlarged, which increases risk of damaging the conduction system and could therefore result in heart block. Surgery for the other listed options does not generally increase the risk of heart block.

▶ Kreutzer C, De Vive J, Oppido G, et al: Twenty-five-year experience with Rastelli repair for transposition of the great arteries. J Thorac Cardiovasc Surg 120:211–223, 2000.

399. A. The venous cannula position should be in the right atrium.

After emergent extracorporeal membrane oxygenation (ECMO) cannulation for presentation of acute congestive heart failure, the venous cannula should be mostly in the right atrium with the tip directed at the inferior vena cava and ports facing the right atrial cavity. The venous cannula should not cross the tricuspid valve. The aortic cannula should be located in the aortic arch with flow directed down the ascending and descending aorta. If the aortic cannula crosses the aortic valve it can cause ventricular dilatation and obstruct flow to the coronary arteries and body. If the aortic cannula goes down the descending aorta it may not provide adequate flow to the coronary arteries and head.

▶ Wong PC, Miller-Hance WC (eds): *Transesophageal Echocardiography for Congenital Heart Disease*, London, Springer-Verlag, 2014, pp 426–427.

ANSWERS

400. B. Intracavitary thrombus.

A ventricular assist device (VAD) mechanically supports the heart of a patient with end-stage heart failure. Patients on VADs are at risk for thrombotic complications and require anti-coagulation therapy to prevent clotting within the device or tubing. In addition, patients are at high risk for clot formation inside the heart itself, due to the low-flow state and disrupted endocardium. The patient in this scenario has likely suffered a stroke, and the echocardiographer should look closely for evidence of intracavitary thrombus. Elevated filling pressures, worsening diastolic function, and worsening systolic function are not risk factors for stroke in this case, since the patient is supported by the VAD.

▶ Wong PC, Miller-Hance WC (eds): *Transesophageal Echocardiography for Congenital Heart Disease*, London, Springer-Verlag, 2014, pp 426–427.

401. A. Thrombus.

Long-standing central lines in the venous system (CVLs) increase the risk of vascular thrombus. It is always important to assess central catheters for evidence of thrombus or vegetation.

▶ Wong PC, Miller-Hance WC (eds): *Transesophageal Echocardiography for Congenital Heart Disease*, London, Springer-Verlag, 2014, p 407.

402. C. LPA stent obstruction.

In this scenario the stent in the left pulmonary artery (LPA) has become obstructed, making it difficult to see flow through it, and due to this obstruction there is now increased ratio of flow through the right pulmonary artery (RPA). Normally there is a 60:40 ratio of flow to the RPA versus the LPA. The increased volume of flow through the RPA in this case is causing it to dilate and have increased Doppler flow velocity across it. A change in cardiac function and a residual ventricular septal defect should not preferentially cause increased flow through the RPA and a decrease in flow seen through the LPA.

▶ Allen HD, Shaddy RE, Penny DJ, et al: *Moss and Adams' Heart Disease in Infants, Children, and Adolescents, Including the Fetus and Young Adult*, 9th edition. Philadelphia, Wolters Kluwer, 2016, p 894.

▶ Wong PC, Miller-Hance WC (eds): *Transesophageal Echocardiography for Congenital Heart Disease*, London, Springer-Verlag, 2014, pp 426–427.

403. D. Sinus venosus ASD with partial anomalous pulmonary venous connection (PAPVC).

Transcatheter device closure is routinely performed for a secundum ASD when there is no associated partial anomalous pulmonary venous connection (PAPVC) or other major concerns. When PAPVC is present, ASD device closure should not be performed and cardiac surgery is indicated. Also, for ASD device closure to be successful there must be adequate atrial rims for the device to be seated well. A large inferior rim is actually helpful for anchoring the device. However, sinus venosus ASDs often have deficient atrial rims that make positioning the ASD device difficult, with an increased risk for residual ASD as well as impingement on or obstruction of adjacent structures. The risk of impingement of the device on surrounding anatomic structures, such as pulmonary veins or the superior vena cava, would prevent ASD device closure as an option and would lead to referral for surgical ASD patch repair. Regarding the other choices in this question, findings of a dilated right atrium and right ventricle are common in the setting of ASD. Also, mild atrioventricular valve regurgitation is common. Neither of these findings would preclude transcatheter ASD device closure.

- Allen HD, Shaddy RE, Penny DJ, et al: *Moss and Adams' Heart Disease in Infants, Children, and Adolescents, Including the Fetus and Young Adult*, 9th edition. Philadelphia, Wolters Kluwer, 2016, p 894.
- Wong PC, Miller-Hance WC (eds): *Transesophageal Echocardiography for Congenital Heart Disease*, London, Springer-Verlag, 2014, pp 438–442.

404. C. Device embolization.

Transcatheter device closures for secundum atrial septal defects (ASDs) are performed routinely, with low rates of complications, but it is important to know what findings on echocardiography, post ASD device closure, need to be addressed immediately. Common findings post device closure include mild atrioventricular valve regurgitation, a small residual ASD, mild pulmonary regurgitation, and residual right atrial and ventricular dilatation. The right heart enlargement does not resolve immediately and may take months or years to normalize, depending on the age of the patient and the size of the defect. More serious complications that require immediate attention are device embolization, intracardiac thrombus formation, and impingement of the device on surrounding anatomic structures such as the pulmonary veins. These may necessitate emergent removal and retrieval of the device and subsequent surgical closure of the ASD.

▶ Allen HD, Shaddy RE, Penny DJ, et al: *Moss and Adams' Heart Disease in Infants, Children, and Adolescents, Including the Fetus and Young Adult*, 9th edition. Philadelphia, Wolters Kluwer, 2016, p 894.

▶ Wong PC, Miller-Hance WC (eds): *Transesophageal Echocardiography for Congenital Heart Disease*, London, Springer-Verlag, 2014, pp 438–442.

405. A. Right pulmonary vein obstruction.

A key assessment of device closure is to evaluate for any obstruction of structures located around the device—for example, the right pulmonary veins or the superior vena cava. Other complications to watch for include device fracture, device migration, a residual shunt, and embolization.

▶ Lai WW, Mertens LL, Cohen MS, et al (eds): *Echocardiography in Pediatric and Congenital Heart Disease: From Fetus to Adult*, 2nd edition. Chichester, UK, Wiley-Blackwell, 2016, p 210.

406. C. Left pulmonary artery.

The patent ductus arteriosus (PDA) is a vascular connection between the descending aorta and main/proximal LPA. A coil or device may protrude into the LPA or descending aorta (isthmus), potentially causing obstruction of the LPA and/or the descending aorta after the PDA occlusion.

▶ Lai WW, Mertens LL, Cohen MS, et al (eds): *Echocardiography in Pediatric and Congenital Heart Disease: From Fetus to Adult*, 2nd edition. Chichester, UK, Wiley-Blackwell, 2016, p 324.

407. A. Coarctation.

The patent ductus arteriosus (PDA) is a vascular connection between the descending aorta and the main/proximal left pulmonary artery (LPA). A coil or device may protrude into the LPA or descending aorta (isthmus), potentially causing LPA and/or descending aortic obstruction after the PDA occlusion.

▶ Lai WW, Mertens LL, Cohen MS, et al (eds): *Echocardiography in Pediatric and Congenital Heart Disease: From Fetus to Adult*, 2nd edition. Chichester, UK, Wiley-Blackwell, 2016, p 324.

408. D. The high-velocity jet represents a possible residual VSD with left ventricle–to–right atrial shunting.

Some studies have shown that a small residual peri-patch ventricular septal defect (VSD) can be seen in up to 38%

of VSD repairs. In this patient the tricuspid regurgitant (TR) jet velocity is high, which indicates an elevated right ventricular pressure and possible pulmonary hypertension, but the ventricular septal contour is not flat, which indicates a normal right ventricular pressure. Given these two conflicting findings, it is more likely that there is a small residual VSD with shunting from the left ventricle to the right atrium. With this type of shunting, the velocity is high because the left ventricular pressure is high but the right atrial pressure is low.

▸ Lai WW, Mertens LL, Cohen MS, et al (eds): *Echocardiography in Pediatric and Congenital Heart Disease: From Fetus to Adult*, 2nd edition. Chichester, UK, Wiley-Blackwell, 2016, p 227.

409. B. Residual VSD.

A residual ventricular septal defect (VSD) is commonly seen following operative closure of a VSD; some studies have found a residual VSD in up to 38% of patients who have undergone VSD closure. Other complications include pericardial effusion and tricuspid valve injury (producing tricuspid regurgitation) due to the surgical approach. However, these complications are much less common. Left ventricular systolic dysfunction can occur postoperatively in some patients, but it is not a common complication.

▸ Lai WW, Mertens LL, Cohen MS, et al (eds): *Echocardiography in Pediatric and Congenital Heart Disease: From Fetus to Adult*, 2nd edition. Chichester, UK, Wiley-Blackwell, 2016, p 228.

410. D. Subcostal sagittal view.

The most common complication after an arterial switch operation is main and branch pulmonary artery obstruction. Due to the LeCompte maneuver that is usually performed with an arterial switch operation, the pulmonary artery is located more anteriorly, and the branch pulmonary arteries straddle the ascending aorta. For these types of patients, the parasternal long- or short-axis view is not as useful for evaluating the right ventricular outflow tract (RVOT), especially in older pediatric patients. If an adequate subcostal sagittal view can be obtained, it offers the best option for evaluating the RVOT.

▸ Lai WW, Mertens LL, Cohen MS, et al (eds): *Echocardiography in Pediatric and Congenital Heart Disease: From Fetus to Adult*, 2nd edition. Chichester, UK, Wiley-Blackwell, 2016, p 459.

411. A. Neoaortic valve regurgitation.

Mild neoaortic valve regurgitation is common after an arterial switch operation, but it can develop into more significant regurgitation in the long term, due to aortic root dilatation. Development of pulmonary hypertension is unlikely, as is the development of neoaortic valve stenosis. Development of a coarctation will not occur if it was not originally present at the time of diagnosis and surgery.

▶ Lai WW, Mertens LL, Cohen MS, et al (eds): *Echocardiography in Pediatric and Congenital Heart Disease: From Fetus to Adult*, 2nd edition. Chichester, UK, Wiley-Blackwell, 2016, p 459.

412. C. Transposition of the great arteries (d-TGA).

Of the options given, only transposition of the great arteries (d-TGA) is an indication for the arterial switch operation. Tricuspid atresia has single-ventricle physiology, and the surgical course to correct it involves a Glenn and Fontan procedure. Severe Ebstein anomaly can also involve single-ventricle physiology and will also require a Glenn and Fontan procedure, although milder forms of Ebstein anomaly may not need surgical palliation. The surgical management of a double aortic arch is division of the smaller arch, with the larger aortic arch becoming the definitive arch; note that the right-sided aortic arch is usually the larger of the two.

▶ Allen HD, Driscoll DJ, Shaddy RE, et al: *Moss and Adams' Heart Disease in Infants, Children, and Adolescents: Including the Fetus and Young Adult*, 8th edition. Philadelphia, Lippincott Williams & Wilkins, 2013, pp 1119–1122.

413. D. Placement of a systemic–to–pulmonary artery shunt.

Stage I palliation for hypoplastic left heart syndrome (HLHS) is a traditional Norwood procedure with some type of systemic–to–pulmonary artery shunt to provide adequate pulmonary artery blood flow. This can be accomplished with a Blalock-Taussig shunt or a central shunt, in which a tube is placed to connect the innominate/subclavian artery (or sometimes the ascending aorta) to the pulmonary artery. Alternatively, a Sano procedure can be performed in which a right ventricle–to–pulmonary artery conduit is placed. All these procedures provide good blood flow to pulmonary arteries after the pulmonary artery becomes the neoaorta.

▶ Lai WW, Mertens LL, Cohen MS, et al (eds): *Echocardiography in Pediatric and Congenital Heart Disease: From Fetus to Adult*, 2nd edition. Chichester, UK, Wiley-Blackwell, 2016, pp 370–376.

414. B. Possible BT shunt obstruction.

Stage I Norwood with either a Blalock-Taussig (BT) shunt or a Sano (right ventricle–to–pulmonary artery) conduit will produce a high-velocity flow of blood to the pulmonary arteries, resulting in a loud shunt murmur. If the shunt has undergone torsion, is kinking, or has become clotted, there will be markedly reduced blood flow through the shunt, leading to hypoperfusion of the pulmonary arteries. The clinical manifestation of this is hypoxemia, and it will be difficult to hear any shunt murmur. To evaluate this, the echocardiographic study should assess BT shunt patency.

▸ Lai WW, Mertens LL, Cohen MS, et al (eds): *Echocardiography in Pediatric and Congenital Heart Disease: From Fetus to Adult*, 2nd edition. Chichester, UK, Wiley-Blackwell, 2016, pp 370–376.

415. C. High velocity through systole with continuation into diastole.

The modified Blalock-Taussig (BT) shunt is a tube that usually connects the innominate (brachiocephalic) artery to the right pulmonary artery. When pulmonary artery pressure is normal, spectral Doppler typically demonstrates high-velocity continuous flow that peaks in systole and extends into diastole, with a gradual decrease in velocity through the cardiac cycle.

▸ Lai WW, Mertens LL, Cohen MS, et al (eds): *Echocardiography in Pediatric and Congenital Heart Disease: From Fetus to Adult*, 2nd edition. Chichester, UK, Wiley-Blackwell, 2016, p 363.

416. A. Connecting the superior vena cava directly to the right pulmonary artery.

Stage II of hypoplastic left heart syndrome palliation is also called bidirectional cavopulmonary anastomosis, or the bidirectional Glenn procedure. With this procedure, the superior vena cava (SVC) is connected directly to the right pulmonary artery. Therefore, SVC return completely bypasses the heart. The SVC/pulmonary artery connection can be unilateral or bilateral, depending on whether the patient has one or two SVCs.

▸ Allen HD, Driscoll DJ, Shaddy RE, et al: *Moss and Adams' Heart Disease in Infants, Children, and Adolescents: Including the Fetus and Young Adult*, 8th edition. Philadelphia, Lippincott Williams & Wilkins, 2013, p 1082.

▸ Lai WW, Mertens LL, Cohen MS, et al (eds): *Echocardiography in Pediatric and Congenital Heart Disease: From Fetus to Adult*, 2nd edition. Chichester, UK, Wiley-Blackwell, 2016, pp 376–377.

417. B. Redirection of inferior vena cava blood directly to the pulmonary arteries.

Stage III of hypoplastic left heart palliation is also called the Fontan procedure. The purpose of this procedure is to redirect inferior vena cava (IVC) flow directly to the pulmonary arteries (generally the right pulmonary artery), such that IVC and hepatic venous return completely bypass the heart. Since its initial description in 1971 by Dr. François Fontan, this procedure has undergone many anatomic modifications: atrioventricular and atriopulmonary connections, lateral tunnel, and most recently an extracardiac conduit. In addition, the lateral tunnel or extracardiac conduit can be fenestrated or nonfenestrated. The purpose of the fenestration is to allow some IVC blood to "pop off" from the Fontan pathway directly back to the heart (thereby maintaining some cardiac output) in the event that the patient has marginal physiology due to lung disease, high pulmonary vascular resistance, borderline pulmonary artery size, or another compromising condition.

▶ Allen HD, Driscoll DJ, Shaddy RE, et al: *Moss and Adams' Heart Disease in Infants, Children, and Adolescents: Including the Fetus and Young Adult*, 8th edition. Philadelphia, Lippincott Williams & Wilkins, 2013, pp 1082–1083.

▶ Lai WW, Mertens LL, Cohen MS, et al (eds): *Echocardiography in Pediatric and Congenital Heart Disease: From Fetus to Adult*, 2nd edition. Chichester, UK, Wiley-Blackwell, 2016, p 377.

418. C. A small hole created between the Fontan pathway/ conduit and the atrium, providing a right-to-left shunt.

The fenestrated Fontan procedure creates a communication between the Fontan pathway/conduit and the atrium. The fenestration is a small hole that the surgeon creates to allow blood to shunt from right to left (desaturated blood to saturated blood). This fenestration can help to decompress elevated venous pressure and maintain cardiac output for some patients with marginal Fontan physiology due to lung disease, elevated pulmonary vascular resistance, borderline pulmonary artery size, marginal ventricular systolic function, significant atrioventricular valve regurgitation, or another compromising condition. The spectral Doppler flow pattern across the fenestration is similar to that of flow across an atrial septal defect.

▶ de Leval MR, Deanfield JE: Four decades of Fontan palliation. Nat Rev Cardiol 7:520–527, 2010.

419. B. No matter whether the flow velocity across the fenestration is high or low, it is difficult to determine pulmonary vascular resistance.

There is specific (but limited) information that can be obtained by the echocardiographic evaluation of a Fontan fenestration. First, the patency of the fenestration can be demonstrated by the presence of a right-to-left shunt from the Fontan conduit into the atrium, which, by color Doppler, will appear as a small jet of red or aliased flow from a standard apical four-chamber view. Second, the approximate width of the fenestration can usually be visualized by 2D imaging and color Doppler, although the color Doppler jet tends to "bleed" over the margins of the fenestration. Third, the mean gradient across the fenestration can be quantified from the spectral Doppler tracing of the flow. However, this gradient gives only an approximation of the pressure difference between the Fontan conduit and atrium. It does not provide direct information about the actual pressures or the pulmonary vascular resistance. For example, a high velocity and high gradient could indicate a high pulmonary artery pressure, suggestive of high pulmonary vascular resistance. However, a high gradient and high velocity could also be seen with a lower atrial pressure. Similarly, a low gradient could indicate a low pulmonary artery pressure and low pulmonary vascular resistance, but it could also indicate an elevated atrial pressure. Of note, the absence of a fenestration jet does not necessarily mean that the fenestration is no longer patent. In some patients, the fenestration is placed in an unusual location, such as more superiorly in the conduit, or with the flow directed into the atrial appendage. In these instances, the fenestration might not be visible with the standard apical four-chamber view.

▸ Lemler MS, Scott WA, Leonard SR, et al: Fenestration improves clinical outcome of the Fontan procedure: a prospective, randomized study. Circulation 105:207–212, 2002.

420. D. Mustard procedure.

Before the arterial switch operation became the standard operation for transposition of the great arteries, a Senning or Mustard procedure was performed. These operations, also known as atrial switch procedures, involve redirection of systemic and pulmonary venous blood flow at the atrial level by means of an intra-atrial baffling procedure. Systemic venous flow from the superior and inferior venae cavae is redirected to the left ventricle, which then pumps the deoxygenated blood to the lungs. Redirected pulmonary venous flow returns to the right ventricle, which then pumps oxygenated blood to the body. With the atrial switch procedure, the morphologic right ventricle remains the systemic ventricle, while the morphologic left ventricle remains the pulmonary ventricle.

▸ Allen HD, Driscoll DJ, Shaddy RE, et al: *Moss and Adams' Heart Disease in Infants, Children, and Adolescents: Including the Fetus and Young Adult*, 8th edition. Philadelphia, Lippincott Williams & Wilkins, 2013, pp 1122–1128.

421. B. Double-inlet left ventricle.

The Fontan procedure is performed for patients with a functional single ventricle in whom a biventricular repair is not possible. A double-inlet left ventricle is an anatomic and functional single ventricle; therefore it will require a Fontan procedure as the ultimate palliation. For the other three options—balanced atrioventricular septal (atrioventricular canal) defect, tetralogy of Fallot, and truncus arteriosus—a biventricular repair is feasible.

▸ Lai WW, Mertens LL, Cohen MS, et al (eds): *Echocardiography in Pediatric and Congenital Heart Disease: From Fetus to Adult*, 2nd edition. Chichester, UK, Wiley-Blackwell, 2016, pp 511–518.

422. C. A rocking PMV is indicative of valve dehiscence.

A prosthetic valve (mechanical or bioprosthetic) that is seen rocking in the position it was sewed into is a major clue to valve dehiscence and is not considered a normal finding. 2D echocardiography is helpful when evaluating valve dehiscence, and off-axis nonstandard views that image around artifacts caused by the prosthesis are frequently used.

▸ Armstrong WF, Ryan T: *Feigenbaum's Echocardiography*, 7th edition. Philadelphia, Lippincott Williams & Wilkins, 2010, pp 385–387.

423. A. Echolucent.

Abscess formation is a complication of prosthetic valves (mechanical or bioprosthetic). Abscesses can appear echolucent (echo-free) or echo-dense on echocardiography. Color Doppler imaging can be helpful when assessing prosthetic valve abscesses, because color Doppler can demonstrate flow into and within the abscess. Moving to additional and non-standard acoustic windows that visualize the area around the artificial valve's sewing ring can also be helpful in assessing abscesses.

▶ Armstrong WF, Ryan T: *Feigenbaum's Echocardiography*, 7th edition. Philadelphia, Lippincott Williams & Wilkins, 2010, pp 414–415.

424. D. Jets seen between the sewing ring and discs are normal.

Jets are engineered to occur as part of the mechanical valve's functioning, and when seen arising between the sewing ring and discs they are normal. These small "washing jets" or "signature jets" are characteristic for each mechanical valve and are designed to help prevent thrombus formation by washing the leaflets. Small perivalvular jets (jets around the sewing ring) may be seen due to technical difficulties during valve implantation, but usually they go away. If no perivalvular leak was visualized post implantation but a perivalvular leak develops after valve implantation, an infectious cause should be suspected.

▶ Armstrong WF, Ryan T: *Feigenbaum's Echocardiography*, 7th edition. Philadelphia, Lippincott Williams & Wilkins, 2010, pp 391, 414.

Refer to video PER-Q425.

425. C. Perivalvular leak.

Video PER-Q425 demonstrates a perivalvular leak in a bioprosthetic mitral valve. Note that the color Doppler region of interest is set around the sewing ring in order to visualize any perivalvular leaks. The prosthetic valve does not rock, and thus dehiscence, based on the findings in this echocardiogram, is not suspected.

▶ Armstrong WF, Ryan T: *Feigenbaum's Echocardiography*, 7th edition. Philadelphia, Lippincott Williams & Wilkins, 2010, p 396.

Refer to video PER-Q426.

426. A. Restricted mechanical mitral leaflet motion.

Refer to video PER-Q426. The spectral Doppler, 2D, and color Doppler flow imaging demonstrates one frozen mitral valve leaflet and the other leaflet with restricted motion. Due to reverberation artifact the left ventricle is not well visualized in this video clip. (In this patient cardiac catheterization also demonstrated abnormal leaflet motion.)

▶ Armstrong, WF & Ryan T: *Feigenbaum's Echocardiography*, 7th edition. Lippincott & Wilkins. Philadelphia, 2010, pp 115–120, 396, 402–409.

427. B. Early post-implantation echocardiography provides baselines for many aspects of valve function, including (and not limited to) gradients, regurgitation, and leaflet motion.

The initial study post valve implantation serves several purposes. During the first echocardiographic study perivalvular leaks can be evaluated if they are present. A trivial perivalvular leak can sometimes be seen soon after implantation due to technical reasons but is considered abnormal only if it develops late after implantation. Pressure gradients will be documented in order to establish a baseline. With a mechanical prosthesis, valve regurgitation (washing jets) is evaluated in order to compare them with future echocardiograms if mechanical dysfunction occurs, which may manifest in a different pattern of regurgitation. Spectral Doppler valve clicks are not generally seen with a normally functioning bioprosthetic valve.

▸ Armstrong WF, Ryan T: *Feigenbaum's Echocardiography*, 7th edition. Philadelphia, Lippincott Williams & Wilkins, 2010, pp 393–394, 414.

428. C. Increased gradients compared to normal native valves.

With a mechanical heart valve, spectral Doppler will demonstrate pressure gradients that are higher than those typically seen in normal native valves, as well as clear valve clicks (opening and closing artifacts). The absence of valve clicks can be a clue to mechanical valvular obstruction. Spectral Doppler valve clicks (opening and closing artifacts) are not usually seen with bioprosthetic valves that have normal function. Small washing jets are a normal finding for mechanical prosthetic valves.

▸ Armstrong WF, Ryan T: *Feigenbaum's Echocardiography*, 6th edition. Philadelphia, Lippincott Williams & Wilkins, 2005, p 410.

▸ Armstrong WF, Ryan T: *Feigenbaum's Echocardiography*, 7th edition. Philadelphia, Lippincott Williams & Wilkins, 2010, pp 388, 395–396.

429. C. Three.

A bileaflet tilting disk valve has three orifices, two semicircular orifices and one central rectangular orifice.

▸ Armstrong WF, Ryan T: *Feigenbaum's Echocardiography*, 7th edition. Philadelphia, Lippincott Williams & Wilkins, 2010, pp 388, 403–406.

430. A. More likely.

Pannus formation is a process in which fibrous tissue ingrowth occurs from a prosthetic valve to the native tissue interface. Pannus ingrowth is not generally seen in native valves in the absence of surgical intervention. By 2D echocardiography pannus appears around the sewing ring, echogenic and not very mobile.

▸ Armstrong WF, Ryan T: *Feigenbaum's Echocardiography*, 7th edition. Philadelphia, Lippincott Williams & Wilkins, 2010, pp 403–406.

431. D. Suture repair of mitral valve regurgitation that may resemble a double orifice.

The Alfieri technique (also known as the "bow-tie" or "edge-to-edge" mitral valve repair) corrects mitral valve regurgitation by suturing the A2 and P2 segments of the mitral valve. If located centrally, the suture can make the mitral valve resemble a double orifice or bow tie.

▸ Armstrong WF, Ryan T: *Feigenbaum's Echocardiography*, 7th edition. Philadelphia, Lippincott Williams & Wilkins, 2010, p 423.

432. C. Parasternal long-axis view in the presence of mechanical aortic and mitral valves, using transthoracic echocardiography.

Of the views listed, the left atrium is most obscured in a transthoracic parasternal long-axis plane in a patient with mechanical aortic and mitral valves. The mechanical aortic valve will obstruct the view of the left atrium, and the mechanical mitral valve will result in shadowing. Transesophageal echocardiography in this scenario should provide the best views of the left atrium.

▸ Armstrong WF, Ryan T: *Feigenbaum's Echocardiography*, 7th edition. Philadelphia, Lippincott Williams & Wilkins, 2010, pp 115–120, 396, 402.

Refer to video PER-Q433.

433. C. 2D imaging of normal mitral leaflet motion of a bileaflet tilting disk valve.

Video PER-Q433 is a 2D image of a bileaflet tilting disk mitral valve prosthesis. The leaflet motion in this image is normal. Notice how both leaflets open simultaneously with no restriction. Due to reverberation artifact, the sewing ring of the prosthetic mitral valve is not well seen and it is difficult

ANSWERS

to rule out small clots in the left atrium. However, the good leaflet motion would suggest that there are no clots on the valve.

▶ Armstrong WF, Ryan T: *Feigenbaum's Echocardiography*, 7th edition. Philadelphia, Lippincott Williams & Wilkins, 2010, pp 387, 394.

434. C. Obstruction of the valve leaflet, as indicated by the increased valve gradient and the diminished valve clicks.

See Color Plate 21 on page xxix.

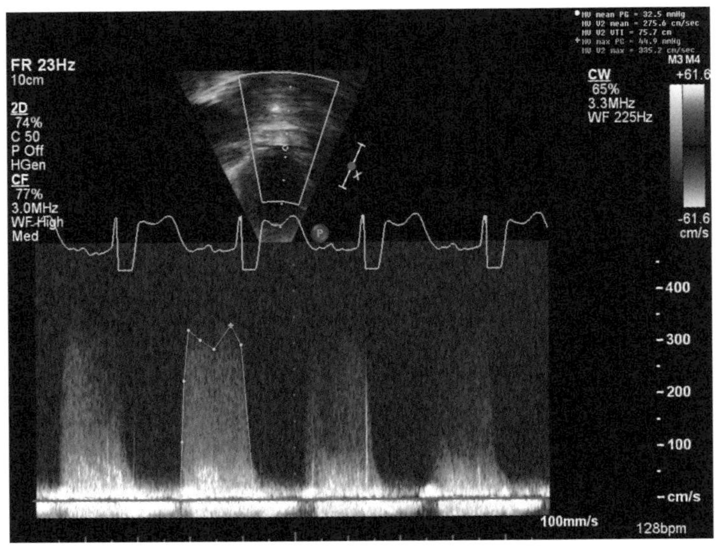

The spectral Doppler image was taken from a patient with thrombus formation on the mechanical mitral valve leaflets, which caused significant obstruction. Note the significantly elevated mean pressure gradient (32.5 mmHg) as well as the diminished valve clicks due to obstruction.

▶ Armstrong WF, Ryan T: *Feigenbaum's Echocardiography*, 6th edition. Philadelphia, Lippincott Williams & Wilkins, 2005, p 410.

▶ Armstrong WF, Ryan T: *Feigenbaum's Echocardiography*, 7th edition. Philadelphia, Lippincott Williams & Wilkins, 2010, pp 388–409.

435. A. Conduit surrounding the ascending aorta, most likely implanted to alleviate dilatation.

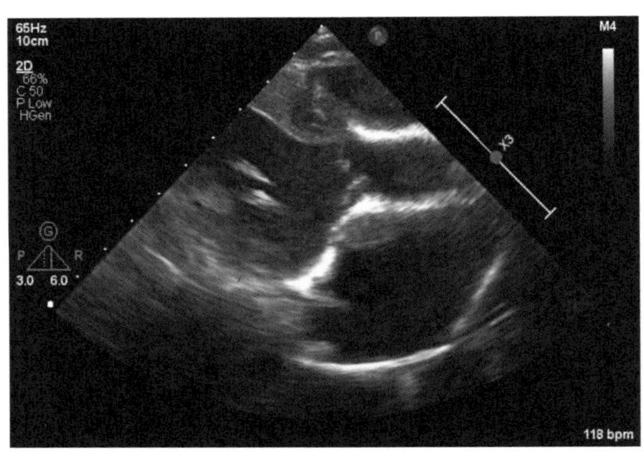

The image depicts a conduit that was implanted in order to relieve ascending aortic dilatation and help support a regurgitant aortic valve with root dilatation. The conduit is ribbed and has a specific acoustic appearance, which creates an artifact below the aorta. The artifact seen in this image can be mistaken for a clot or an abscess. Moving to a different acoustic window and recognizing the reverberation artifact will help you understand why this is not an abscess or clot in this instance.

▶ Armstrong WF, Ryan T: *Feigenbaum's Echocardiography*, 6th edition. Philadelphia, Lippincott Williams & Wilkins, 2005, pp 25–26, 394, 419.

436. C. Right middle lobe pneumonia.

Superior vena cava syndrome (SVC syndrome) is the set of symptoms caused by restricted or blocked SVC blood flow returning from the upper body to the right atrium. This leads to elevated SVC pressure above the level of the obstruction, causing facial and arm swelling. Any clinical situation in which there is external compression or internal obstruction of the SVC will produce SVC syndrome. For example, thrombosis in the SVC or innominate (brachiocephalic) vein, surgical scarring of an SVC cannulation site, a right upper lung mass, and a mediastinal mass can all cause obstruction of the SVC. Right middle lobe pneumonia will not cause compression of the SVC.

PART 5

Clinical Standards and Guidelines

437. D. 12 MHz phased array.

The transducer most appropriate for a small neonate is a phased array transducer. Both the curvilinear and linear array transducers listed in this question have too large a footprint for a small neonate and therefore would not be used. When evaluating cardiac structures in the neonate, it is important to utilize the highest-frequency transducer possible. Higher ultrasound frequencies provide better spatial resolution for measuring critically important structures in a small baby. Therefore, a 12 MHz phased array transducer would be preferable to a 5 MHz phased array transducer. With the use of a high-frequency transducer, there can be a tradeoff in terms of ultrasound penetration; more scattering and absorption of the higher-frequency sound waves can lead to poorer visualization of deeper cardiac structures. However, for parasternal imaging of a neonate, this is generally not a problem due to the thin chest wall and small distance from the transducer to the heart.

▸ Lai WW, Mertens LL, Cohen MS, et al (eds): *Echocardiography in Pediatric and Congenital Heart Disease: From Fetus to Adult*, 2nd edition. Chichester, UK, Wiley-Blackwell, 2016, pp 11–12.

438. A. 12 MHz.

For 2D imaging of a newborn baby, always try to use the highest-frequency transducer possible, especially for the suprasternal view. A higher-frequency transducer has better axial and lateral resolution than a lower-frequency transducer. High resolution is essential for imaging the small cardiac and vascular structures in a newborn with congenital heart disease.

▸ Lai WW, Mertens LL, Cohen MS, et al (eds): *Echocardiography in Pediatric and Congenital Heart Disease: From Fetus to Adult*, 2nd edition. Chichester, UK, Wiley-Blackwell, 2016, p 12.

439. A. Aortic valve stenosis, from the suprasternal notch window.

The blind continuous-wave (CW) Doppler probe is a thin ultrasound transducer with a small footprint and simple design: It consists of two crystals, one that continuously emits low-frequency ultrasound signals and one that continuously receives the returning signals. This probe is used to obtain the maximum Doppler velocity along the line of interrogation. This particular probe can quantify very high-velocity Doppler signals (in excess of 6–7 m/sec), and it is most useful for this purpose. However, no 2D imaging is available for localization, and furthermore, as with all CW Doppler, there is complete range ambiguity—no information is available regarding the origin of the high-velocity Doppler signal along the line of insonation. Therefore, the blind CW probe is best used in combination with 2D imaging and color flow Doppler, so that areas of turbulence can be precisely identified before CW Doppler evaluation is performed. One of the best applications of the blind CW Doppler is to the evaluation of a patient with aortic valve stenosis, using the suprasternal notch window; the small transducer footprint is well suited to evaluation of the high-velocity aortic valve and ascending aortic Doppler signals. The other options—shunting across an atrial septal defect and unobstructed total anomalous pulmonary venous connection to the coronary sinus—involve low-velocity Doppler signals best evaluated by other transducers that can combine 2D imaging with color flow, pulsed-wave, and CW Doppler. Coarctation of the aorta is not well seen from the apical view.

▸ Edelman SK: *Understanding Ultrasound Physics*, 4th edition. The Woodlands, TX, ESP Ultrasound, 2012, pp 312–313.

▸ Lai WW, Mertens LL, Cohen MS, et al (eds): *Echocardiography in Pediatric and Congenital Heart Disease: From Fetus to Adult*, 2nd edition. Chichester, UK, Wiley-Blackwell, 2016, pp 12–13.

440. C. CW Doppler can measure high velocities.

Continuous-wave (CW) Doppler has range ambiguity (cannot determine the exact location of the measured velocity along the line of insonation), but it can measure very high velocities without an aliasing artifact. In contrast, pulsed-wave Doppler has range resolution but is unable to measure high velocities accurately; with pulsed-wave Doppler, high velocities produce aliasing.

▸ Edelman SK: *Understanding Ultrasound Physics*, 4th edition. The Woodlands, TX, ESP Ultrasound, 2012, pp 312–314.

ANSWERS

441. D. Change to a 5 MHz transducer.

A lower-frequency transducer has better penetration and generates a smaller Doppler shift. As a result it will obtain a better-quality spectral and color flow Doppler signal, and there will be a reduced amount of aliasing.

▶ Lai WW, Mertens LL, Cohen MS, et al (eds): *Echocardiography in Pediatric and Congenital Heart Disease: From Fetus to Adult*, 2nd edition. Chichester, UK, Wiley-Blackwell, 2016, pp 16–17.

442. B. Use a lower-frequency transducer.

The best approach to improving the image quality in this scenario is to use a lower-frequency transducer. Lower-frequency ultrasound waves have better tissue penetration, thereby providing improved 2D visualization and color flow Doppler depiction of cardiac structures. However, the tradeoff is reduced 2D spatial resolution compared to higher-frequency transducers. Of the other options, decreasing overall 2D imaging gain will not result in an improved color flow Doppler signal. Decreasing the Nyquist limit might enhance the visualization of lower-velocity color flow signals (such as venous flow), but the flow across the aortic arch and coarctation of the aorta will be higher-velocity, and in fact lowering the Nyquist limit will merely produce aliasing of the color flow signal, particularly through the coarctation. Narrowing the sector width will improve temporal resolution (with higher frame rates) but will not improve the color flow Doppler signal.

▶ Lai WW, Mertens LL, Cohen MS, et al (eds): *Echocardiography in Pediatric and Congenital Heart Disease: From Fetus to Adult*, 2nd edition. Chichester, UK, Wiley-Blackwell, 2016, pp 16–17.

443. A. Obstetric/fetal imaging.

A curvilinear array probe has a convex transducer surface, which provides a larger field of view that is suitable for obstetric and fetal imaging. Its large, rounded footprint makes it unsuitable for neonatal imaging, and imaging of vascular structures should be performed with a linear sequential array transducer with a smaller footprint and much higher frequency (at least 12–15 MHz or even more). If an adult has a limited transthoracic window, the larger footprint of the curvilinear array transducer would not provide better imaging.

▶ Callen PW: *Ultrasonography in Obstetrics and Gynecology*, 5th edition. Philadelphia, Saunders Elsevier, 2008, pp 8–12.

444. D. Matrix array probe.

The transducer that is currently used for 3D/4D is known as a matrix array probe, in which individual transducer elements are arranged in a 2D matrix. One of the most common arrangements is a 50 × 50 matrix, yielding 2500 elements in total; some transducers have more than 3000 elements. This arrangement enables the collection of a pyramidal dataset that includes ultrasonic information in all three planes—axial, lateral, and elevational—and this information can be used to produce a 3D rendering of the heart. Furthermore, the 3D images can be displayed in real time, resulting in a "4D" image. None of the other options in this question will collect a 3D ultrasonic dataset.

▶ Eidem BW, O'Leary PW, Cetta F: *Echocardiography in Pediatric and Adult Congenital Heart Disease*, 2nd edition. Philadelphia, Wolters Kluwer, 2015, pp 62–70.

▶ Simpson J, Lopez L, Acar P, et al: Three-dimensional echocardiography in congenital heart disease: an expert consensus document from the European Association of Cardiovascular Imaging and the American Society of Echocardiography. J Am Soc Echocardiogr 30:1–27, 2017.

445. C. Dynamic range/compression.

Dynamic range and compression act to increase or decrease the number of shades of gray that are displayed. A narrow dynamic range reduces the number of shades of gray, resulting in high contrast. Conversely, a wide dynamic range increases the number of shades of gray and produces low contrast. For visualization of the coronary arteries, a narrow dynamic range (increased contrast) is preferable. None of the other parameters listed for this question affects image contrast. Persistence serves to superimpose previous frames on the most current frame, resulting in a smoother image and reduced noise, but with a reduced frame rate. Transmit power will increase the amplitude of the transmitted echo signals and therefore increase visualization from weaker signal reflectors, but at the expense of the patient being exposed to greater acoustic energy. Line density will change the number of scan lines; a larger number of scan lines (with the same sector size) will improve lateral resolution, but at the expense of temporal resolution.

▶ Edelman SK: *Understanding Ultrasound Physics*, 4th edition. The Woodlands, TX, ESP Ultrasound, 2012, pp 256, 265–258.

▶ Lai WW, Mertens LL, Cohen MS, et al (eds): *Echocardiography in Pediatric and Congenital Heart Disease: From Fetus to Adult*, 2nd edition. Chichester, UK, Wiley-Blackwell, 2016, pp 5–6.

▶ Wong PC, Miller-Hance WC (eds): *Transesophageal Echocardiography for Congenital Heart Disease*, London, Springer-Verlag, 2014, pp 41–42.

ANSWERS

446. B. A high-frequency transducer for the suprasternal view, because it provides better lateral resolution.

Higher-frequency transducers have a small focal zone and provide better spatial (lateral and axial) resolution. That is why using a high-frequency transducer is better for imaging a small baby and for imaging more superficial structures; higher-frequency ultrasound does not penetrate as deeply due to greater absorption and scattering. In contrast to spatial resolution, temporal resolution is dependent upon frame rate, not transducer frequency. Frame rate is in turn dependent upon sector width and depth—the wider and longer the sector, the lower the frame rate.

▸ Edelman SK: *Understanding Ultrasound Physics*, 4th edition. The Woodlands, TX, ESP Ultrasound, 2012, pp 113–128.

447. D. Decreasing transducer frequency.

In the generation of an echocardiographic image, an ultrasonic pulse must be emitted and the returning ultrasonic information collected along the line of insonation. A series of adjacent lines collected sequentially forms the characteristic pie-shaped echocardiographic image, and the process must be repeated continually to produce a moving image. Temporal resolution (determined by frame rate, given in frames per second) represents the speed at which these images can be repeated. The faster the frame rate, the better the temporal resolution. Temporal resolution depends upon both the depth of the image sector and the width of the sector. The deeper the sector, the longer it takes for ultrasound waves to travel from the transducer to the selected depth and then return to the transducer. Therefore, decreasing the depth will reduce the time required to produce an image and improve temporal resolution. Similarly, decreasing sector width generally means that fewer scan lines will be required to generate an image; therefore frame rates will increase. When color Doppler information is added to a 2D image, the increased amount of information will slow the frame rate; hence temporal resolution decreases. Removing the color Doppler will improve the frame rate. Changing transducer frequency will not change temporal resolution, because the speed of sound in tissue remains constant, irrespective of sonic frequency.

▸ Lai WW, Mertens LL, Cohen MS, et al (eds): *Echocardiography in Pediatric and Congenital Heart Disease: From Fetus to Adult*, 2nd edition. Chichester, UK, Wiley-Blackwell, 2016, p 11.

448. C. Reducing the color flow Doppler scale.

Reducing the color Doppler scale—i.e., adjusting the Nyquist limit—will enhance very low-velocity color flow Doppler signals such as those found in the pulmonary veins in some patients with total anomalous pulmonary venous connection (TAPVC). Conversely, it will cause higher-velocity color flow signals to alias. Increasing color flow Doppler gains might help to visualize the lower-velocity pulmonary venous flow, but it will also enhance higher-velocity flows and produce significant color flow "noise." Decreasing 2D imaging gains will not improve visualization or low-flow color Doppler signals. Similarly, changing from brightness to variance mode might improve display of turbulence but will not improve low-flow color Doppler signals.

▶ Lai WW, Mertens LL, Cohen MS, et al (eds): *Echocardiography in Pediatric and Congenital Heart Disease: From Fetus to Adult*, 2nd edition. Chichester, UK, Wiley-Blackwell, 2016, pp 16–17.

449. B. Improving endocardial border definition.

Tissue harmonic imaging relies on the fact that relatively high-pressure sound waves traveling through tissue at a given frequency will generate sound waves at harmonic frequencies that are multiples of the original frequency. For example, if the fundamental frequency is 2.5 MHz, the second harmonic frequency will be 5.0 MHz, the third harmonic frequency will be 7.5 MHz, etc. In tissue harmonic imaging the focal point becomes the second harmonic frequency. The advantage of this type of imaging is that artifacts—which all arise from the fundamental frequency—are reduced or eliminated because the focus is on the second harmonic. Thus signal-to-noise ratio is increased, resulting in enhanced contrast resolution and border delineation (during visualization of endocardial borders, for example). Tissue harmonic imaging specifically applies to 2D imaging, not M-mode imaging, color flow Doppler, or spectral Doppler.

▶ Edelman SK: *Understanding Ultrasound Physics*, 4th edition. The Woodlands, TX, ESP Ultrasound, 2012, pp 269–274.

450. D. Compensate for attenuation by boosting signal amplitudes at different depths.

Time gain compensation (TGC) allows for gain adjustments at different depths and therefore can be used to compensate for attenuation of ultrasound signals with depth. Most ultrasound machines have a set of "slider bars" that can be adjusted to increase the amplitude of ultrasound signals returning from greater depths, thereby providing more uniformity in the echogenicity of similar tissues regardless of their distance from the transducer. None of the other answer choices correctly describes what TGC adjustment accomplishes.

▶ Edelman SK: *Understanding Ultrasound Physics*, 4th edition. The Woodlands, TX, ESP Ultrasound, 2012, pp 226–228.

▶ Lai WW, Mertens LL, Cohen MS, et al (eds): *Echocardiography in Pediatric and Congenital Heart Disease: From Fetus to Adult*, 2nd edition. Chichester, UK, Wiley-Blackwell, 2016, p 5.

451. D. Reduce image sector size.

In pediatric patients, the heart rate is usually higher than the normal adult heart rate, so a higher temporal resolution is generally required. Better temporal resolution by definition means an increased frame rate. Of the choices for this question, only reducing the image sector size will increase the frame rate. Changing the focus improves lateral resolution and using a higher-frequency transducer improves spatial resolution, but neither of these maneuvers improves the temporal resolution. Changing the gain range will also not affect temporal resolution.

▶ Edelman SK: *Understanding Ultrasound Physics*, 4th edition. The Woodlands, TX, ESP Ultrasound, 2012, pp 198–199.

▶ Lai WW, Mertens LL, Cohen MS, et al (eds): *Echocardiography in Pediatric and Congenital Heart Disease: From Fetus to Adult*, 2nd edition. Chichester, UK, Wiley-Blackwell, 2016, pp 10–12.

452. A. Poor angle of insonation.

See Color Plate 22 on page xxix.

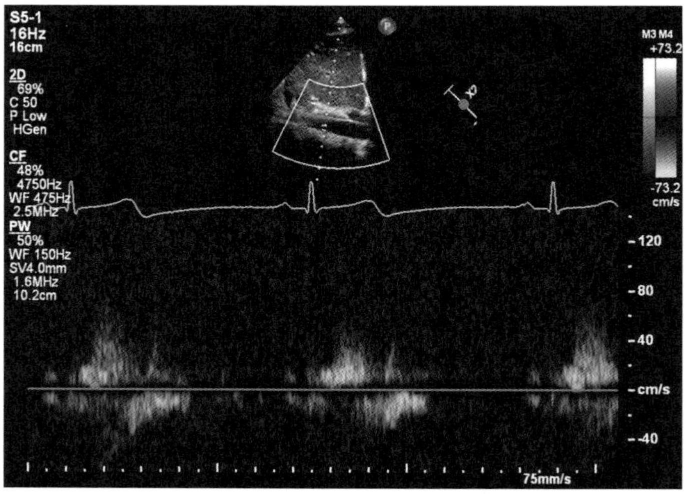

Optimal Doppler interrogation of a blood vessel requires that the angle of insonation be as parallel as possible to the direction of blood flow. According to the Doppler equation, as

the angle of insonation approaches 90° (i.e., as the ultrasound beam gets closer to being perpendicular to the direction of blood flow), the calculated velocity decreases considerably, approaching zero. In this spectral tracing of the descending aorta, the angle of insonation is nearly 90° to the direction of blood flow, and this produces a poor Doppler waveform.

- Edelman SK: *Understanding Ultrasound Physics*, 4th edition. The Woodlands, TX, ESP Ultrasound, 2012, pp 309–310.
- Lai WW, Mertens LL, Cohen MS, et al (eds): *Echocardiography in Pediatric and Congenital Heart Disease: From Fetus to Adult*, 2nd edition. Chichester, UK, Wiley-Blackwell, 2016, pp 12–16.

453. B. Image dropout artifact.

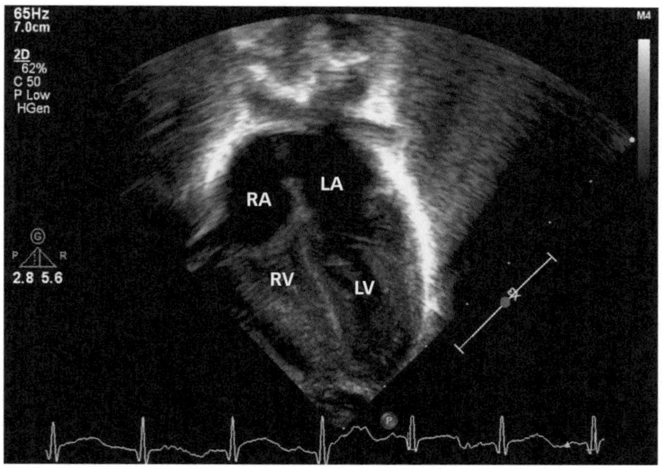

This image demonstrates a dropout artifact. The plane of the thin atrial septum is located parallel to the ultrasound beam, and the thinness of the septum, as well as its constant motion, can result in "dropout" that gives the appearance of an atrial septal defect. To confirm the presence of the defect, the atrial septum should be visualized in other planes, such as the subcostal long- and short-axis planes. In the subcostal views, the plane of the atrial septum will be perpendicular to the ultrasound beam, resulting in a much clearer (and more reliable) visualization of atrial septal anatomy. Slice-thickness artifacts are beam-width artifacts resulting from objects within the elevational plane of the ultrasound beam and appear to be in the same tomographic scan plane as the currently visualized cardiac structures. Side lobe artifacts are phantom structures resulting from energy falling outside the main beam and generally are seen adjacent to the main beam. RA = right atrium, LA = left atrium, RV = right ventricle, LV = left ventricle.

- Lai WW, Mertens LL, Cohen MS, et al (eds): *Echocardiography in Pediatric and Congenital Heart Disease: From Fetus to Adult*, 2nd edition. Chichester, UK, Wiley-Blackwell, 2016, pp 7, 203.

454. D. When a strong reflector is located behind an object along the path of the primary ultrasound beam.

Mirror-image artifacts occur when you are interrogating a structure that is located in front of a strong reflector, along the path of the primary ultrasound beam. When a transmit pulse encounters the structure at your focal point (the object of your study), some energy is reflected back to the transducer, producing the first image. However, some sound energy is transmitted through the structure of interest and then continues to the interface of the strong reflector, beyond the structure. The sound that returns from that interface undergoes partial reflection at the structure, and this secondary echo returns back to the strong reflector interface, where it is reflected again and eventually returns back to the transducer. Because of the added time required for this multiply reflected signal to return to the transducer, a longer distance is calculated for the signal, giving rise to a secondary object that appears to be beyond the interface, and on the echocardiogram it appears as a mirror image of original structure. In other words, the object and its mirror image are on opposite sides and equal distances from the reflector. Mirror-image artifacts can also occur with color flow Doppler. None of the other options for answering this question describes the setting for a mirror-image artifact.

▸ Edelman SK: *Understanding Ultrasound Physics*, 4th edition. The Woodlands, TX, ESP Ultrasound, 2012, p 363.

455. A. Aliasing.

See Color Plate 23 on page xxx.

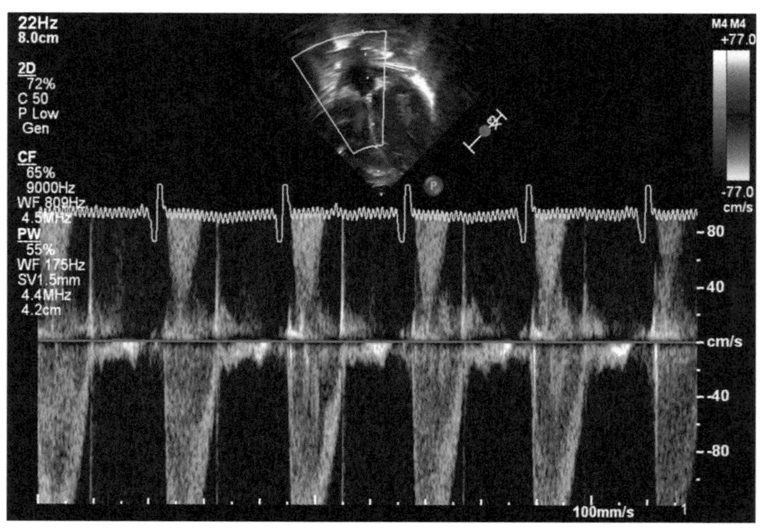

The tracing shows the typical "wraparound" effect associated with aliasing. This can be noted on a pulsed-wave spectral Doppler tracing when the velocity is too high and the pulse

repetition frequency (or half the Nyquist limit) is exceeded. To obtain an accurate measurement, one can try increasing the pulse repetition frequency (PRF) or moving the spectral baseline up or down (depending on the direction of flow) to assign the entire spectral range to the velocity in question. However, if aliasing still occurs, continuous-wave Doppler evaluation might be necessary to quantify the velocity accurately. Other techniques to avoid aliasing include the use of a lower-frequency transducer and interrogation from a window with reduced depth from the transducer to the area of interest (not always possible). In this question, the main flow on the spectral display is systolic and higher-velocity, not continuous low-velocity as would be expected with venous flow, so choice C, "typical venous spectral Doppler flow pattern," would not be correct. The flow in question is not diastolic; therefore it is not mitral, and choice D, "flow across the mitral valve," is incorrect. Choice B is incorrect because excessive gain would not produce the spectral Doppler wraparound waveform seen in this tracing.

▸ Edelman SK: *Understanding Ultrasound Physics*, 4th edition. The Woodlands, TX, ESP Ultrasound, 2012, pp 319–323.

▸ Lai WW, Mertens LL, Cohen MS, et al (eds): *Echocardiography in Pediatric and Congenital Heart Disease: From Fetus to Adult*, 2nd edition. Chichester, UK, Wiley-Blackwell, 2016, pp 15–16.

456. D. Large acoustic impedance mismatch between two objects.

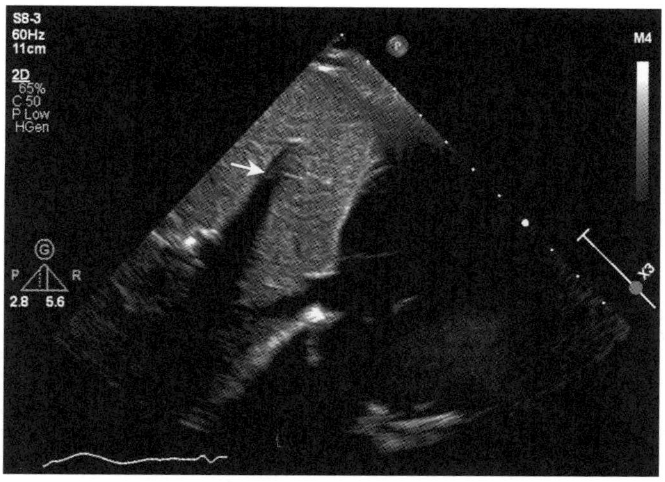

The artifact shown, known as acoustic shadowing, is a dark area that results from acoustic impedance mismatching between two structures. When sound waves traveling through one medium encounter a structure or interface with markedly different acoustic impedance, most of the incident sound is reflected and little to none is transmitted beyond that interface.

ANSWERS

This produces a signal void or area of acoustic shadowing beyond the interface, represented by a dark, hypoechoic or anechoic band (arrow) in which no acoustic information is available. This acoustic void is known as a dropout artifact.

▶ Lai WW, Mertens LL, Cohen MS, et al (eds): *Echocardiography in Pediatric and Congenital Heart Disease: From Fetus to Adult*, 2nd edition. Chichester, UK, Wiley-Blackwell, 2016, p 8.

457. D. The artifact appears deeper than the real structure.

A mirror-image artifact is the appearance of the mirror image of the real object on the opposite side of a strong reflector (hence the name "mirror image"). Reflectors that commonly cause mirror-image artifacts include the pericardium, the diaphragm, and the pleura. Incident ultrasound beams from the transducer that pass through the structure of interest to the reflector are reflected back to the structure and then are reflected from the structure back to the reflector. This ultrasonic energy is then reflected off the reflector and back to the transducer. The returning signal produces a mirror image of the real object of interest and, because of the time delay, the mirror image appears to be deeper—i.e., on the other side of the reflector. Therefore, the artifactual image always appears deeper than the image of the real structure of interest. Incorrect time gain compensation will cause a focal enhancement artifact, and a mechanical mitral valve can cause comet-tail and shadow artifacts. Neither causes a mirror-image artifact.

▶ Edelman SK: *Understanding Ultrasound Physics*, 4th edition. The Woodlands, TX, ESP Ultrasound, 2012, p 363.

458. B. Angle the sound beam so it is more parallel to the direction of flow.

See Color Plate 24 on page xxx.

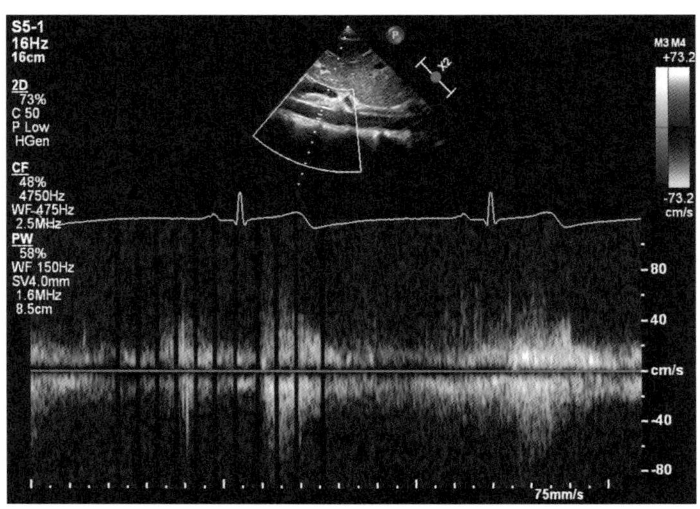

The artifact shown on the image represents spectral Doppler mirroring. It is seen when the angle of insonation is perpendicular (approximately 90°) to the direction of flow. In theory, when there is a perpendicular angle of insonation, the calculated returning velocity should be 0. In practice, however, the entire beam emerging from a transducer will not be at an exact 90° angle to the flow in the sample volume; some parts of the beam will have an angle slightly greater than 90° and some slightly less than 90°. Hence, spectral Doppler signals can be obtained above and below the baseline. The other methods listed—changing to a lower-frequency transducer, changing the spectral Doppler baseline, and increasing the spectral Doppler scale—can be used to reduce or eliminate Doppler aliasing but will not affect spectral Doppler mirroring. Note that the spectral Doppler mirror artifact is different from a mirror-image artifact.

▶ Zagzebski JA: *Essentials of Ultrasound Physics*. St Louis, Mosby, 1996, pp 129–131.

459. A. Suprasternal coronal view.

The suprasternal coronal view, also referred to as the "crab view," is the best view to demonstrate the four individual pulmonary veins. Other imaging views from the subcostal, apical, and even parasternal windows can also demonstrate some pulmonary veins, but not all can be well visualized in the same image using these other views.

▶ Snider AR, Silverman NH: Suprasternal notch echocardiography: a two-dimensional technique for evaluating congenital heart disease. Circulation 63:165–173, 1981.

460. A. Position of the azygos and hemiazygos veins.

The subcostal long-axis (transverse) view is obtained with the transducer located in the upper abdomen, just below the xiphoid process, and directed posteriorly toward the spine with the transducer notch/dot at the 3 o'clock position and the apex of the imaging sector seen at the top of the screen. For normal visceroatrial situs, the liver and the inferior vena cava (IVC) will be located to the right of midline and the stomach to the left of midline. The morphologic right atrial appendage is broad-based and triangular, while the morphologic left atrial appendage is narrow and "finger-like." The azygos vein is generally located to the right of midline and posterior; however, when the IVC is patent, the azygos vein can be very difficult to visualize. Furthermore, absence of the azygos vein (and presence of the hemiazygos vein) will not provide information regarding visceroatrial situs.

- Eidem BW, O'Leary PW, Cetta F: *Echocardiography in Pediatric and Adult Congenital Heart Disease*, 2nd edition. Philadelphia, Wolters Kluwer, 2015, pp 24–26.
- Ezon DS, Goldberg JF, Kyle WB: *Atlas of Congenital Heart Disease Nomenclature: An Illustrated Guide to the Van Praagh and Anderson Approaches to Describing Congenital Cardiac Pathology*. Houston, Ezon Educational Services/CreateSpace, 2015, pp 4–5.
- Lai WW, Mertens LL, Cohen MS, et al (eds): *Echocardiography in Pediatric and Congenital Heart Disease: From Fetus to Adult*, 2nd edition. Chichester, UK, Wiley-Blackwell, 2016, p 46.

461. C. Invert the image and rotate the transducer notch to 6 o'clock.

A

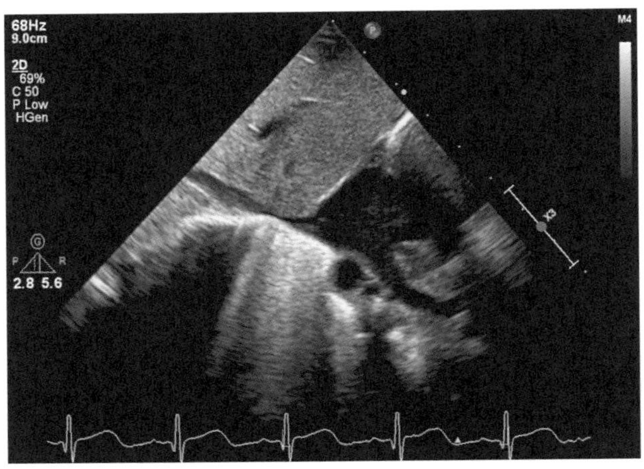

B

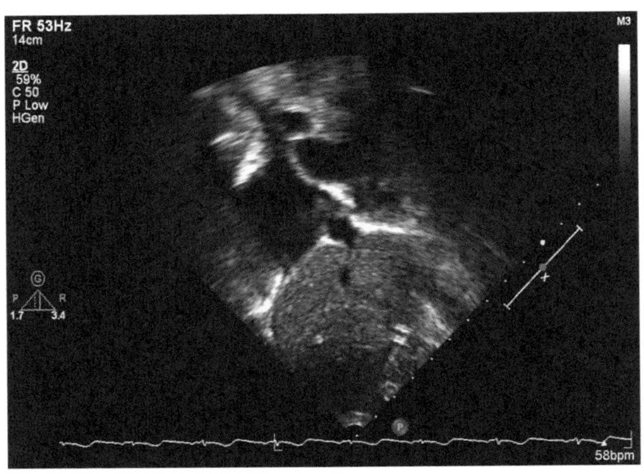

***A** This image was obtained from a subcostal short-axis view in the conventional manner for adult echocardiographic display, but this view is incorrect for pediatric echocardiography and pediatric subcostal short-axis sweeps. **B** The correct display is in the "anatomically correct" position with the image*

ANSWERS

inverted so that the apex is at the bottom of the screen. The transducer notch/dot should be at 6 o'clock so that the inferior structures will be at the bottom of the screen and the superior structures at the top of the screen.

▶ Lai WW, Mertens LL, Cohen MS, et al (eds): *Echocardiography in Pediatric and Congenital Heart Disease: From Fetus to Adult*, 2nd edition. Chichester, UK, Wiley-Blackwell, 2016, pp 46–50.

Refer to video PER-Q462.

462. D. Nothing, based on this sweep.

The subcostal short-axis sweep seen in video PER-Q462 is not (by itself) diagnostic for evaluation of cardiac position and visceroatrial situs, because the same sweep can be obtained with situs solitus and situs inversus. In situs solitus, the transducer is swept to the left; in situs inversus (with otherwise normal anatomy, also known as mirror-image dextrocardia), it is swept to the right. In both cases, an identical sweep will be obtained unless information is provided as to which side the transducer is angled toward. The important point is that this sweep alone should not be used for establishment of left-right orientation; the subcostal long-axis sweep must be performed to determine left-right cardiac orientation.

▶ Lai WW, Mertens LL, Cohen MS, et al (eds): *Echocardiography in Pediatric and Congenital Heart Disease: From Fetus to Adult*, 2nd edition. Chichester, UK, Wiley-Blackwell, 2016, pp 46–48.

463. B. Infradiaphragmatic TAPVC.

Infradiaphragmatic total anomalous pulmonary venous connection (infradiaphragmatic TAPVC) can be a difficult diagnosis to establish. The subcostal long- and short-axis views are essential for visualization of the vertical vein that drains the pulmonary vein confluence and then returns below the diaphragm to the portal vein, inferior vena cava, or hepatic vein(s). No other echocardiographic view will demonstrate so clearly the vertical vein drainage and its connection with the systemic veins below the diaphragm, which is why this sweep is important for the initial evaluation of any patient with suspected CHD. Supracardiac TAPVC can be suspected from evidence seen in the subcostal sweeps, but the site of pulmonary venous drainage is best evaluated from other echocardiographic windows, such as the parasternal and suprasternal. A double aortic arch and coarctation of the aorta are not well seen from the subcostal windows and require suprasternal imaging.

▶ Lai WW, Mertens LL, Cohen MS, et al (eds): *Echocardiography in Pediatric and Congenital Heart Disease: From Fetus to Adult*, 2nd edition. Chichester, UK, Wiley-Blackwell, 2016, pp 46–49, 171–172.

464. A. Subcostal long-axis sweep.

The cardiac position in the right chest has a number of different etiologies, including the following:

- *Dextroposition—normal cardiac anatomy/orientation, but the cardiac mass is shifted to the right due to pneumothorax, diaphragmatic hernia, or another condition.*
- *Situs inversus—mirror-image dextrocardia.*
- *Situs solitus with congenital heart disease—such as congenitally corrected transposition of the great arteries.*
- *Situs ambiguus—heterotaxy.*

Therefore, the first question that must be asked is whether there is normal visceroatrial situs, and if so, what the segmental anatomy is. The subcostal long-axis sweep (with transducer notch/dot pointed to the left) provides the left-right orientation and information that is critical for determining visceroatrial situs and cardiac orientation. Using this view and sweeping superiorly from below the diaphragm into the thorax, you can systematically evaluate the liver and cardiac position, location of systemic and pulmonary venous return, and cardiac segments and connections (as well as the cardiac base-to-apex orientation). While the other views mentioned in the choices—the subcostal short-axis, parasternal long-axis, and parasternal short-axis sweeps—are also important for the evaluation of dextrocardia, they will not provide the same initial overview of left-right orientation and understanding of visceroatrial situs, systemic/pulmonary venous return, and segmental anatomy.

▶ Lai WW, Mertens LL, Cohen MS, et al (eds): *Echocardiography in Pediatric and Congenital Heart Disease: From Fetus to Adult*, 2nd edition. Chichester, UK, Wiley-Blackwell, 2016, pp 46–49, 560–563.

Refer to video PER-Q465.

465. C. Subcostal short-axis, right ventricular outflow tract.

Video PER-Q465 demonstrates the subcostal short-axis visualization of the right ventricular outflow tract (RVOT), with both 2D imaging and color flow Doppler. This view is part of the subcostal short-axis (sagittal) sweep and provides some of the best and most complete echocardiographic images of the RVOT. The subcostal short-axis window is very useful for demonstrating cardiac defects that involve this area, including various types of conotruncal abnormalities (such as double-outlet right ventricle) and defects that result in subpulmonary stenosis (such as double-chambered right ventricle and tetralogy of Fallot).

▶ Lai WW, Mertens LL, Cohen MS, et al (eds): *Echocardiography in Pediatric and Congenital Heart Disease: From Fetus to Adult*, 2nd edition. Chichester, UK, Wiley-Blackwell, 2016, pp 45–49.

Refer to video PER-Q466.

466. A. Right pulmonary artery.

From the subcostal long-axis sweep (video PER-Q466), the right pulmonary artery can be visualized superior to the right upper pulmonary vein and just prior to visualizing the more anterior ascending aorta. It can be distinguished from pulmonary venous flow by its pulsatile nature and the direction of flow toward the right lung. With the sweep, the right pulmonary artery can be seen to arise from the main pulmonary artery and posterior to the ascending aorta; therefore it is not a right aortic arch. The location is too inferior for a normal innominate (brachiocephalic) vein; furthermore, the usual flow pattern in the innominate vein is continuous, lower-velocity, phasic venous flow—different from the flow pattern demonstrated in this video.

▶ Lai WW, Mertens LL, Cohen MS, et al (eds): *Echocardiography in Pediatric and Congenital Heart Disease: From Fetus to Adult*, 2nd edition. Chichester, UK, Wiley-Blackwell, 2016, pp 45–49.

467. C. Move the "tail" of the transducer toward the feet (more inferiorly).

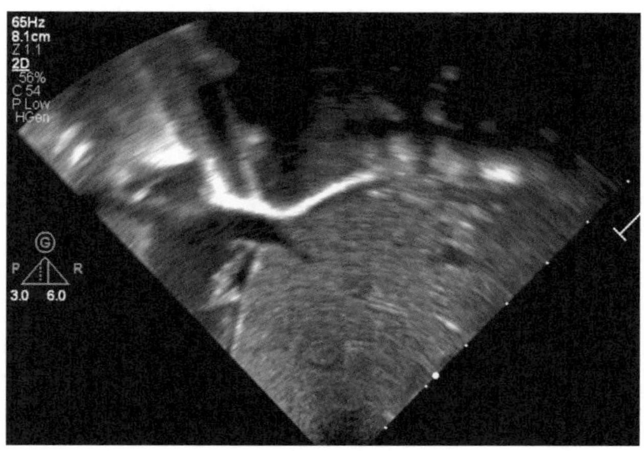

In this subcostal short-axis image, the heart is too far to the right of the screen and part of the image is not visible. To center the image, the transducer "tail" must be moved toward the feet (more inferiorly) in order to place the entire heart in the center of the screen. From that position, the transducer

can be angled to the left to perform a subcostal short-axis sweep. Centering the image also provides the best angles of insonation for Doppler evaluation of superior/inferior vena caval flow, as well as the pulmonary and aortic outflow tracts.

▶ Lai WW, Mertens LL, Cohen MS, et al (eds): *Echocardiography in Pediatric and Congenital Heart Disease: From Fetus to Adult*, 2nd edition. Chichester, UK, Wiley-Blackwell, 2016, pp 48–49.

ANSWERS

468. A. Right and left ventricular outflow tracts.

In addition to imaging many important intracardiac structures, the subcostal long-axis sweep is very useful for visualizing the right and left ventricular outflow tracts (RVOT and LVOT). This can be very useful for the evaluation of important cardiac defects such as tetralogy of Fallot, double-outlet right ventricle, truncus arteriosus, and d- and l-transposition of the great arteries. In some instances, counterclockwise rotation of the transducer notch to 2 o'clock (right anterior oblique view) or clockwise to 4–5 o'clock (left anterior oblique view) can provide additional imaging that is useful to separate the aortic and pulmonary outflows and determine additional important anatomic features such as conal septal malalignment and straddling atrioventricular valves. Of the other choices, the individual pulmonary veins and ductus arteriosus are better visualized from parasternal or suprasternal views. The semilunar valves can be seen from subcostal imaging and color flow/spectral Doppler, but visualization of semilunar valve morphology is better from the parasternal views because the valves are closer to the transducer and therefore en face views of the valves can often be obtained.

▶ Lai WW, Mertens LL, Cohen MS, et al (eds): *Echocardiography in Pediatric and Congenital Heart Disease: From Fetus to Adult*, 2nd edition. Chichester, UK, Wiley-Blackwell, 2016, pp 46–49.

469. B. Apex down, transducer notch/dot at 3 o'clock.

For pediatric echocardiography, the apical four-chamber view should be displayed in the "anatomically correct" position with the apex at the bottom and the transducer notch/dot at 3 o'clock so that the patient's left is on the right side of the screen and the patient's right is on the left side of the screen. This differs from the way the apical four-chamber view is displayed in adult echocardiography; for adults, the apex is at the top, with the transducer notch/dot at 3 o'clock.

▶ Lai WW, Mertens LL, Cohen MS, et al (eds): *Echocardiography in Pediatric and Congenital Heart Disease: From Fetus to Adult*, 2nd edition. Chichester, UK, Wiley-Blackwell, 2016, pp 49–50.

470. A. Atrial septum.

The apical four-chamber view provides excellent anatomic detail of the atrioventricular valves (mitral and tricuspid), as well as optimal angles of insonation for color flow and spectral Doppler evaluation. Similarly, with anterior angulation, the apical five-chamber view provides excellent anatomic detail and optimal Doppler angles for evaluation of the left ventricular outflow tract (LVOT), suitable for assessment of subaortic and aortic valve pathology. While the atrial septum is visible from the apical four-chamber view, it can be difficult to evaluate atrial septal morphology and accurately diagnose atrial septal defects (ASDs) from this window, because the parallel orientation of the ultrasound beam to the atrial septum can lead to false dropout. For optimal evaluation of the atrial septum, other echocardiographic views (subcostal long-axis or short-axis and high right parasternal views) should be used.

▸ Lai WW, Mertens LL, Cohen MS, et al (eds): *Echocardiography in Pediatric and Congenital Heart Disease: From Fetus to Adult*, 2nd edition. Chichester, UK, Wiley-Blackwell, 2016, pp 49–50.

471. C. Left ventricular circumferential strain.

Left ventricular circumferential strain (LVCS) is best evaluated from the parasternal short-axis view. The other measurements listed in this question can all be performed from the apical four-chamber view. In the case of left ventricular ejection fraction (LVEF), the apical two-chamber view can also be added for the biplane modified Simpson's measurement of ejection fraction.

▸ Lai WW, Mertens LL, Cohen MS, et al (eds): *Echocardiography in Pediatric and Congenital Heart Disease: From Fetus to Adult*, 2nd edition. Chichester, UK, Wiley-Blackwell, 2016, pp 96–131.

472. A. Clockwise rotation, transducer marker pointing to the patient's left hip.

The rule when scanning for dextrocardia is that the transducer marker is always pointed to the patient's left, never to the patient's right. Usually the transducer is located on the patient's right chest, with the transducer marker pointed to the patient's left shoulder to obtain a parasternal long-axis view. From that position, the transducer is rotated clockwise approximately 90° to point the marker toward the patient's left hip in order to obtain a parasternal short-axis view.

▸ Lai WW, Mertens LL, Cohen MS, et al (eds): *Echocardiography in Pediatric and Congenital Heart Disease: From Fetus to Adult*, 2nd edition. Chichester, UK, Wiley-Blackwell, 2016, pp 560–561.

ANSWERS

473. D. Rotation of the transducer clockwise with the notch/dot at 4 o'clock.

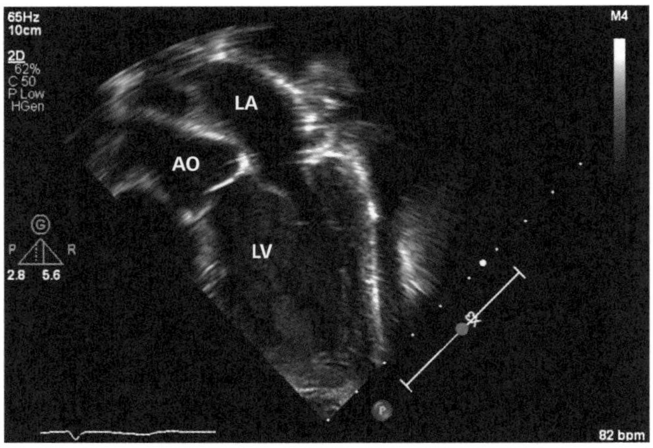

This image was taken from the apical three-chamber view, obtained from the apical four-chamber view by clockwise rotation of the transducer to 4 o'clock. No transducer angulation is necessary. In addition to allowing visualization of the left atrium and parts of the right and left ventricles, the apical three-chamber window is very useful for the evaluation of the left ventricular outflow tract, particularly subaortic structures oriented perpendicular to the plane of insonation. This also enables optimal Doppler evaluation (using spectral and color flow Doppler) of the left ventricular outflow tract and ascending aorta. Of note, angling the transducer anteriorly from the apical four-chamber view (as opposed to rotating clockwise) will produce the apical five-chamber view. AO = aorta, LA = left atrium, LV = left ventricle.

▶ Lai WW, Mertens LL, Cohen MS, et al (eds): *Echocardiography in Pediatric and Congenital Heart Disease: From Fetus to Adult*, 2nd edition. Chichester, UK, Wiley-Blackwell, 2016, p 50.

474. B. Rotate the transducer counterclockwise with the notch/dot at 12–1 o'clock.

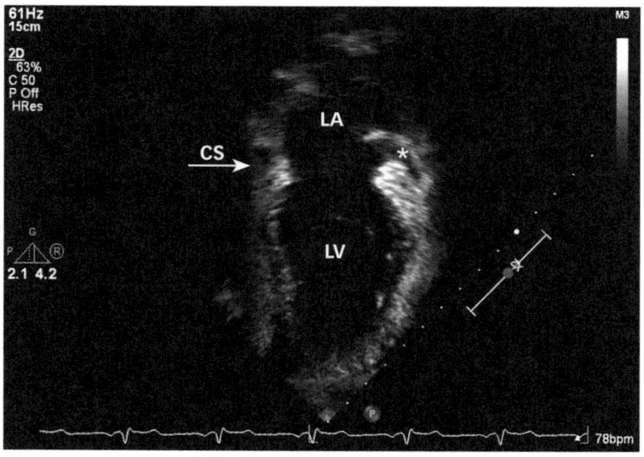

This image was obtained from the apical two-chamber view, suitable for assessment of left atrial size, global left ventricular function, and left ventricular regional wall motion abnormalities. From the apical four-chamber view, the transducer should be rotated counterclockwise so that the notch/dot is at 12–1 o'clock. No transducer angulation should be performed. The anterior wall should be displayed on the right side of the screen and the inferior wall on the left side of the screen. The coronary sinus (CS) can also be seen from this view: It appears as a small circle on the left of the screen (arrow). The left atrial appendage can sometimes be imaged from the apical two-chamber window and is seen here on the right of the screen (asterisk). LA = left atrium, LV = left ventricle.

- Lai WW, Mertens LL, Cohen MS, et al (eds): *Echocardiography in Pediatric and Congenital Heart Disease: From Fetus to Adult*, 2nd edition. Chichester, UK, Wiley-Blackwell, 2016, p 50.

Refer to video PER-Q475.

475. A. Angulation to patient's right, then left.

Video PER-Q475 demonstrates the typical parasternal long-axis sweep to the right and then to the left. First, the standard parasternal long-axis view is shown, displaying the left atrium (LA), mitral valve, left ventricle (LV), aortic valve, ascending aorta (Ao), and a portion of the right ventricle (RV). With rightward angulation of the transducer, the right-sided inflow structures are visualized, including the right atrium (RA), tricuspid valve, and RV inflow. With leftward angulation of the transducer, the anterior ventricular septum, right ventricular outflow tract (RVOT), pulmonary valve, and main pulmonary artery (MPA) are seen. The left coronary artery system can also be seen, including the left main coronary artery (LMCA) and its bifurcation into the left anterior descending (LAD) and left circumflex (LCX) coronary arteries. Once a standard parasternal long-axis view is obtained, the transducer should be angled only right and left; it should not be moved or rotated.

- Lai WW, Mertens LL, Cohen MS, et al (eds): *Echocardiography in Pediatric and Congenital Heart Disease: From Fetus to Adult*, 2nd edition. Chichester, UK, Wiley-Blackwell, 2016, pp 50–51.

476. C. The right upper pulmonary vein.

The coronary sinus and mid to distal right coronary artery, as well as a part of the right atrial appendage, can be visualized from a parasternal long-axis sweep when the transducer is tilted or angled to the right. The right upper pulmonary vein will not be visible because it is more superior and empties into the left atrium, which is also not seen in this particular view.

- Lai WW, Mertens LL, Cohen MS, et al (eds): *Echocardiography in Pediatric and Congenital Heart Disease: From Fetus to Adult*, 2nd edition. Chichester, UK, Wiley-Blackwell, 2016, p 50.

Refer to video PER-Q477.

477. C. Move the transducer superiorly toward the right shoulder.

Refer to video PER-Q477. The transducer is positioned too inferiorly, toward the cardiac apex, and must be moved superiorly one or two rib spaces to obtain a standard parasternal long-axis view. To determine the proper location, look for the following: The aortic valve and mitral valve should be in the middle of the screen, and a portion of the right ventricle, as well as the left atrium and ascending aorta, should be visible. None of the other maneuvers mentioned in this question will enable you to acquire a standard parasternal long-axis view.

- Lai WW, Mertens LL, Cohen MS, et al (eds): *Echocardiography in Pediatric and Congenital Heart Disease: From Fetus to Adult*, 2nd edition. Chichester, UK, Wiley-Blackwell, 2016, pp 50–51.

478. D. Suprasternal sagittal view.

Placing the transducer in the suprasternal notch and angling or tilting slightly toward the patient's right with the notch/dot at the 12 o'clock position, you can demonstrate the azygos vein draining into the right superior vena cava (SVC) just superior to the right pulmonary artery. This view is also good to see partial or total pulmonary veins returning to the SVC. An alternative view that provides very similar visualization is the high right parasternal parasagittal view.

- Lai WW, Mertens LL, Cohen MS, et al (eds): *Echocardiography in Pediatric and Congenital Heart Disease: From Fetus to Adult*, 2nd edition. Chichester, UK, Wiley-Blackwell, 2016, pp 55–57, 182, 187–188.
- Snider AR, Silverman NH: Suprasternal notch echocardiography: a two-dimensional technique for evaluating congenital heart disease. Circulation 63:165–173, 1981.

Refer to video PER-Q479.

479. A. High right parasternal parasagittal.

Video PER-Q479 is taken from a high right parasternal parasagittal view with the transducer located on the right chest, to the right of the sternum, and the notch/dot pointed superiorly toward the right neck (12 o'clock). This view provides excellent visualization of the superior vena cava

(SVC), azygos vein, right atrium (RA), left atrium (LA), and the superior portion of the atrial septum. The right pulmonary artery (RPA) can be also be seen above the LA. With increased depth, inferior vena cava (IVC) inflow can also be seen. This view is useful for visualization of atrial septal defects, particularly sinus venosus atrial septal defects, as well as partial or total anomalous pulmonary venous connection (TAPVC) to the SVC. When there is an interrupted IVC (as in polysplenia/left isomerism), the azygos vein is much larger and flow is higher-velocity and more prominent.

▶ Lai WW, Mertens LL, Cohen MS, et al (eds): *Echocardiography in Pediatric and Congenital Heart Disease: From Fetus to Adult*, 2nd edition. Chichester, UK, Wiley-Blackwell, 2016, p 55.

480. D. Suprasternal coronal view.

Placing the transducer in the suprasternal notch position with the marker point at 3 o'clock can help you obtain a coronal plane displaying the heart and vascular structures. This view will enable you to visualize both a right and a left superior vena cava, as well as the individual pulmonary veins, innominate vein (if present), transverse aortic arch, and right pulmonary artery.

▶ Snider AR, Silverman NH: Suprasternal notch echocardiography: a two-dimensional technique for evaluating congenital heart disease. Circulation 63:165–173, 1981.

481. B. Parasternal short-axis view at level of the aortic valve.

The parasternal short-axis window provides the best view for visualization of the origins of the right and left coronary arteries. Particularly in children, the close proximity of the transducer to the aorta allows for the use of higher-frequency transducers and color Doppler evaluation of coronary flow. With small degrees of clockwise and counterclockwise rotation, the proximal courses of the left and right coronary arteries can be well visualized, and the bifurcation of the left main coronary artery into the left anterior descending and circumflex coronary arteries can also be demonstrated. This view is particularly useful for visualization of intramural coronary arteries, as well as coronary artery aneurysms that can be associated with Kawasaki disease. Of note, the parasternal long-axis view is also useful for visualizing the proximal coronary arteries as well as the left coronary artery bifurcation, but it can be more difficult to visualize and separate the origins of the individual coronary arteries in the parasternal long-axis plane. The apical four-chamber view can provide some additional information regarding the coronary arteries arising from the aorta but should not serve as the primary plane for evaluating the coronary artery origins. The subcostal short-axis view does not demonstrate coronary artery origins well; furthermore, the spatial resolution needed for coronary artery visualization in this plane is often not as good as that from the parasternal views. The high right parasternal parasagittal view generally does not provide optimal visualization of the coronary arteries.

- Lai WW, Mertens LL, Cohen MS, et al (eds): *Echocardiography in Pediatric and Congenital Heart Disease: From Fetus to Adult*, 2nd edition. Chichester, UK, Wiley-Blackwell, 2016, pp 51–52, 584–608, 739–747.

Refer to video PER-Q482.

482. D. High left parasternal parasagittal view.

Video PER-Q482 demonstrates a high left parasternal parasagittal view, also known as a "ductal view." It was obtained from a high left parasternal window, below the left clavicle, and with the transducer notch/dot pointed superiorly to 12 o'clock. In this video, a sweep is first performed with 2D imaging and then repeated with color Doppler. First the transducer is angled to the right to visualize the ascending aorta (Asc Ao), right pulmonary artery (RPA), and left atrium (LA). Then leftward angulation visualizes the aortic arch, followed by the main pulmonary artery (MPA), RPA, left pulmonary artery (LPA), patent ductus arteriosus (PDA), and descending aorta (Desc Ao). The latter view is also known as a "three-finger view," with the three fingers comprising the RPA, LPA, and (when present) PDA. Of note, this transducer position can also be used to visualize a left superior vena cava (sagittal view), as well as the vertical vein from supracardiac total anomalous pulmonary venous connection that drains to the leftward aspect of the innominate (brachiocephalic) vein.

- Lai WW, Mertens LL, Cohen MS, et al (eds): *Echocardiography in Pediatric and Congenital Heart Disease: From Fetus to Adult*, 2nd edition. Chichester, UK, Wiley-Blackwell, 2016, pp 52–53.

483. C. Place a pillow under the patient's neck and shoulders and try to reimage from the suprasternal window.

Suprasternal imaging of the distal aortic arch/aortic isthmus can be difficult. When one is having difficulty imaging from the suprasternal window, elevation of the neck and shoulders can be attempted. This maneuver will allow the transducer to be angulated more inferiorly, which can provide improved imaging of the distal aortic arch as well as better angles of insonation for spectral and color Doppler evaluation. Moving the transducer to a lower parasternal position might provide adequate imaging of the distal aortic arch, but the anatomy of the coarctation might not be well seen, and there will likely be a suboptimal angle of insonation for spectral Doppler assessment. The other maneuvers listed in this question will not provide improved imaging of the distal aortic arch.

▸ Lai WW, Mertens LL, Cohen MS, et al (eds): *Echocardiography in Pediatric and Congenital Heart Disease: From Fetus to Adult*, 2nd edition. Chichester, UK, Wiley-Blackwell, 2016, pp 53–55.

484. B. Suprasternal coronal view with the transducer notch/dot at 3 o'clock; transducer should be angled anteriorly.

The best view to visualize the entire innominate (brachiocephalic) vein and its drainage to the right superior vena cava is the suprasternal notch coronal view, with the transducer notch/dot at 3 o'clock. It must be remembered that the innominate vein lies anterior to the aortic arch and therefore, from the suprasternal window, the transducer needs to be angled quite anteriorly in order to visualize it. Elevation of the patient's shoulders and neck can help move away the patient's chin, thereby enabling the anterior angulation needed to image the innominate vein. From this view it is important to inspect the leftward extent of the innominate vein to exclude a left superior vena cava or anomalous pulmonary venous return. Of the other options, the suprasternal sagittal view will display the innominate vein in cross section and therefore will not provide a complete picture of the vessel. Similarly, the high right parasternal parasagittal view described will also display the innominate vein only in cross section (when the transducer is angled to the patient's right side). For the high left parasternal view, the transducer must be angled quite superiorly to visualize the innominate vein, but the resulting image will generally not be as good as that obtained from suprasternal imaging.

▸ Lai WW, Mertens LL, Cohen MS, et al (eds): *Echocardiography in Pediatric and Congenital Heart Disease: From Fetus to Adult*, 2nd edition. Chichester, UK, Wiley-Blackwell, 2016, pp 53–55.

Refer to video PER-Q485.

485. D. Left atrial appendage.

Video PER-Q485 demonstrates a suprasternal coronal view, specifically focusing on the left atrium and individual pulmonary veins. It is also known as the "crab view" because the individual pulmonary veins resemble the legs of a crab extending into the body (left atrium). The arrow points to the left atrial appendage, which can be visualized just superior to the left upper pulmonary vein. This structure should not be confused with a left pulmonary vein, and color flow Doppler can help distinguish the two structures: For the left pulmonary veins, continuous venous flow will be seen entering the left atrium, whereas for the left atrial appendage bidirectional low-velocity flow can be seen entering and exiting the appendage throughout the cardiac cycle. The left pulmonary artery will be located superior to the left atrial appendage. The coronary sinus is not well seen in this view.

▸ Eidem BW, O'Leary PW, Cetta F: *Echocardiography in Pediatric and Adult Congenital Heart Disease*, 2nd edition. Philadelphia, Wolters Kluwer, 2015, pp 16–19.

Refer to video PER-Q486.

486. A. Left aortic arch, normal head and neck artery branching pattern.

Video PER-Q486 is a suprasternal coronal sweep, with the transducer placed in the suprasternal notch and the notch/dot pointed toward the patient's left (3 o'clock). The initial coronal view provides imaging of the superior vena cava (SVC) and ascending aorta (Ao). As the transducer is angled superiorly toward the head, the innominate, or brachiocephalic, vein (Inn vein), aortic arch (Arch), and individual head and neck arterial branches are visualized. The aortic arch shown in this video is a left-sided arch, as defined by its position to the left of the trachea and the fact that it crosses over the left mainstem bronchus. In addition, the head and neck artery branching pattern is normal for a left aortic arch: The first branch from the aorta gives rise to the (rightward) innominate artery, which then divides into the right subclavian artery (RSCA) and right common carotid artery (RCCA); the second branch gives rise to the left common carotid artery (LCCA), and the third branch gives rise to the left subclavian artery (LSCA). The reverse would be true for a right aortic arch: The aortic arch would be located to the right of the trachea, crossing over the right mainstem bronchus, and the first vessel would be the (leftward) innominate artery, giving rise to the left subclavian and left carotid arteries (followed by the right carotid and then right subclavian arteries). A double aortic arch would show the ascending aorta bifurcating into right and left aortic arches, and there is no right aortic arch seen in this video clip.

▸ Lai WW, Mertens LL, Cohen MS, et al (eds): *Echocardiography in Pediatric and Congenital Heart Disease: From Fetus to Adult*, 2nd edition. Chichester, UK, Wiley-Blackwell, 2016, pp 53–55, 609–623.

487. C. Appearance of the aortic arch.

With a suprasternal sagittal view of the aortic arch, the appearance of the aortic arch will be identical whether it is a left or right arch. To determine arch sidedness when using the sagittal view, you must first locate the trachea and then systematically tilt/angle the transducer to the right or left to determine on which side of the trachea the aortic arch is located. With further angulation of the transducer, the division of the first head and neck artery can be visualized. With a left aortic arch, the first branch, the innominate (brachiocephalic) artery, is seen with rightward angulation, and it divides into a right subclavian and right carotid artery; with a right aortic arch, the first branch (innominate artery) is seen with leftward angulation, and it divides into a left subclavian and left carotid artery.

▶ Lai WW, Mertens LL, Cohen MS, et al (eds): *Echocardiography in Pediatric and Congenital Heart Disease: From Fetus to Adult*, 2nd edition. Chichester, UK, Wiley-Blackwell, 2016, pp 53–55.

PART 6

Measurement Techniques and Quantification

488. C. 3.

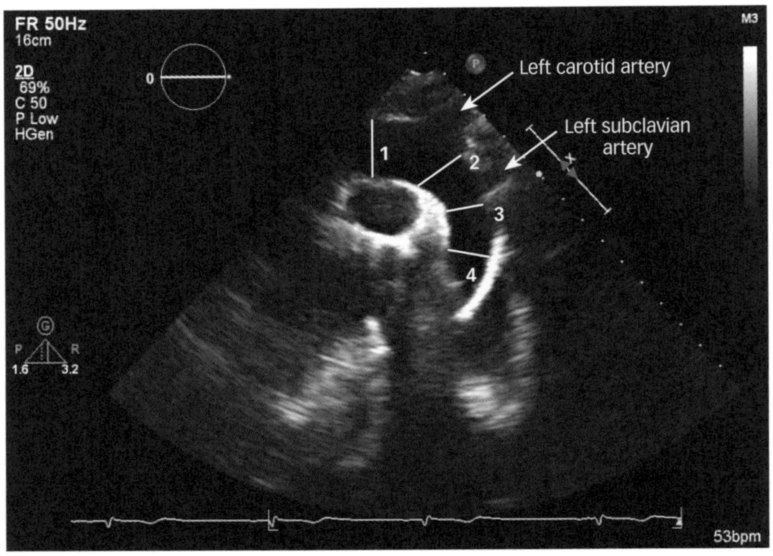

The aortic arch has three segments, numbered in this image as follows:

(1) the proximal arch, located between the innominate (brachiocephalic) artery and the left carotid artery

(2) the distal arch, located between the left carotid artery and the left subclavian artery

(3) the isthmus, located between the left subclavian artery and the ductus arteriosus or the ligamentum arteriosum

The item that is being measured (see the calipers) is #3, the aortic isthmus. The beginning portion of the descending aorta corresponds to #4.

▸ Lai WW, Mertens LL, Cohen MS, et al (eds): *Echocardiography in Pediatric and Congenital Heart Disease: From Fetus to Adult*, 2nd edition. Chichester, UK, Wiley-Blackwell, 2016, p 383.

489. A. 7 mm.

The normal aortic arch criteria include the following:

- *Proximal aorta diameter is greater than 60% of the ascending aorta diameter.*
- *Distal arch diameter is greater than 50% of the ascending aorta diameter.*
- *Aortic isthmus diameter is greater than 40% of the ascending aorta diameter.*

Another method for evaluating aortic (Ao) measurements is the calculation of the diameter Z-score. A Z-score less than –2 is considered abnormal. This corresponds to a value less than 2 standard deviations below the normal population mean. Normal Z-scores are available for the important Ao arch measurements. (See also the answer to question 516.)

- Lai WW, Mertens LL, Cohen MS, et al (eds): *Echocardiography in Pediatric and Congenital Heart Disease: From Fetus to Adult*, 2nd edition. Chichester, UK, Wiley-Blackwell, 2016, p 382.
- Lopez L, Colan SD, Stylianou M, et al: Echo Z- scores adjusted for body surface area are not affected by age, sex, or race: the Pediatric Heart Network Normal Echo Database. Circulation 136:A15546, 2017.

490. C. 48 mmHg.

The modified Bernoulli equation is used when multiple obstructions are present. The formula is: $\Delta P_{max} = 4 \times (V_{max}^2 - V_{proximal}^2)$*. In this case, using the modified Bernoulli equation yields the following:* $4 \times (4^2 - 2^2) = 48$*.*

- Lai WW, Mertens LL, Cohen MS, et al (eds): *Echocardiography in Pediatric and Congenital Heart Disease: From Fetus to Adult*, 2nd edition. Chichester, UK, Wiley-Blackwell, 2016, pp 80, 386.
- Lewin MB, Stout K (eds): *Echocardiography in Congenital Heart Disease*. Philadelphia, Elsevier Saunders, 2012, p 177.

491. D. Coarctation of the aorta.

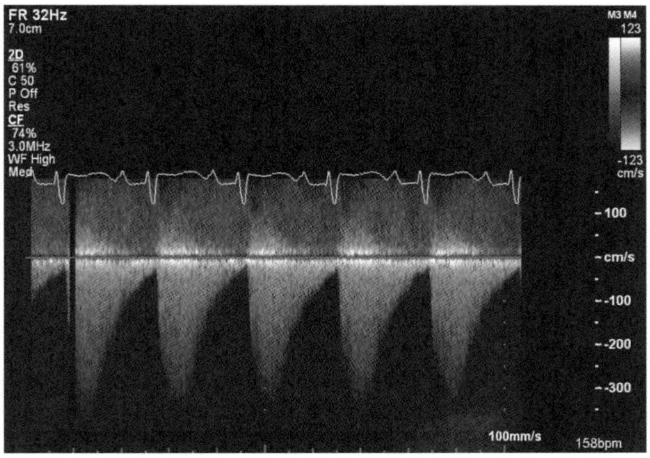

The typical continuous-wave spectral Doppler in severe coarctation has a high peak systolic velocity and continuous antegrade flow throughout diastole. Aortic valve stenosis, pulmonary valve stenosis, and subaortic stenosis might have a high systolic velocity, but they do not have antegrade flow throughout diastole.

- Lai WW, Mertens LL, Cohen MS, et al (eds): *Echocardiography in Pediatric and Congenital Heart Disease: From Fetus to Adult*, 2nd edition. Chichester, UK, Wiley-Blackwell, 2016, p 386.

ANSWERS

492. B. Pulmonary valve stenosis.

The formula for the modified Bernoulli equation is $\Delta P_{max} = 4 \times (V_{max}^2 - V_{proximal}^2)$. *If the proximal velocity is small compared to the distal velocity, the proximal velocity can be ignored, so the equation can be condensed and simplified to* $\Delta P_{max} = 4 \times V_{distal}^2$. *For situations in which there is multilevel obstruction or long segment narrowing, the simplified Bernoulli equation cannot be used and instead the modified equation must be used.*

▶ Lai WW, Mertens LL, Cohen MS, et al (eds): *Echocardiography in Pediatric and Congenital Heart Disease: From Fetus to Adult*, 2nd edition. Chichester, UK, Wiley-Blackwell, 2016, p 80.

493. C. Mild pulmonary valve stenosis.

A large patent ductus arteriosus (PDA) in the presence of anemia will increase preload volume in the left atrium and left ventricle, so there will be a larger ejected stroke volume from the left ventricle that can increase the measured gradient and overestimate aortic valve stenosis. Conversely, poor left ventricular function will result in a smaller than normal ejected stroke volume, resulting in a reduced gradient and underestimation of the degree of aortic valve stenosis. Right-sided heart obstruction will not affect your measurement of the degree of aortic valve stenosis.

▶ Allen HD, Driscoll DJ, Shaddy RE, et al: *Moss and Adams' Heart Disease in Infants, Children, and Adolescents: Including the Fetus and Young Adult*, 8th edition. Philadelphia, Lippincott Williams & Wilkins, 2013, p 1029.

Refer to video PER-Q494.

494. B. It is underestimated.

Refer to video PER-Q494. When a large ventricular septal defect (VSD) coexists with aortic valve stenosis, the stroke volume across the aortic valve will be reduced due to the large amount of left-to-right shunting across the VSD serving as a "popoff." In that setting, the velocity across the aortic valve, and thus the severity of aortic valve stenosis, will be underestimated.

▶ Allen HD, Driscoll DJ, Shaddy RE, et al: *Moss and Adams' Heart Disease in Infants, Children, and Adolescents: Including the Fetus and Young Adult*, 8th edition. Philadelphia, Lippincott Williams & Wilkins, 2013, p 1029.

495. C. Potential coarctation of the aorta.

The presence of a posterior "shelf" (infolding) at the level of the aortic isthmus indicates a potential coarctation of the aorta. However, the diagnosis of coarctation cannot be ruled in or ruled out until the patent ductus arteriosus (PDA) closes, even if it is a small PDA, because there might be associated ductal tissue in the area that could constrict with PDA closure, causing progressive aortic arch obstruction or coarctation. Even if the Doppler velocity across the aortic isthmus is low at this time, after spontaneous closure of a small PDA there can be progressive coarctation of the aorta leading to a significantly higher Doppler velocity across the isthmus. This patient does not have a hypoplastic aortic arch because the question notes that it is "good-sized."

▸ Awasthy N, Tomar M, Radhakrishnan S, et al: Constriction of juxta-ductal aorta and rapid progression of obstruction in a newborn. Ann Pediatr Cardiol 3:181–183, 2010.

496. B. Parasternal short-axis view.

The parasternal short-axis sweep of the left ventricle is the best view to evaluate a muscular ventricular septal defect (VSD), especially an anterior muscular defect. Color flow and spectral Doppler angle are almost parallel to the left-to-right blood flow across the muscular VSD, so an accurate velocity and gradient across the VSD can be obtained. The parasternal long-axis window can also provide an excellent view of the anterior muscular VSD. The other echocardiographic views mentioned in this question are not as useful for the evaluation of an anterior muscular VSD.

▸ Lai WW, Mertens LL, Cohen MS, et al (eds): *Echocardiography in Pediatric and Congenital Heart Disease: From Fetus to Adult*, 2nd edition. Chichester, UK, Wiley-Blackwell, 2016, p 224.

497. D. 64 mmHg.

Using the simplified Bernoulli equation, $\Delta P_{max} = 4V_{max}^2$, yields the following result: $4 \times 4^2 = 64$ mmHg.

▸ Lai WW, Mertens LL, Cohen MS, et al (eds): *Echocardiography in Pediatric and Congenital Heart Disease: From Fetus to Adult*, 2nd edition. Chichester, UK, Wiley-Blackwell, 2016, p 80.

498. D. 56 mmHg.

The patient's systolic blood pressure is 120 mmHg, which means the left ventricular systolic pressure is about 120 mmHg. The velocity is 4 m/sec through the ventricular septal defect; using the simplified Bernoulli equation to calculate the peak gradient between the left ventricle and right ventricle, the value obtained is 64 mmHg, so the estimated right ventricular systolic pressure is 120 mmHg − 64 mmHg = 56 mmHg.

▶ Lai WW, Mertens LL, Cohen MS, et al (eds): *Echocardiography in Pediatric and Congenital Heart Disease: From Fetus to Adult*, 2nd edition. Chichester, UK, Wiley-Blackwell, 2016, pp 80, 221.

499. B. Use continuous-wave spectral Doppler. If the flow is systolic, a VSD is possible.

Sometimes it can be difficult to separate tricuspid valve inflow from ventricular septal defect (VSD) flow, especially when the VSD flow is low-velocity left-to-right shunting (as would be the case with pulmonary hypertension). The better way to distinguish the two blood flows is by using spectral Doppler and an electrocardiogram to determine the timing of the flow during the cardiac cycle: A VSD with left-to-right shunting produces systolic flow, while tricuspid valve inflow is diastolic.

500. C. Moderate.

A parachute mitral valve is a type of congenital heart defect (CHD) that can be seen in association with other forms of congenital heart disease, but it can also occur in isolation, as noted in this scenario. Parachute mitral valves can be associated with varying degrees of stenosis (from none to severe). The mean mitral pressure gradient in this patient is 8 mmHg, which is between 6 and 12 mmHg, the range generally considered to classify the degree of mitral stenosis as moderate. Mild mitral valve stenosis is considered to be present when the mean pressure gradient is approximately 4–5 mmHg, and severe mitral valve stenosis is considered to be present when the mean gradient is greater than 13 mmHg.

▶ Allen HD, Shaddy RE, Penny DJ, et al: *Moss and Adams' Heart Disease in Infants, Children, and Adolescents, Including the Fetus and Young Adult*, 9th edition. Philadelphia, Wolters Kluwer, 2016, pp 1003–1010, 1019.

▶ Park MK: *Park's Pediatric Cardiology for Practitioners*, 6th edition. Philadelphia, Saunders, 2014, pp 375–376.

501. B. Transposition of the great arteries (d-TGA) with intact ventricular septum.

When a patient has an atrial septal defect (ASD) as an isolated cardiac defect, the size of the ASD and the volume of atrial shunting are the most important factors in making clinical management decisions. The mean gradient is less useful; with moderate to large ASDs, there is usually a low-velocity left-to-right shunt. Congenitally corrected transposition of the great arteries has "normal" physiology; there is sometimes an ASD and a ventricular septal defect (VSD), but the mean gradient across the ASD is not generally a key point for clinical management. Instead, the morphology and competency of the systemic atrioventricular valve, the degree of subpulmonary stenosis (if present), and the size of the VSD (if present) are much more important factors that are used to decide clinical management and possible timing for surgery. For double-inlet left ventricle, an ASD is not necessary for survival in most patients, except in the rare case of stenosis of one of the atrioventricular valves. However, in transposition of the great arteries (d-TGA) with intact ventricular septum, an ASD is essential for survival: There needs to be adequate mixing between the deoxygenated systemic venous circulation and the oxygenated pulmonary venous circulation, and this is accomplished most effectively at the atrial level. Echocardiography is important to assess the size of the ASD, as well as the mean gradient across the ASD. A high mean gradient indicates a restrictive ASD; a restrictive ASD can prohibit adequate mixing and produce significant (and sometimes life-threatening) cyanosis. In these cases, a balloon atrial septostomy is necessary to create an ASD that is large enough for adequate mixing.

- Lai WW, Mertens LL, Cohen MS, et al (eds): *Echocardiography in Pediatric and Congenital Heart Disease: From Fetus to Adult*, 2nd edition. Chichester, UK, Wiley-Blackwell, 2016, pp 512–518.
- Lewin MB, Stout K (eds): *Echocardiography in Congenital Heart Disease*. Philadelphia, Elsevier Saunders, 2012, pp 64–65, 104.

502. D. The peak pressure gradient between the left and right atrium is 4 mmHg.

Pulsed-wave or continuous-wave Doppler does not measure the absolute peak pressure at a defect or valve; instead, it measures the pressure difference between two points. Therefore, the velocity of 1 m/sec across the atrial septal defect (ASD) means that there is a 4 mmHg peak gradient between the left and right atria. We do not know the exact pressure in either the left or right atrium. Both atrial pressures can be high, low, or normal. The only conclusion that can be made is that the pressure difference is 4 mmHg.

- Lai WW, Mertens LL, Cohen MS, et al (eds): *Echocardiography in Pediatric and Congenital Heart Disease: From Fetus to Adult*, 2nd edition. Chichester, UK, Wiley-Blackwell, 2016, p 79.

ANSWERS

503. C. Severe aortic valve stenosis.

With normal left ventricular function, aortic valve stenosis is evaluated as follows:

- *Mild stenosis: Peak velocity across the valve < 3 m/sec, mean gradient < 25 mmHg.*
- *Moderate stenosis: Peak velocity = 3–4 m/sec, mean gradient = 25–40 mmHg.*
- *Severe stenosis: Peak velocity > 4 m/sec, mean gradient > 40 mmHg.*

▶ Allen HD, Driscoll DJ, Shaddy RE, et al: *Moss and Adams' Heart Disease in Infants, Children, and Adolescents: Including the Fetus and Young Adult*, 8th edition. Philadelphia, Lippincott Williams & Wilkins, 2013, p 1029.

▶ Lai WW, Mertens LL, Cohen MS, et al (eds): *Echocardiography in Pediatric and Congenital Heart Disease: From Fetus to Adult*, 2nd edition. Chichester, UK, Wiley-Blackwell, 2016, p 341.

504. B. Moderate.

See the answer to question 503.

▶ Allen HD, Driscoll DJ, Shaddy RE, et al: *Moss and Adams' Heart Disease in Infants, Children, and Adolescents: Including the Fetus and Young Adult*, 8th edition. Philadelphia, Lippincott Williams & Wilkins, 2013, p 1029.

▶ Lai WW, Mertens LL, Cohen MS, et al (eds): *Echocardiography in Pediatric and Congenital Heart Disease: From Fetus to Adult*, 2nd edition. Chichester, UK, Wiley-Blackwell, 2016, p 341.

505. C. Severely stenotic.

In the normal fully grown young adult, aortic valve area is evaluated as follows:

- *Normal aortic valve area > 3–4 cm^2*
- *Mild stenosis = 1.5–3 cm^2*
- *Moderate stenosis = 1.0–1.5 cm^2*
- *Severe stenosis < 1.0 cm^2*

For children, the normal aortic valve area is ≥ 2 cm^2/m^2.

▶ Allen HD, Driscoll DJ, Shaddy RE, et al: *Moss and Adams' Heart Disease in Infants, Children, and Adolescents: Including the Fetus and Young Adult*, 8th edition. Philadelphia, Lippincott Williams & Wilkins, 2013, p 1029.

▶ Lai WW, Mertens LL, Cohen MS, et al (eds): *Echocardiography in Pediatric and Congenital Heart Disease: From Fetus to Adult*, 2nd edition. Chichester, UK, Wiley-Blackwell, 2016, p 342.

506. A. Aortic pressure half-time (PHT) became shorter.

When the aortic valve has an increased amount of regurgitation, the difference in diastolic pressure between the ascending aorta and the left ventricle will decrease more rapidly, so it will take a shorter time to reach the pressure half-time (PHT). A PHT less than 200–250 milliseconds (ms) signifies severe aortic regurgitation; moderate regurgitation is between 200 and 400 ms, and mild regurgitation is greater than 400 ms.

- Allen HD, Driscoll DJ, Shaddy RE, et al: *Moss and Adams' Heart Disease in Infants, Children, and Adolescents: Including the Fetus and Young Adult*, 8th edition. Philadelphia, Lippincott Williams & Wilkins, 2013, p 185.
- Lai WW, Mertens LL, Cohen MS, et al (eds): *Echocardiography in Pediatric and Congenital Heart Disease: From Fetus to Adult*, 2nd edition. Chichester, UK, Wiley-Blackwell, 2016, p 87.

507. A. Severe aortic valve regurgitation.

See Color Plate 25 on page xxxi.

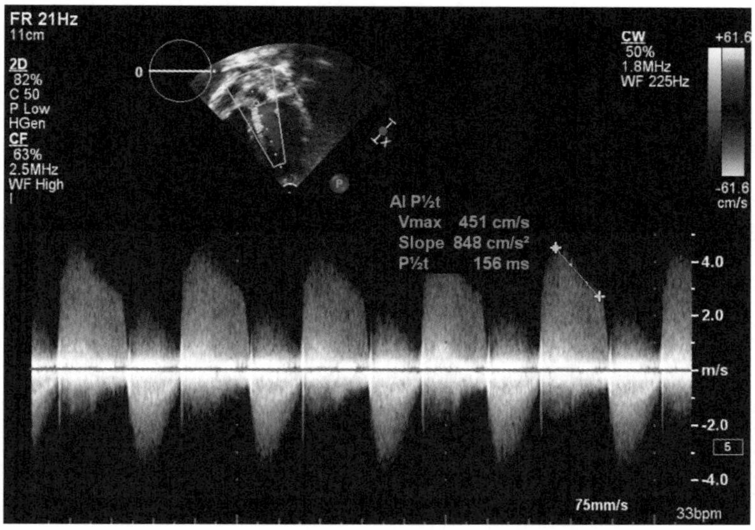

An Austin Flint murmur is best heard at the cardiac apex and is associated with significant aortic valve regurgitation. This severe aortic valve regurgitation, with a pressure half-time of 156 ms, is seen above the baseline, as demonstrated by the spectral Doppler tracing. Mild aortic valve stenosis is also seen on the Doppler profile below the baseline.

- Allen HD, Driscoll DJ, Shaddy RE, et al: *Moss and Adams' Heart Disease in Infants, Children, and Adolescents: Including the Fetus and Young Adult*, 8th edition. Philadelphia, Lippincott Williams & Wilkins, 2013, p 185.
- Lai WW, Mertens LL, Cohen MS, et al (eds): *Echocardiography in Pediatric and Congenital Heart Disease: From Fetus to Adult*, 2nd edition. Chichester, UK, Wiley-Blackwell, 2016, p 87.

508. C. Aortic valve regurgitation.

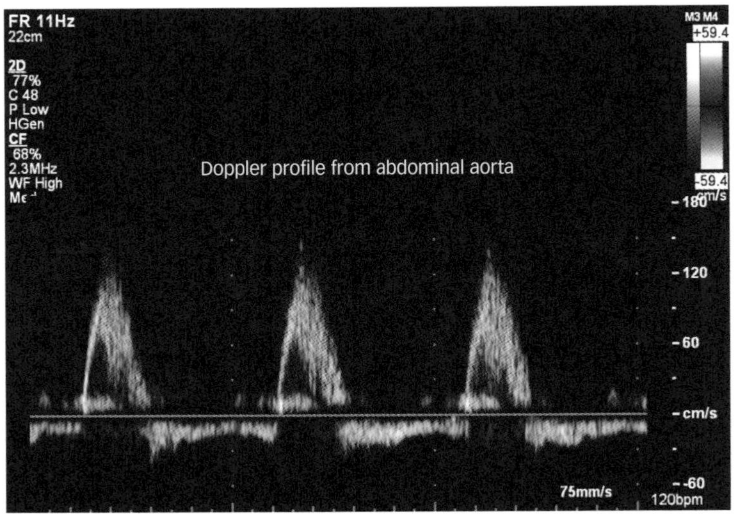

This spectral Doppler waveform shows diastolic reversal of flow in the descending abdominal aorta, which is not a normal finding. Diastolic reversal of flow in the abdominal aorta can be seen when there is hemodynamically significant (at least moderate) aortic valve regurgitation. Aortitis would not have this characteristic. Coarctation of the aorta would have a blunted descending aortic waveform.

▶ Allen HD, Driscoll DJ, Shaddy RE, et al: *Moss and Adams' Heart Disease in Infants, Children, and Adolescents: Including the Fetus and Young Adult*, 8th edition. Philadelphia, Lippincott Williams & Wilkins, 2013, p 185.

▶ Lai WW, Mertens LL, Cohen MS, et al (eds): *Echocardiography in Pediatric and Congenital Heart Disease: From Fetus to Adult*, 2nd edition. Chichester, UK, Wiley-Blackwell, 2016, pp 87–89.

509. D. Reversal of flow in the descending aorta.

When aortic valve regurgitation becomes acutely worse, the left ventricle dimension and left ventricular ejection fraction can remain unchanged for a short period of time, depending on left ventricle compliance. Reversal of flow in the descending aorta is an early and reliable echocardiographic sign of more hemodynamically significant aortic regurgitation. However, it is important to remember that descending aortic diastolic reversal of flow can be produced by other types of heart disease (such as truncus arteriosus or aortopulmonary window), so it is important to use color flow Doppler of the descending aorta in combination with direct visualization of the aortic valve to establish the diagnosis. Tissue Doppler is not a good method of evaluating the severity of aortic valve regurgitation.

▶ Lai WW, Mertens LL, Cohen MS, et al (eds): *Echocardiography in Pediatric and Congenital Heart Disease: From Fetus to Adult*, 2nd edition. Chichester, UK, Wiley-Blackwell, 2016, pp 88–89.

Refer to video PER-Q510.

510. A. A small patent ductus arteriosus.

The feature indicated by color flow Doppler (video PER-Q510) is retrograde diastolic flow in the distal aortic arch and proximal descending aorta. An aortopulmonary window, a large cerebral arteriovenous malformation (such as a vein of Galen malformation), and a Blalock-Taussig shunt can all cause reversal flow in this area; this occurs because of the prominent diastolic runoff of flow that occurs in each of these different conditions, resulting in retrograde diastolic flow in the distal aortic arch and proximal descending aorta. A small patent ductus arteriosus is the only choice that will not produce significant diastolic runoff of blood from the aorta to the pulmonary artery.

511. D. Moderate to severe pulmonary valve regurgitation.

When a patient has moderate to severe pulmonary valve regurgitation, diastolic reversal of flow can be seen in both pulmonary arteries. None of the other abnormalities given in the choices will have this spectral Doppler finding. In a moderate-sized patent ductus arteriosus or an aortopulmonary window, continuous diastolic antegrade flow can actually be found.

- Lai WW, Mertens LL, Cohen MS, et al (eds): *Echocardiography in Pediatric and Congenital Heart Disease: From Fetus to Adult*, 2nd edition. Chichester, UK, Wiley-Blackwell, 2016, p 88.

512. B. Peak velocity across the aortic valve.

The equation for calculating cardiac output is:

$$TVI \times CSA \times heart\ rate$$

where TVI is the measured time velocity integral across the aortic valve and CSA is aortic valve cross-sectional area (calculated from the aortic valve annulus diameter). Peak velocity across the aortic valve is not required to calculate cardiac output.

- Lai WW, Mertens LL, Cohen MS, et al (eds): *Echocardiography in Pediatric and Congenital Heart Disease: From Fetus to Adult*, 2nd edition. Chichester, UK, Wiley-Blackwell, 2016, p 78.

513. B. SF increases.

The shortening fraction (SF) is a measurement of left ventricular (LV) systolic function. SF is expressed as a percentage and is calculated using this equation:

$$SF = \frac{LVEDD - LVESD}{LVEDD} \times 100$$

ANSWERS

where LVEDD = left ventricular end-diastolic diameter and LVESD = left ventricular end-systolic diameter. Both LVEDD and LVESD can be measured by either M-mode or 2D imaging, usually from the parasternal short-axis view, although the parasternal long-axis view can also be used. The shortening fraction is load dependent and can be affected by changes in both preload and afterload. When LV volume acutely increases, preload and stroke volume are increased, LV end-diastolic volume increases, and more blood is ejected by the LV per beat (assuming that LV myocardial contractility is normal); thus the LV volume at the end of ejection remains unchanged. Therefore using the SF equation above, LVEDD is increased, LVESD remains unchanged, and the left ventricular SF increases.

▶ Lai WW, Mertens LL, Cohen MS, et al (eds): *Echocardiography in Pediatric and Congenital Heart Disease: From Fetus to Adult*, 2nd edition. Chichester, UK, Wiley-Blackwell, 2016, p 101.

514. C. 28%–38%.

The normal range for the resting left ventricular shortening fraction (LVSF) is 28%–38%, although in certain hyperdynamic states (such as exercise) LVSF can exceed 40%. In general, the LVSF serves as a reasonable proxy for the left ventricular ejection fraction (LVEF), which is usually about twice the LVSF. However, care must be taken when interpreting LVSF in the presence of left ventricular dyskinesis, pulmonary hypertension, or an abnormality of ventricular septal position. In these types of conditions, the LVSF might not accurately represent left ventricular systolic function, and calculation of ejection fraction might be indicated using another method, such as the modified Simpson's method by 2D.

▶ Allen HD, Driscoll DJ, Shaddy RE, et al: *Moss and Adams' Heart Disease in Infants, Children, and Adolescents: Including the Fetus and Young Adult*, 8th edition. Philadelphia, Lippincott Williams & Wilkins, 2013, p 176.

▶ Lai WW, Mertens LL, Cohen MS, et al (eds): *Echocardiography in Pediatric and Congenital Heart Disease: From Fetus to Adult*, 2nd edition. Chichester, UK, Wiley-Blackwell, 2016, p 101.

515. C. Reduced global ventricular wall motion.

Use of M-mode to calculate shortening fraction (SF) is limited to a small region of the left ventricle. If the ventricular septum is dyskinetic but the remainder of the wall motion is normal, the SF will be underestimated. A similar underestimation of SF will occur with paradoxical systolic motion of the ventricular septum. When a patient has premature ventricular contractions with bigeminy, left ventricular volume is not the same between the heartbeats, so SF can be inaccurate. However, when global left ventricular wall motion is reduced, SF presents a generally accurate representation of the reduced left ventricular systolic function.

▶ Allen HD, Driscoll DJ, Shaddy RE, et al: *Moss and Adams' Heart Disease in Infants, Children, and Adolescents: Including the Fetus and Young Adult*, 8th edition. Philadelphia, Lippincott Williams & Wilkins, 2013, pp 176–177.

516. A. A value based on the standard deviation around a mean value for that particular cardiac structure which varies by body surface area.

Z-scores were developed to compare specific cardiac structural measurements for pediatric patients of different ages and different body surface areas. Z-scores are the numbers derived from the standard deviation around the mean measurement in a normal population and are based on the specific structure measured as well as the specific body surface area (BSA). In other words, for any cardiac structure (such as aortic valve annulus) and any given BSA, there are certain "normal" mean values based on the normal population. Using statistical analysis, a standard deviation can be calculated for each mean value, and one Z-score unit represents one standard deviation above or below the "normal" mean value. The Z-score can be positive or negative: A positive number means that the value is above the mean measurement for a normal population, and a negative number means that the value is below the mean measurement in normal population. Z-scores greater than +2 or less than −2 are considered outside the range of normal. For example, an aortic valve annulus diameter Z-score of −3.5 means that the size of the aortic valve annulus is below the mean measurement by 3.5 standard deviations for the normal population with the same BSA. This would be considered a hypoplastic aortic valve annulus.

▶ Allen HD, Driscoll DJ, Shaddy RE, et al: *Moss and Adams' Heart Disease in Infants, Children, and Adolescents: Including the Fetus and Young Adult*, 8th edition. Philadelphia, Lippincott Williams & Wilkins, 2013, p 172.

517. C. Heart rate.

The most common formula for calculating left ventricular mass is

$$0.8 \times [1.04 \times (LVEDD + IVSd + PWd)^3 - LVEDD^3] + 0.6\ g$$

where LVEDD is left ventricular end-diastolic dimension, IVSd is interventricular septum wall thickness in end diastole, PWd is posterior left ventricular wall thickness in end diastole, and g stands for gram.

- Allen HD, Driscoll DJ, Shaddy RE, et al: *Moss and Adams' Heart Disease in Infants, Children, and Adolescents: Including the Fetus and Young Adult*, 8th edition. Philadelphia, Lippincott Williams & Wilkins, 2013, p 174.

518. A. Ventricular contractility.

The dP/dt value is a measure of ventricular contractility and systolic function. It is calculated from the spectral Doppler tracing of mitral (or tricuspid) regurgitation and measures the rate of ventricular pressure rise in systole during the time period between the regurgitant jet velocities of 1 m/sec to 3 m/sec. (The ventricular pressure is calculated from mitral/tricuspid regurgitant jet velocity by the simplified Bernoulli equation.) The reported unit is in mmHg/sec. The equation is:

$$dp/dt = 32/T$$

where T = the time period from 1 to 3 m/sec on the MR or TR regurgitant jet, and the result is in mmHg per second. The dP/dT value is ventricular geometry and afterload independent, but it is preload dependent, and has limited reproducibility on a very short time interval.

- Lai WW, Mertens LL, Cohen MS, et al (eds): *Echocardiography in Pediatric and Congenital Heart Disease: From Fetus to Adult*, 2nd edition. Chichester, UK, Wiley-Blackwell, 2016, pp 105–106.
- Lang RM, Goldstein SA, Kronzon I, et al (eds): *ASE's Comprehensive Echocardiography*, 2nd edition. Philadelphia, Sauders, 2016, p 122.

519. A. Use a Doppler sweep speed of 150 cm/sec.

When measuring distance or time between two points, an enlarged graph will improve precision and reproducibility compared to a smaller graph. Using a higher sweep speed will provide an expanded spectral Doppler tracing and an enlarged graph, thereby providing greater details of the spectral Doppler waveform compared to a lower sweep speed. To calculate dP/dt, it is necessary only to show the spectral Doppler tracing between the time points corresponding to 1 m/sec and 3 m/sec; it is not necessary to show the peak Doppler velocity (unless the peak velocity happens to correspond to 3 m/sec).

▸ Lai WW, Mertens LL, Cohen MS, et al (eds): *Echocardiography in Pediatric and Congenital Heart Disease: From Fetus to Adult*, 2nd edition. Chichester, UK, Wiley-Blackwell, 2016, pp 105–106.

▸ Lang RM, Goldstein SA, Kronzon I, et al (eds): *ASE's Comprehensive Echocardiography*, 2nd edition. Philadelphia, Sauders, 2016, p 122.

520. D. Inject agitated saline into a vein in the left arm.

Usually a left superior vena cava (SVC) drains into the coronary sinus (CS) and then to the right atrium; this is why the CS is dilated. However, in some cases a patient is found to have a left SVC but the CS is not dilated. In such cases there is a strong possibility that the left SVC drains directly into the left atrium. This direct drainage of the left SVC to the left atrium may be difficult to visualize with 2D imaging and color Doppler echocardiography, even from the suprasternal coronal and subcostal views. In this situation, a contrast study can be very helpful, offering a simple method to demonstrate the abnormality. Agitated saline should be injected into a vein in the left arm. The test is positive if the contrast agent is seen first entering the left atrium. Agitated saline injection into a vein in the right arm will probably not be useful, because if there are bilateral SVCs (which is usually the case), there is generally not an innominate (brachiocephalic) vein connecting the two SVCs. Therefore, the agitated saline injected into the right arm will enter the right atrium directly and will provide no information regarding the drainage of the left SVC.

▸ Allen HD, Driscoll DJ, Shaddy RE, et al: *Moss and Adams' Heart Disease in Infants, Children, and Adolescents: Including the Fetus and Young Adult*, 8th edition. Philadelphia, Lippincott Williams & Wilkins, 2013, pp 164–165.

521. D. Aortopulmonary collaterals.

Contrast echo with agitated saline (also known as a "bubble" study) is performed by injecting agitated saline into a systemic vein. In a patient with normal anatomy, the agitated saline (microbubbles) will return to the right side of the heart without crossing to the left side. Agitated saline contrast should not appear on the left side of the heart because the lungs will filter out the microbubbles, as well as absorb these microbubbles. Any contrast seen in the left side of the heart signifies that there is an intracardiac and/or intrapulmonary right-to-left shunt. Because of their ability to detect right-to-left shunting, bubble studies are useful in cases of suspected unroofed coronary sinus and pulmonary arteriovenous fistulae. The bubble study is also helpful for visualizing the atrial septum, which can sometimes be difficult to visualize due to a poor subcostal view. Aortopulmonary collaterals result in a left-to-right (not right-to-left) shunt, so when this condition is suspected an agitated contrast study is not helpful. Furthermore, aortopulmonary collaterals are easily detected by color Doppler on a standard pediatric echocardiogram.

▸ Allen HD, Driscoll DJ, Shaddy RE, et al: *Moss and Adams' Heart Disease in Infants, Children, and Adolescents: Including the Fetus and Young Adult*, 8th edition. Philadelphia, Lippincott Williams & Wilkins, 2013, pp 164–165.

522. B. Echocardiogram with contrast (bubble study).

A small proportion of patients who have undergone the Glenn or Fontan procedure can develop arteriovenous malformations (AVMs), which can cause hypoxemia due to intrapulmonary right-to-left shunting. A contrast injection study using agitated saline (bubble study) is the best and easiest way to detect this problem. Contrast should be injected into a systemic vein or, during cardiac catheterization, directly into one of the pulmonary arteries. Normally, the microbubbles present in the contrast will be filtered by the pulmonary arterial-capillary bed and will not appear in the pulmonary veins. However, when a pulmonary AVM is present, contrast will be seen prominently in the pulmonary veins, returning to the heart.

▸ Allen HD, Driscoll DJ, Shaddy RE, et al: *Moss and Adams' Heart Disease in Infants, Children, and Adolescents: Including the Fetus and Young Adult*, 8th edition. Philadelphia, Lippincott Williams & Wilkins, 2013, pp 164–165.

523. D. Blalock-Taussig shunt patency.

The indication for contrast echocardiography using agitated saline is to rule out a possible intracardiac or intrapulmonary right-to-left shunt in patients in whom a shunt cannot be definitively demonstrated by standard 2D and color Doppler echocardiography. Examples of this include an unroofed coronary sinus, a thromboembolic stroke (due to a possible small interatrial communication or atrial septal defect), poor echocardiographic windows to detect an atrial septal defect after a Glenn or Fontan procedure with persistent hypoxemia, an intra-atrial baffle leak following an atrial switch operation, and liver disease potentially causing the development of arteriovenous malformations. A Blalock-Taussig (BT) shunt, however, results in a left-to-right shunt (from the subclavian or innominate/ brachiocephalic artery to the pulmonary artery), not a right-to-left shunt, so contrast injection is not useful for evaluation of a BT shunt.

▶ Allen HD, Driscoll DJ, Shaddy RE, et al: *Moss and Adams' Heart Disease in Infants, Children, and Adolescents: Including the Fetus and Young Adult*, 8th edition. Philadelphia, Lippincott Williams & Wilkins, 2013, pp 164–165.

524. D. 4.

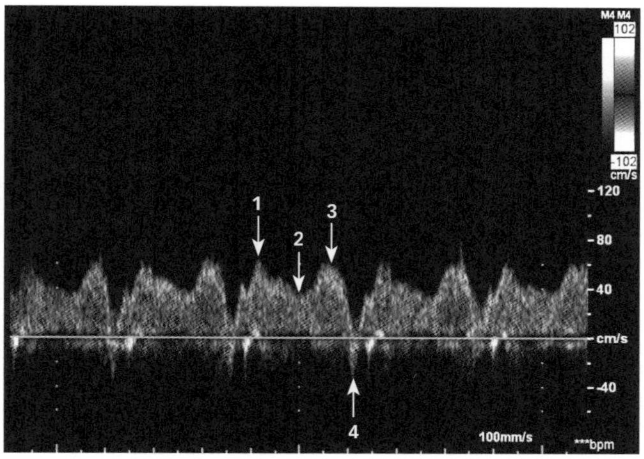

On spectral Doppler normal pulmonary veins demonstrate one or two systolic S waves (marked 1 and 2 on this waveform) and a diastolic D wave (number 3). Atrial contraction follows the P wave as noted on the electrocardiogram; there is a small reversal of flow back into pulmonary veins below the baseline, called the Ar wave (number 4), that corresponds to atrial contraction.

▶ Allen HD, Driscoll DJ, Shaddy RE, et al: *Moss and Adams' Heart Disease in Infants, Children, and Adolescents: Including the Fetus and Young Adult*, 8th edition. Philadelphia, Lippincott Williams & Wilkins, 2013, p 190.

525. A. S wave.

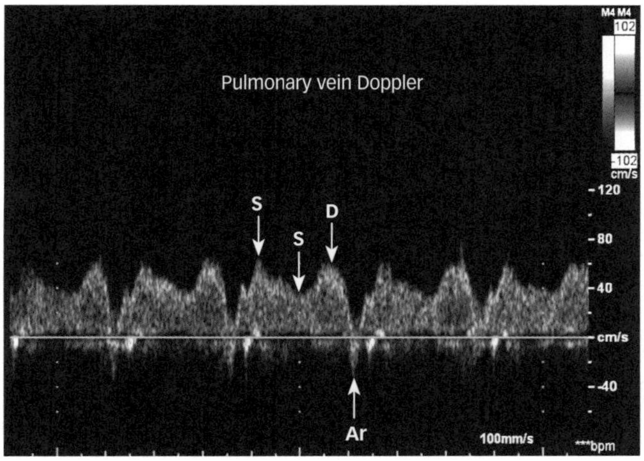

Spectral Doppler of the normal pulmonary vein has a systolic S wave, a diastolic D wave, and (following the P wave on the electrocardiogram) atrial contraction, with a small reversal of flow back into the pulmonary veins called the Ar wave. An E wave is not seen on the pulmonary vein tracing; E waves appear on mitral valve inflow tracings and correspond to early ventricular filling.

▶ Allen HD, Driscoll DJ, Shaddy RE, et al: *Moss and Adams' Heart Disease in Infants, Children, and Adolescents: Including the Fetus and Young Adult*, 8th edition. Philadelphia, Lippincott Williams & Wilkins, 2013, p 190.

526. A. 1.

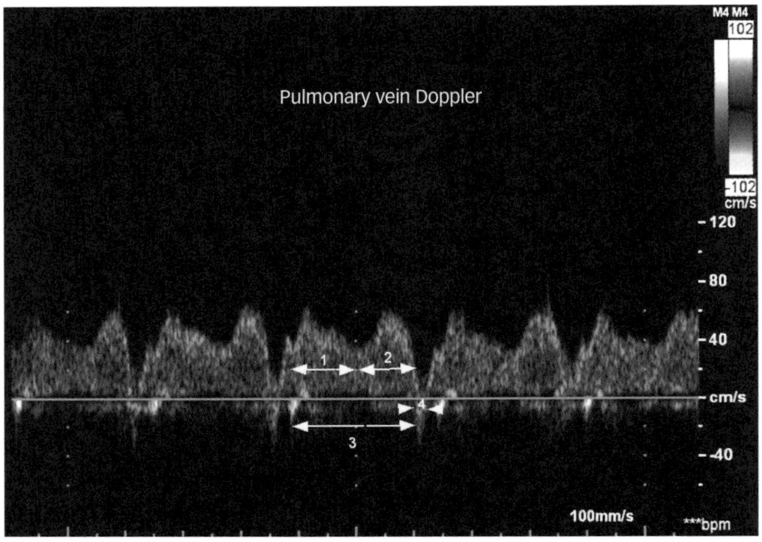

The area marked by 1 corresponds to systole, the area marked by 2 corresponds to early diastole (ventricular filing), the area marked by 3 represents the combined portions of 1 and 2, and the area marked by 4 represents atrial contraction (causing a small reversal of flow back into the pulmonary vein called the Ar wave).

▶ Allen HD, Driscoll DJ, Shaddy RE, et al: *Moss and Adams' Heart Disease in Infants, Children, and Adolescents: Including the Fetus and Young Adult*, 8th edition. Philadelphia, Lippincott Williams & Wilkins, 2013, p 190.

527. A. Reduce color Doppler sector.

To optimize the color flow Doppler evaluation of the pulmonary veins, place the color flow sector on the region of interest and select an appropriate size. A smaller color box (sector) yields a better frame rate and thus better color sensitivity. Increasing the Nyquist limit might actually reduce the sensitivity to low-velocity color flow signals, and using color flow Doppler comparison (dual mode) will not enhance the color

ANSWERS

flow Doppler. Increasing the Doppler gain will increase all signal sensitivity, including display of noise, which could reduce the image quality.

▶ Edelman SK: *Understanding Ultrasound Physics*, 4th edition. The Woodlands, TX, ESP Ultrasound, 2012, pp 198–201.

▶ Lai WW, Mertens LL, Cohen MS, et al (eds): *Echocardiography in Pediatric and Congenital Heart Disease: From Fetus to Adult*, 2nd edition. Chichester, UK, Wiley-Blackwell, 2016, pp 16–17.

528. A. Deeper atrial reversal Ar wave.

The atrial reversal Ar wave will disappear (not become deeper) with pulmonary vein stenosis. All of the other options listed—an increased peak velocity and mean gradient, loss of phasic variation in the spectral Doppler signal, and turbulent flow demonstrated by color Doppler—are typically seen in the presence of pulmonary vein stenosis during Doppler interrogation.

▶ Lai WW, Mertens LL, Cohen MS, et al (eds): *Echocardiography in Pediatric and Congenital Heart Disease: From Fetus to Adult*, 2nd edition. Chichester, UK, Wiley-Blackwell, 2016, pp 164–165.

529. D. Atrial septal defect.

An atrial septal defect (ASD) allows blood to flow from the left to the right atrium, serving as a "popoff" in the setting of mitral valve stenosis and reducing the amount of blood that crosses the mitral valve. This will, in turn, decrease the mitral valve gradient and result in underestimation of the degree of mitral valve stenosis. All of the other cardiac defects listed—ventricular septal defect, patent ductus arteriosus, and mitral valve regurgitation—increase the amount of blood in the left atrium and left ventricle, thereby increasing left atrial volume and left ventricular preload. As a result the apparent gradient across the mitral valve is higher, potentially producing an overestimation of the degree of mitral valve stenosis.

▶ Lai WW, Mertens LL, Cohen MS, et al (eds): *Echocardiography in Pediatric and Congenital Heart Disease: From Fetus to Adult*, 2nd edition. Chichester, UK, Wiley-Blackwell, 2016, pp 251–253.

530. A. Becomes longer.

As mitral valve stenosis worsens, it takes longer for the left atrium to empty into the left ventricle. Therefore mitral valve pressure half-time (PHT) lengthens. This is reflected in this equation for mitral valve area (MVA):

$$MVA\ (cm^2) = 220/PHT\ (ms)$$

ANSWERS

There is an inverse relationship between calculated MVA and PHT: As PHT becomes longer, the calculated MVA becomes smaller.

- Armstrong WF, Ryan T: *Feigenbaum's Echocardiography*, 7th edition. Philadelphia, Lippincott Williams & Wilkins, 2010, pp 304–307.
- Lai WW, Mertens LL, Cohen MS, et al (eds): *Echocardiography in Pediatric and Congenital Heart Disease: From Fetus to Adult*, 2nd edition. Chichester, UK, Wiley-Blackwell, 2016, pp 251–253.

531. D. Body surface area.

Pressure half-time (PHT) is the time it takes the peak pressure gradient across the mitral valve to decrease to half of the original pressure gradient. In the pediatric population, many factors can affect PHT, including left atrial pressure and left ventricular diastolic pressure, as well as changes in heart rate. Body surface area (BSA) does not affect PHT.

- Armstrong WF, Ryan T: *Feigenbaum's Echocardiography*, 7th edition. Philadelphia, Lippincott Williams & Wilkins, 2010, pp 304–307.
- Lai WW, Mertens LL, Cohen MS, et al (eds): *Echocardiography in Pediatric and Congenital Heart Disease: From Fetus to Adult*, 2nd edition. Chichester, UK, Wiley-Blackwell, 2016, pp 251–253.

532. A. >3 mmHg.

Authorities vary on what reference values correspond to the beginnings of mitral valve stenosis, but a mean gradient greater than 3 mmHg or a peak gradient greater than 12 mmHg is commonly accepted as the definition of significant mitral valve stenosis in native mitral valves.

- LaCorte M, Harada K, Williams RG: Echocardiographic features of congenital left ventricular inflow obstruction. Circulation 54:562–566, 1976.
- Lai WW, Mertens LL, Cohen MS, et al (eds): *Echocardiography in Pediatric and Congenital Heart Disease: From Fetus to Adult*, 2nd edition. Chichester, UK, Wiley-Blackwell, 2016, p 253.
- Moore P, Adatia I, Spevak PJ, et al: Severe congenital mitral stenosis in infants. Circulation 89:2099–2106, 1994.

533. B. Parasternal short-axis view.

With the parasternal short-axis view of the left ventricle, the mitral valve leaflets can be seen en face (a 3D echocardiographic view also known as a "surgical view"), thereby demonstrating a cleft in the anterior leaflet of the mitral valve. In addition, chordal attachments to the ventricular septum can be clearly seen. The other views in this question—the parasternal long-axis, apical four-chamber, and subcostal long-axis views—do not display the mitral valve leaflet anatomy as distinctly and are more useful in visualizing leaflet and chordal motion, as well as the severity of mitral valve regurgitation (if present).

▸ Lai WW, Mertens LL, Cohen MS, et al (eds): *Echocardiography in Pediatric and Congenital Heart Disease: From Fetus to Adult*, 2nd edition. Chichester, UK, Wiley-Blackwell, 2016, p 245.

534. C. Mitral valve displaced >2 mm in systole.

Mitral valve prolapse should be evaluated from the parasternal long-axis view. The definition of prolapse is systolic displacement of the mitral leaflet that exceeds 2 mm above the plane of the annulus.

▸ Freed LA, Levy D, Levine RA, et al: Prevalence and clinical outcome of mitral valve prolapse. N Engl J Med 341:1–7, 1999.

▸ Lai WW, Mertens LL, Cohen MS, et al (eds): *Echocardiography in Pediatric and Congenital Heart Disease: From Fetus to Adult*, 2nd edition. Chichester, UK, Wiley-Blackwell, 2016, p 243.

535. B. 70 mmHg.

When a large ventricular septal defect (VSD) is present, both ventricles have equal systolic pressure. This patient's blood pressure is 70/50 mmHg, so the left systolic ventricle pressure is 70 mmHg; therefore the right ventricular (RV) systolic pressure is 70 mmHg. The tricuspid regurgitant velocity measurement is unreliable for this patient because of the incomplete spectral Doppler signal, but this information is also not necessary, because the presence of the large VSD provides the information necessary to estimate RV systolic pressure.

▸ Nichols DG, Ungerleider RM, Spevak PJ, et al: *Critical Heart Disease in infants and Children*, 2nd edition. Philadelphia, Mosby Elsevier, 2006, p 587.

536. B. Parasternal short-axis view.

The parasternal short-axis view best demonstrates the relationship of the great arteries, allowing visualization of side-by-side arteries, the anterior and posterior relationship of the arteries, and the position of the aorta to the left or right of the pulmonary artery. The other views listed in the answer choices—the parasternal long-axis, apical four- and five-chamber, and subcostal long- and short-axis views—will also display the relationship of great arteries. However, these views are best interpreted by the sonographer, not necessarily by the reader of the echocardiogram, unless precise, protocolized sweeps are performed and recorded.

- Lai WW, Mertens LL, Cohen MS, et al (eds): *Echocardiography in Pediatric and Congenital Heart Disease: From Fetus to Adult*, 2nd edition. Chichester, UK, Wiley-Blackwell, 2016, pp 44–58.

537. B. Pulmonary blood flow to systemic blood flow.

Qp/Qs is the ratio of pulmonary blood flow to systemic blood flow.

- Bergersen L, Foerster S, Marshall AC, et al (eds): *Congenital Heart Disease: The Catheterization Manual*. New York, Springer, 2009, p 9.
- Reynolds T: *The Pediatric Echocardiographer's Pocket Reference*, 3rd edition. Phoenix, Arizona Heart Foundation, 2013, pp 336–337.

538. C. 1.

The Qp/Qs ratio is the ratio of pulmonary to systemic blood flow. For both pediatric and adult patients, the normal Qp/Qs ratio is 1.

- Bergersen L, Foerster S, Marshall AC, et al (eds): *Congenital Heart Disease: The Catheterization Manual*. New York, Springer, 2009, p 9.
- Reynolds T: *The Pediatric Echocardiographer's Pocket Reference*, 3rd edition. Phoenix, Arizona Heart Foundation, 2013, pp 336–337.

539. A. 1.5:1.

The patient has an atrial septal defect (ASD) with left-to-right shunting. Therefore pulmonary blood flow is greater than systemic flow, so the Qp/Qs ratio should be greater than 1. Choice A is the only option greater than 1; all the other options—1:1, 1:1.3, and 0.7:1—are equal to or less than 1 and therefore incorrect.

- Bergersen L, Foerster S, Marshall AC, et al (eds): *Congenital Heart Disease: The Catheterization Manual*. New York, Springer, 2009, p 9.
- Reynolds T: *The Pediatric Echocardiographer's Pocket Reference*, 3rd edition. Phoenix, Arizona Heart Foundation, 2013, pp 336–337.

540. B. 87 mmHg.

Given measurements of both a systolic and a diastolic blood pressure, mean blood pressure can be calculated using the following equation:

$$MAP = 1/3 \times (SBP - DBP) + DBP$$

where MAP = mean arterial pressure, SBP = systolic blood pressure, and DBP = diastolic blood pressure. In this patient, the systolic blood pressure is 120 mmHg, the diastolic blood pressure 70 mmHg. Therefore

$$\begin{aligned} MAP &= 1/3 \times (120 - 70) + 70 \\ &= 50/3 + 70 \\ &= 16.67 + 70 \\ &= 86.67 \text{ mmHg} \end{aligned}$$

Rounding up, the answer is choice B, 87 mmHg.

▶ Klabunde RE: *Cardiovascular Physiology Concepts*, 2nd edition. Baltimore, Lippincott Williams & Wilkins, 2012, pp 93–123.

541. B. Rare among all pediatric patients.

Diastolic heart disease is not often seen in pediatric patients and is considered rare. When it is found it is most often associated with pediatric disease processes such as hypertrophic cardiomyopathy, type 1 diabetes mellitus, chronic kidney disease, and restrictive cardiomyopathy.

▶ Lai WW, Mertens LL, Cohen MS, et al (eds): *Echocardiography in Pediatric and Congenital Heart Disease: From Fetus to Adult*, 2nd edition. Chichester, UK, Wiley-Blackwell, 2016, pp 132, 145–147.

542. D. They vary by age.

When assessing for diastolic dysfunction in pediatric populations, echocardiographers apply the same Doppler techniques as those used for the adult population, but the normal values are different. These normal values vary according to age and become less reliable with tachycardic infants and children.

▶ Lai WW, Mertens LL, Cohen MS, et al (eds): *Echocardiography in Pediatric and Congenital Heart Disease: From Fetus to Adult*, 2nd edition. Chichester, UK, Wiley-Blackwell, 2016, pp 132, 134, 143.

543. D. Abnormally decreased due to spectral gate position.

See Color Plate 26 on page xxxi.

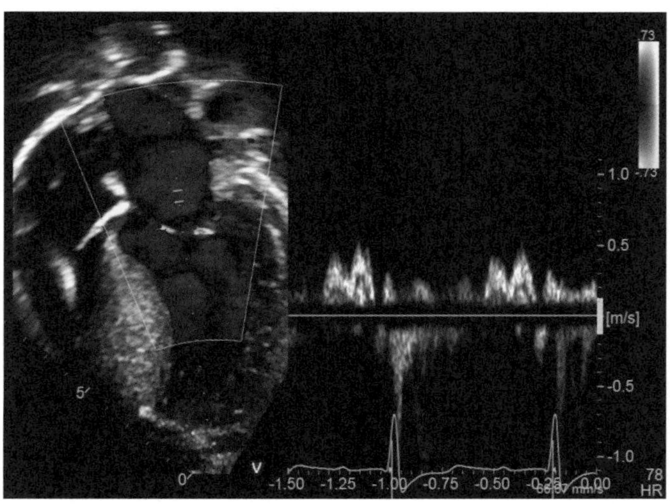

The spectral Doppler gate in this image is placed in the left atrium, which can decrease the recorded velocities. When evaluating the mitral inflow pattern, care should be taken to place the pulsed-wave Doppler gate at the leaflet tips.

▶ Lai WW, Mertens LL, Cohen MS, et al (eds): *Echocardiography in Pediatric and Congenital Heart Disease: From Fetus to Adult*, 2nd edition. Chichester, UK, Wiley-Blackwell, 2016, p 133.

544. B. Isovolumic relaxation time.

See Color Plate 27 on page xxxii.

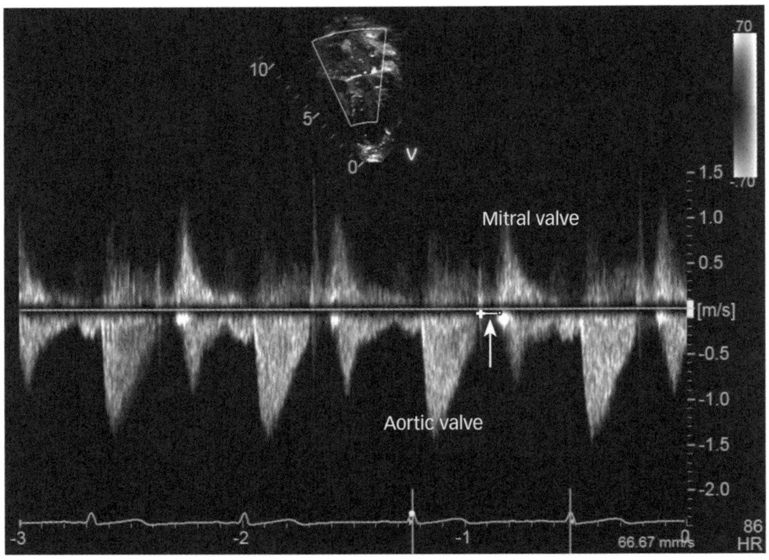

These two waveforms correspond to mitral valve inflow and aortic valve outflow. Isovolumic relaxation time can be determined by using calipers to measure the time from the closure of the aortic valve to the beginning of the mitral valve E wave (arrow).

▶ Lai WW, Mertens LL, Cohen MS, et al (eds): *Echocardiography in Pediatric and Congenital Heart Disease: From Fetus to Adult*, 2nd edition. Chichester, UK, Wiley-Blackwell, 2016, pp 134–137.

545. C. Increased with impaired left ventricular relaxation and normal left atrial pressure.

Ventricular "compliance" and "relaxation" represent different components of diastolic function and should not be used interchangeably. Isovolumic relaxation time is increased in the presence of impaired ventricular relaxation and normal left atrial pressure and can be measured by using continuous-wave Doppler to record the time between aortic valve closure and mitral valve opening. Conversely, ventricular compliance is a reflection of ventricular chamber rigidity or stiffness. Note that isovolumic relaxation time can be shortened in patients with abnormal left ventricular compliance and increased left atrial pressures.

▶ Lai WW, Mertens LL, Cohen MS, et al (eds): *Echocardiography in Pediatric and Congenital Heart Disease: From Fetus to Adult*, 2nd edition. Chichester, UK, Wiley-Blackwell, 2016, pp 134, 138, 141–142.

546. D. E-wave deceleration time is decreased.

Increased E-wave deceleration time is seen with abnormal relaxation and normal left atrial pressure; however, this measure is affected by heart rate and is not useful in the setting of tachycardia. E-wave deceleration time shortens with an increase in heart rate. With tachycardia, the E and A waves have a tendency to fuse together.

▶ Lai WW, Mertens LL, Cohen MS, et al (eds): *Echocardiography in Pediatric and Congenital Heart Disease: From Fetus to Adult*, 2nd edition. Chichester, UK, Wiley-Blackwell, 2016, p 134.

547. D. Findings are not reliable; diastolic function cannot be assessed in this setting.

The mitral valve inflow pattern in the setting of mitral stenosis is not a reliable indicator of diastolic function. The inflow patterns seen in both mitral and tricuspid valve stenosis reveal more about the valvular stenosis than they do about diastolic function.

▶ Lai WW, Mertens LL, Cohen MS, et al (eds): *Echocardiography in Pediatric and Congenital Heart Disease: From Fetus to Adult*, 2nd edition. Chichester, UK, Wiley-Blackwell, 2016, p 135.

548. B. Tricuspid E wave, early right ventricular filling.

Right ventricular filling is relatively preload dependent, and inspiration can cause tricuspid valve inflow (E-wave and A-wave) velocities to vary. Tissue Doppler imaging is preload independent, and varying velocities are not seen with inspiration. Under normal circumstances, mitral valve inflow velocities do not vary as much with respiration. However, processes like pericardial effusion and arrhythmias (atrial fibrillation) can affect mitral valve inflow velocities.

▶ Lai WW, Mertens LL, Cohen MS, et al (eds): *Echocardiography in Pediatric and Congenital Heart Disease: From Fetus to Adult*, 2nd edition. Chichester, UK, Wiley-Blackwell, 2016, pp 135, 711.

ANSWERS

549. A. A.

See Color Plate 28 on page xxxii.

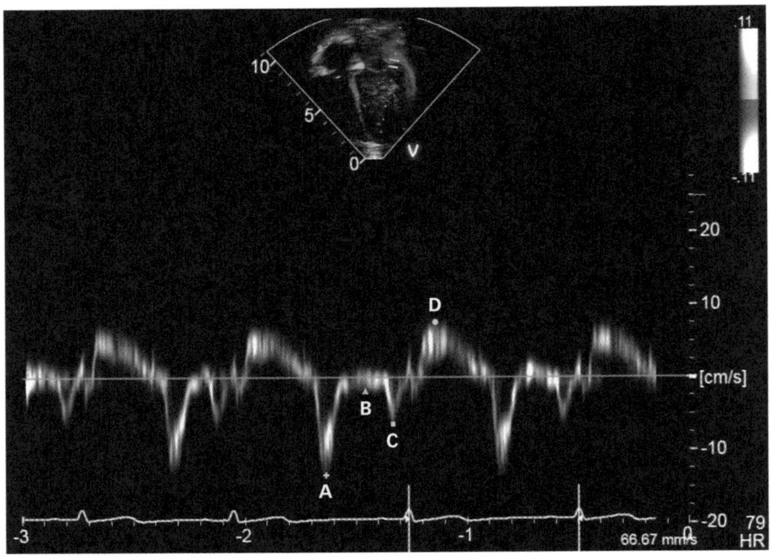

This image displays tissue Doppler imaging of the mitral valve lateral annulus. Letter A marks early diastolic filling as represented by the e′ wave. An easy way to differentiate an e′ wave from an a′ wave is to examine the ECG tracing and notice that the a′ wave occurs slightly after the atrial contraction (P wave), while the e′ wave occurs in early diastole, before the onset of atrial contraction.

▶ Lai WW, Mertens LL, Cohen MS, et al (eds): *Echocardiography in Pediatric and Congenital Heart Disease: From Fetus to Adult*, 2nd edition. Chichester, UK, Wiley-Blackwell, 2016, p 136.

550. B. Chronic left ventricular diastolic dysfunction.

An increase in left atrial volume is a good marker for chronic left ventricular diastolic dysfunction in the absence of mitral valve disease. Normal values for children are categorized by body surface area and were originally obtained by the use of 3D echocardiography. Both Simpson's method and the area-length method are used to measure left atrial volume.

▶ Lai WW, Mertens LL, Cohen MS, et al (eds): *Echocardiography in Pediatric and Congenital Heart Disease: From Fetus to Adult*, 2nd edition. Chichester, UK, Wiley-Blackwell, 2016, p 138.

551. C. Simpson's method.

Although Simpson's method and the area-length method are good ways of measuring left atrial (LA) volume, they both underestimate LA volume on echocardiography as compared to computed tomography (CT) and magnetic resonance imaging (MRI). Choices B and D are technical pitfalls that should be avoided.

▶ Lai WW, Mertens LL, Cohen MS, et al (eds): *Echocardiography in Pediatric and Congenital Heart Disease: From Fetus to Adult*, 2nd edition. Chichester, UK, Wiley-Blackwell, 2016, p 139.

552. C. Decreased E-wave/A-wave ratio as compared to that of older children.

In the neonatal heart it is normal to see a decreased E-wave velocity as compared to the A wave. The myocardium of the infant heart is thought to be immature, with diastolic function that is not fully developed compared to that of older children and adults. This is typified by the finding of an E-wave velocity lower than the A-wave velocity, representing impaired diastolic relaxation.

▶ Lai WW, Mertens LL, Cohen MS, et al (eds): *Echocardiography in Pediatric and Congenital Heart Disease: From Fetus to Adult*, 2nd edition. Chichester, UK, Wiley-Blackwell, 2016, p 143.

553. A. Abnormal left ventricular relaxation with normal left atrial pressure.

In early diastolic dysfunction, the left ventricular relaxation is abnormal, and this is represented by a lower E-wave velocity as compared to the A-wave velocity. In this early form of diastolic dysfunction, left ventricular compliance is normal and therefore left atrial pressure is considered normal.

▶ Lai WW, Mertens LL, Cohen MS, et al (eds): *Echocardiography in Pediatric and Congenital Heart Disease: From Fetus to Adult*, 2nd edition. Chichester, UK, Wiley-Blackwell, 2016, pp 139–143.

554. A. Abnormal relaxation and slower heart rates.

In hearts with abnormal relaxation and a normal left atrial pressure (representing the earliest form of diastolic dysfunction), an L wave can sometimes be seen on spectral Doppler during slow heart rates. This L wave occurs during diastasis, which represents the time during diastole between the E and A waves (as noted by spectral Doppler), when no left ventricular filling normally occurs. However, markedly delayed relaxation can create a mid-diastolic pressure gradient across the mitral valve, resulting in additional filling during diastasis, as demonstrated by the presence of the L wave.

- Lai WW, Mertens LL, Cohen MS, et al (eds): *Echocardiography in Pediatric and Congenital Heart Disease: From Fetus to Adult*, 2nd edition. Chichester, UK, Wiley-Blackwell, 2016, p 140.
- Nagueh SF, Smiseth OA, Appleton CP, et al: Recommendations for the evaluation of left ventricular diastolic function by echocardiography: an update from the American Society of Echocardiography and the European Association of Cardiovascular Imaging. J Am Soc Echocardiogr 29:277–314, 2016.

555. C. Increased left ventricular filling pressure.

An increased Ar wave duration, as compared to the mitral valve inflow A wave duration, is a good marker of elevated left atrial and left ventricular end-diastolic pressures, representing diastolic dysfunction. This is a known finding in adults with diastolic dysfunction and has also been documented in pediatric patients by a study performed at the Mayo Clinic (O'Leary et al. 1998).

- Lai WW, Mertens LL, Cohen MS, et al (eds): *Echocardiography in Pediatric and Congenital Heart Disease: From Fetus to Adult*, 2nd edition. Chichester, UK, Wiley-Blackwell, 2016, p 140.
- Nagueh SF, Smiseth OA, Appleton CP, et al: Recommendations for the evaluation of left ventricular diastolic function by echocardiography: an update from the American Society of Echocardiography and the European Association of Cardiovascular Imaging. J Am Soc Echocardiogr 29:277–314, 2016.
- O'Leary PW, Durongpisitkul K, Cordes TM, et al: Diastolic ventricular function in children: a Doppler echocardiographic study establishing normal values and predictors of increased ventricular end-diastolic pressure. Mayo Clin Proc 73:616–628, 1998.

556. D. E/e′ ratio of 12.

In an adult echocardiographic study (Nagueh et al. 1997) performed to estimate left ventricular filling pressures, an E/e′ ratio greater than 10 predicted an LVEDP greater than 12 mmHg.

- Lai WW, Mertens LL, Cohen MS, et al (eds): *Echocardiography in Pediatric and Congenital Heart Disease: From Fetus to Adult*, 2nd edition. Chichester, UK, Wiley-Blackwell, 2016, p 141.
- Nagueh SF, Appleton CP, Gillebert TC, et al: Recommendations for the evaluation of left ventricular diastolic function by echocardiography. J Am Soc Echocardiogr 22:107–133, 2009.
- Nagueh SF, Middleton KJ, Kopelen HA, et al: Doppler tissue imaging: a noninvasive technique for evaluation of left ventricular relaxation and estimation of filling pressures. J Am Coll Cardiol 30:1527–1533, 1997.
- Nagueh SF, Smiseth OA, Appleton CP, et al: Recommendations for the evaluation of left ventricular diastolic function by echocardiography: an update from the American Society of Echocardiography and the European Association of Cardiovascular Imaging. J Am Soc Echocardiogr 29:277–314, 2016.

557. C. Abnormal left ventricular diastolic compliance.

See Color Plate 29 on page xxxiii.

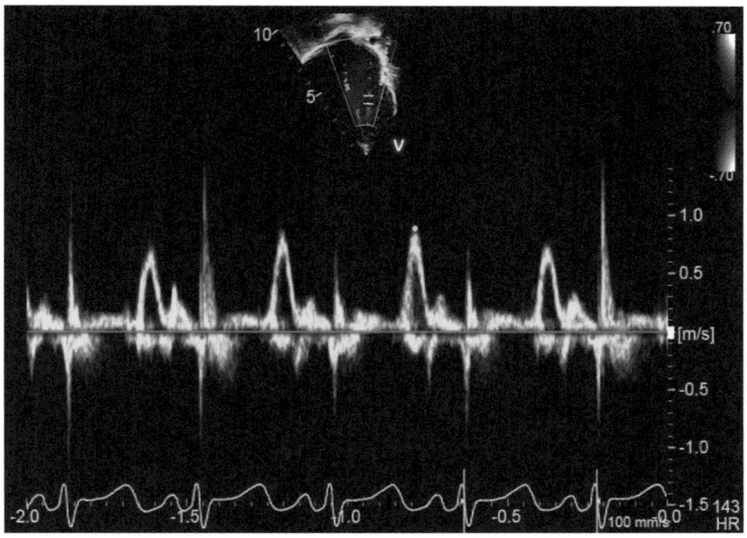

This spectral Doppler tracing is taken from a patient with restrictive cardiomyopathy. The spectral Doppler pattern across the mitral valve shows an increased E wave, with rapid deceleration time and a very low-velocity A wave. An E/A ratio greater than 2 is often seen in restrictive cardiomyopathy. Causes of restrictive cardiomyopathy include (but are not limited to) amyloidosis, hemochromatosis, hypereosinophilia, and idiopathic causes.

▶ Lai WW, Mertens LL, Cohen MS, et al (eds): *Echocardiography in Pediatric and Congenital Heart Disease: From Fetus to Adult*, 2nd edition. Chichester, UK, Wiley-Blackwell, 2016, pp 139–146, 694–695, 702.

558. B. 36%.

It is important that a distinction be made between an athletic (or athlete's) heart—which can be hypertrophied but with a normal spectral Doppler profile—and a heart with increased left ventricular mass like that encountered in the setting of systemic hypertension. The latter type of heart will likely have an abnormal diastolic filling pattern. In a study of pediatric patients with essential hypertension (Border et al. 2007), 36% of patients with essential hypertension had diastolic filling abnormalities. Elevated ventricular mass was found to be the most important independent predictor of pathologic diastolic function.

▶ Border WL, Kimball TR, Witt SA, et al: Diastolic filling abnormalities in children with essential hypertension. J Pediatr 150:503–509, 2007.

▶ Lai WW, Mertens LL, Cohen MS, et al (eds): *Echocardiography in Pediatric and Congenital Heart Disease: From Fetus to Adult*, 2nd edition. Chichester, UK, Wiley-Blackwell, 2016, pp 146–147.

ANSWERS

559. D. Measuring atrial lengths in both the apical four-chamber and apical two-chamber views.

In order to avoid left atrial foreshortening when assessing left atrial volume, one must obtain an image that is neither too posterior (visualizing the coronary sinus is a sign of being too posterior) nor too anterior (visualizing the outflow tracts is a clue that the image is too anterior). In the area-length method, you measure in two different views—the apical two-chamber and apical four-chamber views—and use the shortest (not longest) length to estimate the volume. However, these left atrial lengths should not differ by more than 5 mm, and the closer these length measurements are to each other, the more likely it is that the estimate of left atrial volume will be accurate. Both the pulmonary vein ostia and the left atrial appendage should be excluded, not included, in the left atrial trace.

▶ Lai WW, Mertens LL, Cohen MS, et al (eds): *Echocardiography in Pediatric and Congenital Heart Disease: From Fetus to Adult*, 2nd edition. Chichester, UK, Wiley-Blackwell, 2016, pp 138–139.

560. C. Triphasic pulmonary venous inflow waves are seen during atrial filling and do not indicate diastolic disease.

See Color Plate 30 on page xxxiii.

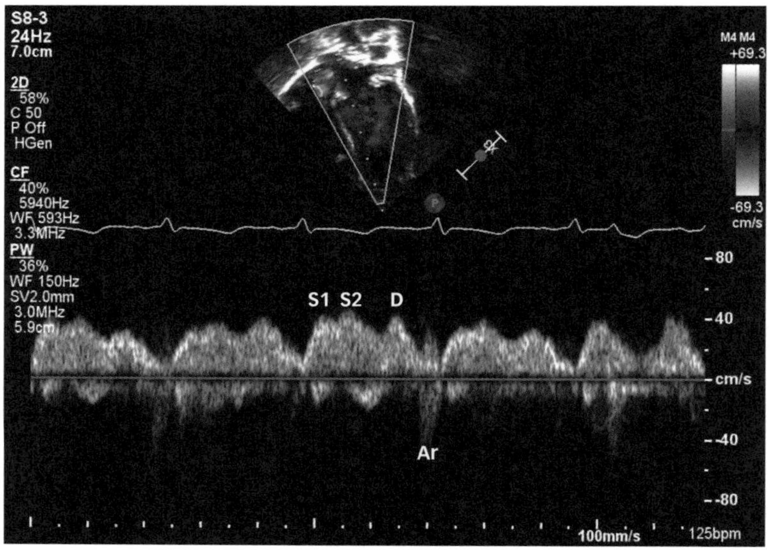

A triphasic waveform is a normal pulmonary venous Doppler finding in infants and does not indicate diastolic dysfunction.

▶ Lai WW, Mertens LL, Cohen MS, et al (eds): *Echocardiography in Pediatric and Congenital Heart Disease: From Fetus to Adult*, 2nd edition. Chichester, UK, Wiley-Blackwell, 2016, pp 134–135.

561. D. Diastasis.

An L wave is observed between the E and A waves, the period known as diastasis, when pressures in the atria and ventricles have equalized and usually no flow can be detected between the two chambers. However, an L wave can be seen in patients with slow heart rates and markedly abnormal relaxation, in which the significantly delayed relaxation produces a mid-diastolic pressure gradient across the mitral valve during diastasis, resulting in additional filling during this period and manifesting as the L wave.

▸ Lai WW, Mertens LL, Cohen MS, et al (eds): *Echocardiography in Pediatric and Congenital Heart Disease: From Fetus to Adult*, 2nd edition. Chichester, UK, Wiley-Blackwell, 2016, p 140.

562. C. C.

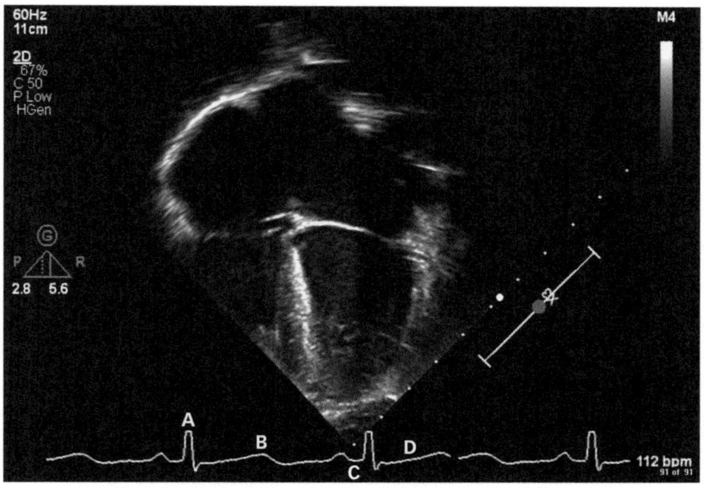

Late ventricular filling occurs during atrial contraction, which is shown beginning with the P wave on the electrocardiogram, which is marked as C in this image.

▸ Lai WW, Mertens LL, Cohen MS, et al (eds): *Echocardiography in Pediatric and Congenital Heart Disease: From Fetus to Adult*, 2nd edition. Chichester, UK, Wiley-Blackwell, 2016, pp 132–133.

563. A. With abnormal relaxation and normal left atrial pressure.

With abnormal relaxation and normal left atrial pressure (the mildest form of diastolic dysfunction), the E wave has a lower velocity than the A wave. This occurs because impaired relaxation prolongs the decrease in left ventricular filling pressure, resulting in a lower pressure gradient across the mitral valve (during early left ventricular filling) and less ventricular filling

ANSWERS

in early diastole (seen on spectral Doppler as a lower E wave). More diastolic filling must occur in late diastole/atrial contraction, resulting in a higher A wave. This produces E/A reversal, with a resultant E/A ratio that is less than 1.

▶ Lai WW, Mertens LL, Cohen MS, et al (eds): *Echocardiography in Pediatric and Congenital Heart Disease: From Fetus to Adult*, 2nd edition. Chichester, UK, Wiley-Blackwell, 2016, p 140.

564. C. Noncompliant, stiff left ventricle.

The spectral Doppler values listed in the question are consistent with restrictive physiology in a noncompliant, stiff left ventricle. Note that deceleration time is dependent on heart rate and in a patient with tachycardia would not be a very useful measure to assess diastolic function.

▶ Lai WW, Mertens LL, Cohen MS, et al (eds): *Echocardiography in Pediatric and Congenital Heart Disease: From Fetus to Adult*, 2nd edition. Chichester, UK, Wiley-Blackwell, 2016, pp 139–143, 695.

565. D. Diastolic dysfunction.

In a pediatric study performed by the Mayo Clinic (O'Leary et al. 1998), prolongation of the Ar wave (atrial reversal with atrial contraction) was found to be an indicator of diastolic dysfunction. Duration of the Ar wave should not exceed the duration of the mitral inflow A wave by more than 1.2 times nor by more than 29 msec. In patients with a pseudonormalized mitral inflow pattern, a prolonged Ar wave duration compared to the mitral inflow A wave duration can be useful in identifying patients with elevated left ventricular filling pressure and elevated left atrial pressure.

▶ Lai WW, Mertens LL, Cohen MS, et al (eds): *Echocardiography in Pediatric and Congenital Heart Disease: From Fetus to Adult*, 2nd edition. Chichester, UK, Wiley-Blackwell, 2016, p 140.

▶ O'Leary PW, Durongpisitkul K, Cordes TM, et al: Diastolic ventricular function in children: a Doppler echocardiographic study establishing normal values and predictors of increased ventricular end-diastolic pressure. Mayo Clin Proc 73:616–628, 1998.

566. D. Measure in both the apical two-chamber and apical four-chamber planes using biplane Simpson's method (summation of disks).

As compared to M-mode, which correlates poorly with angiography, biplane Simpson's method (summation of disks) is best when assessing left atrial volume (LAV). Both the apical four-chamber and apical two-chamber views should be used to accurately assess LAV. The biplane area-length method, using both two-chamber and four-chamber views, is also a good way to assess LAV, but it is not given as one of the answer choices. Care should be taken in both biplane Simpson's method and the area-length method not to foreshorten the atria, as that will result in underestimation of LAV. Clinical situations in which the calculation of LAV is useful include diastolic dysfunction and mitral regurgitation.

▶ Lopez L, Colan SD, Frommelt PC, et al: Recommendations for quantification methods during the performance of a pediatric echocardiogram: a report from the Pediatric Measurements Writing Group of the American Society of Echocardiography Pediatric and Congenital Heart Disease Council. J Am Soc Echocardiogr 23:465–495, 2010.

567. B. At end systole before mitral valve opening.

It is recommended that left atrial volume measurements be made at end systole, before mitral valve opening. The left atrial tracings should not include the left atrial appendage or the pulmonary veins.

▶ Lai WW, Mertens LL, Cohen MS, et al (eds): *Echocardiography in Pediatric and Congenital Heart Disease: From Fetus to Adult*, 2nd edition. Chichester, UK, Wiley-Blackwell, 2016, pp 132–139.

▶ Lopez L, Colan SD, Frommelt PC, et al: Recommendations for quantification methods during the performance of a pediatric echocardiogram: a report from the Pediatric Measurements Writing Group of the American Society of Echocardiography Pediatric and Congenital Heart Disease Council. J Am Soc Echocardiogr 23:465–495, 2010.

568. D. Go to the apical four-chamber view and measure the mitral valve annulus from inner edge to inner edge.

The mitral valve annulus should be measured at its largest diameter during early diastole from inner edge to inner edge and a Z-score calculated. In pediatric patients mitral valve pathology (e.g., supramitral valve ring, cleft mitral valve, or double orifice mitral valve) varies significantly, so an en face mitral valve measurement can be unreliable—in contrast to the echocardiographic measurements that are obtained for adults, which are generally well established.

▶ Baumgartner H, Hung J, Bermejo J, et al: Echocardiographic assessment of valve stenosis: EAE/ASE recommendations for clinical practice. J Am Soc Echoccardiogr 22:1–23, 2009.

▶ Lai WW, Mertens LL, Cohen MS, et al (eds): *Echocardiography in Pediatric and Congenital Heart Disease: From Fetus to Adult*, 2nd edition. Chichester, UK, Wiley-Blackwell, 2016, pp 63–72, 893–894.

▶ Lopez L, Colan SD, Frommelt PC, et al: Recommendations for quantification methods during the performance of a pediatric echocardiogram: a report from the Pediatric Measurements Writing Group of the American Society of Echocardiography Pediatric and Congenital Heart Disease Council. J Am Soc Echocardiogr 23:465–495, 2010.

ANSWERS

569. A. Incorrect for measurement of the mitral valve annulus because the mitral valve is closed.

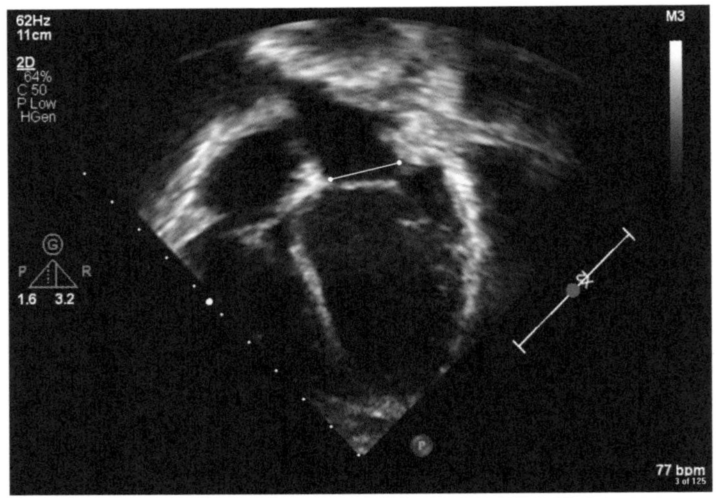

This image demonstrates incorrect caliper placement for measuring the mitral valve annulus because the mitral valve is closed. The mitral valve annulus should be measured from inner edge to inner edge when the valve is open and at its largest diameter during early diastole. The angulation of the calipers is not an important consideration when measuring the mitral valve annulus.

▶ Lopez L, Colan SD, Frommelt PC, et al: Recommendations for quantification methods during the performance of a pediatric echocardiogram: a report from the Pediatric Measurements Writing Group of the American Society of Echocardiography Pediatric and Congenital Heart Disease Council. J Am Soc Echocardiogr 23:465–495, 2010.

570. C. Mean mitral valve gradient with continuous-wave Doppler.

The most useful measurement in assessing the mitral valve stenosis in this patient would be the mean mitral valve gradient acquired with continuous-wave Doppler. 2D planimetry and pressure half-time are not generally used to evaluate mitral valve stenosis in pediatric patients due to the complexity of the different types of mitral valve stenosis, such as that associated with supramitral rings, parachute mitral valves, and poor correlation with cardiac catheterization. A mean gradient of 4–5 mmHg is seen in mild congenital mitral stenosis, and a mean gradient greater than 13 mmHg is seen in severe mitral stenosis.

▶ Lai WW, Mertens LL, Cohen MS, et al (eds): *Echocardiography in Pediatric and Congenital Heart Disease: From Fetus to Adult*, 2nd edition. Chichester, UK, Wiley-Blackwell, 2016, pp 246–253.

▶ Lopez L, Colan SD, Frommelt PC, et al: Recommendations for quantification methods during the performance of a pediatric echocardiogram: a report from the Pediatric Measurements Writing Group of the American

Society of Echocardiography Pediatric and Congenital Heart Disease Council. J Am Soc Echocardiogr 23:465–495, 2010.

▶ Park MK: *Park's Pediatric Cardiology for Practitioners*, 6th edition. Philadelphia, Saunders, 2014, pp 375–378.

571. D. Severe mitral valve stenosis.

See Color Plate 31 on page xxxiv.

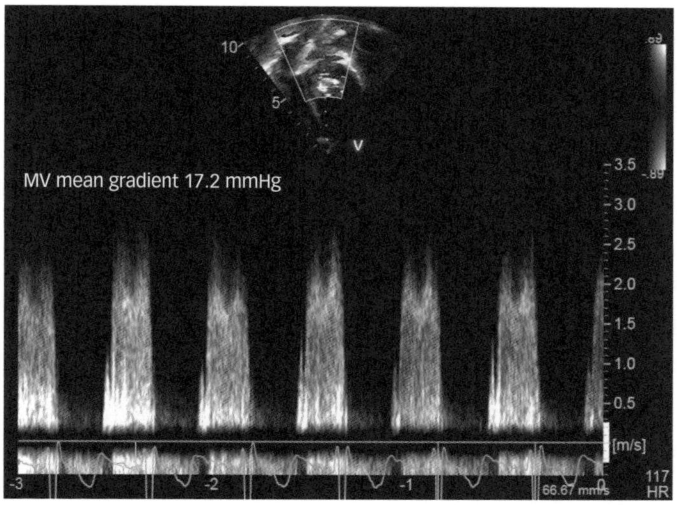

This image demonstrates an increased mean mitral valve gradient (greater than 13 mmHg), which can be seen in severe mitral valve stenosis.

▶ Lopez L, Colan SD, Frommelt PC, et al: Recommendations for quantification methods during the performance of a pediatric echocardiogram: a report from the Pediatric Measurements Writing Group of the American Society of Echocardiography Pediatric and Congenital Heart Disease Council. J Am Soc Echocardiogr 23:465–495, 2010.

▶ Park MK: *Park's Pediatric Cardiology for Practitioners*, 6th edition. Philadelphia, Saunders, 2014, pp 375–376.

572. B. Anterior–posterior diameter.

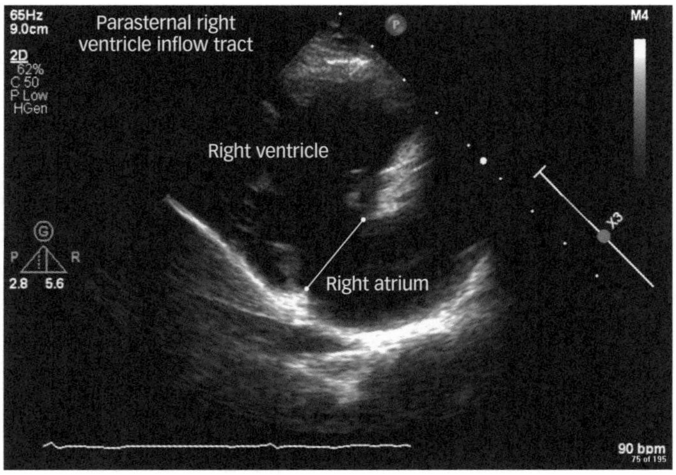

This view is of the right ventricular inflow tract in a normal pediatric heart. It was acquired in the parasternal long-axis view by tilting the transducer toward the patient's right. This

particular view demonstrates the tricuspid valve anterior–posterior diameter. It can be helpful for the assessment of the posterior tricuspid valve leaflet in Ebstein anomaly of the tricuspid valve, for evaluation of tricuspid valve dysplasia, and for ruling out tricuspid valve endocarditis.

▸ Lai WW, Mertens LL, Cohen MS, et al (eds): *Echocardiography in Pediatric and Congenital Heart Disease: From Fetus to Adult*, 2nd edition. Chichester, UK, Wiley-Blackwell, 2016, pp 132, 231–241.

▸ Lopez L, Colan SD, Frommelt PC, et al: Recommendations for quantification methods during the performance of a pediatric echocardiogram: a report from the Pediatric Measurements Writing Group of the American Society of Echocardiography Pediatric and Congenital Heart Disease Council. J Am Soc Echocardiogr 23:465–495, 2010.

ANSWERS

Refer to video PER-Q573.

573. A. Left-sided atrioventricular valve (AV valve) at the widest diameter in early diastole.

Video PER-Q573 demonstrates L-looped (inverted) ventricles, with the morphologic right ventricle on the left side and the morphologic left ventricle on the right side. Because the AV valves are always associated with their respective ventricles (tricuspid valve with right ventricle and mitral valve with left ventricle), the left-sided AV valve in this patient is the tricuspid valve, and it should be measured at its widest diameter in early diastole.

▸ Lai WW, Mertens LL, Cohen MS, et al (eds): *Echocardiography in Pediatric and Congenital Heart Disease: From Fetus to Adult*, 2nd edition. Chichester, UK, Wiley-Blackwell, 2016, pp 37–38.

▸ Lopez L, Colan SD, Frommelt PC, et al: Recommendations for quantification methods during the performance of a pediatric echocardiogram: a report from the Pediatric Measurements Writing Group of the American Society of Echocardiography Pediatric and Congenital Heart Disease Council. J Am Soc Echocardiogr 23:465–495, 2010.

574. C. The mean mitral pressure gradient is underestimated due to the presence of an ASD.

See Color Plate 32 on page xxxiv.

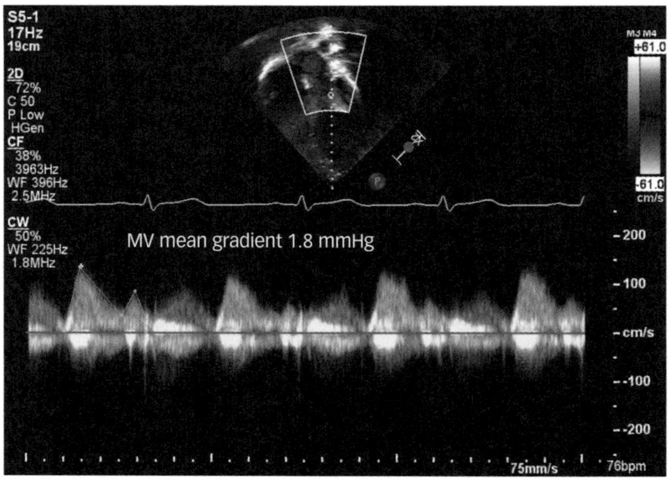

In this patient, there is shunting of some left atrial blood to the right atrium through the atrial septal defect (ASD). This shunting reduces the flow across the mitral valve, thereby lowering the transvalvular gradient. In this setting, therefore, the mean mitral valve pressure gradient underestimates mitral valve stenosis. Instead, closer anatomic inspection of mitral valve leaflets, chordae tendineae, papillary muscles, and mitral annular Z-scores should be undertaken to determine whether the patient has mitral valve stenosis.

- Lai WW, Mertens LL, Cohen MS, et al (eds): *Echocardiography in Pediatric and Congenital Heart Disease: From Fetus to Adult*, 2nd edition. Chichester, UK, Wiley-Blackwell, 2016, p 253.
- Lopez L, Colan SD, Frommelt PC, et al: Recommendations for quantification methods during the performance of a pediatric echocardiogram: a report from the Pediatric Measurements Writing Group of the American Society of Echocardiography Pediatric and Congenital Heart Disease Council. J Am Soc Echocardiogr 23:465–495, 2010.

Refer to video PER-Q575.

575. C. Displacement index.

Video PER-Q575 is taken from a patient with Ebstein anomaly of the tricuspid valve. The displacement index is used to determine if the tricuspid valve fits in the category of Ebstein anomaly. Using the apical four-chamber view, it is a measure of apical displacement of the septal leaflet of the tricuspid valve when compared to the level of the anterior leaflet of mitral valve. The linear distance between septal insertions of the septal tricuspid valve leaflet and anterior mitral valve leaflet is divided by the patient's body surface area, measured in square meters, to determine this index, and if the result is greater than 8 mm/m^2 the diagnosis of Ebstein anomaly of the tricuspid valve is established. The Celermajer index helps determine the prognosis for a patient already diagnosed with Ebstein anomaly.

- Lai WW, Mertens LL, Cohen MS, et al (eds): *Echocardiography in Pediatric and Congenital Heart Disease: From Fetus to Adult*, 2nd edition. Chichester, UK, Wiley-Blackwell, 2016, pp 234–239.

576. D. Poor prognosis in the setting of Ebstein anomaly of the tricuspid valve.

The Celermajer index is used in the setting of Ebstein anomaly to assess prognosis. A value greater than 1 is associated with a poor prognosis. The Celermajer index is obtained by calculating the planimetered area of the right atrium (which includes the atrialized portion of right ventricle) and dividing it by the sum of the planimetered areas of the functional right ventricle (which excludes the atrialized portion of the right ventricle), left atrium, and left ventricle. Celermajer introduced this technique in 1992. Ebstein anomaly affects the tricuspid valve, not the mitral valve.

- Lai WW, Mertens LL, Cohen MS, et al (eds): *Echocardiography in Pediatric and Congenital Heart Disease: From Fetus to Adult*, 2nd edition. Chichester, UK, Wiley-Blackwell, 2016, pp 234–239.

577. D. Obligatory left-to-right atrial shunting.

Hepatomegaly, right atrial hypertrophy, and right ventricular outflow tract obstruction are associated with tricuspid valve stenosis. There is no known association between tricuspid valve stenosis and an obligatory left-to-right atrial shunt.

- Allen HD, Shaddy RE, Penny DJ, et al: *Moss and Adams' Heart Disease in Infants, Children, and Adolescents, Including the Fetus and Young Adult*, 9th edition. Philadelphia, Wolters Kluwer, 2016, pp 877–879, 885–886.

578. B. At end diastole.

The right ventricular free wall thickness should be measured at end diastole using the subcostal long-axis, parasternal short-axis, or parasternal long-axis plane. Care should be taken to exclude heavy trabeculations when measuring the right ventricle free wall. The right ventricle in a normal heart is complex and composed of an inlet region, sinus body, and outflow tract. It is difficult to view the entire normal right ventricle at once by echocardiography. Understanding that different echocardiographic views are required to visualize different right ventricular segments is important when obtaining right ventricular measurements.

- Ezon DS, Goldberg JF, Kyle WB: *Atlas of Congenital Heart Disease Nomenclature: An Illustrated Guide to the Van Praagh and Anderson Approaches to Describing Congenital Cardiac Pathology*. Houston, Ezon Educational Services/CreateSpace, 2015, p 6.
- Lopez L, Colan SD, Frommelt PC, et al: Recommendations for quantification methods during the performance of a pediatric echocardiogram: a report from the Pediatric Measurements Writing Group of the American Society of Echocardiography Pediatric and Congenital Heart Disease Council. J Am Soc Echocardiogr 23:465–495, 2010.

579. A. Endocardial fibroelastosis.

Endocardial fibroelastosis (EFE), in which there is thickening of the endocardium by collagen and elastic fibers, probably represents a nonspecific endocardial reaction to a significant underlying disease process that affects the heart. Examples of such disease processes include dilated cardiomyopathy, infections (such as mumps), metabolic disease, and congenital heart disease—notably the left-sided obstructive lesions, such as aortic stenosis, Shone's variants, and hypoplastic left heart syndrome (HLHS). In patients with HLHS, left ventricular EFE is most commonly found in the anatomic variant with mitral stenosis and aortic atresia (MS/AA), possibly signifying an endocardial reaction to the very high left ventricular pressures found in this variant. The appearance of a bright hyperechoic endocardium can be echocardiographic evidence for EFE. However, even with careful inspection, EFE can be missed by echocardiography.

- Lai WW, Mertens LL, Cohen MS, et al (eds): *Echocardiography in Pediatric and Congenital Heart Disease: From Fetus to Adult*, 2nd edition. Chichester, UK, Wiley-Blackwell, 2016, p 365.
- Lurie P: Changing concepts of endocardial fibroelastosis. Cardiol Young 20:115–123, 2010.
- Rudolph AM: *Congenital Diseases of the Heart: Clinical-Physiological Considerations*, 3rd edition. Chichester, UK, Wiley Blackwell, 2009, p 258.

ANSWERS

580. B. Right ventricular length.

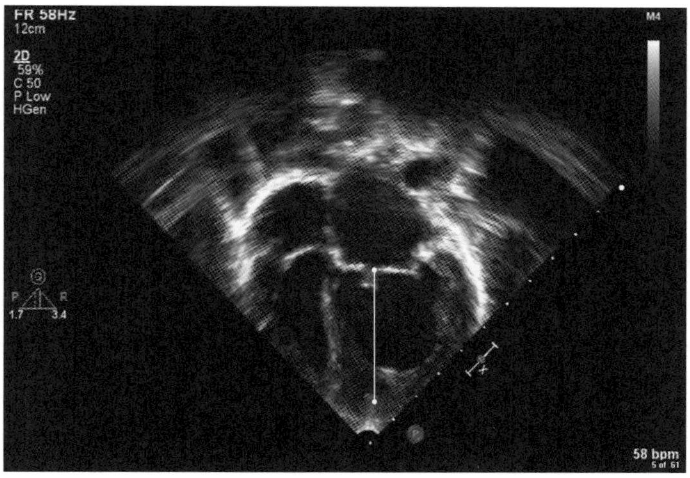

The apical four-chamber view seen in this image has been taken from a patient with L-looped ventricles. Therefore, the right-sided ventricle is the morphologic left ventricle, and the left-sided ventricle is the morphologic right ventricle. The measurement being performed is the right ventricular length at end diastole.

- Lai WW, Mertens LL, Cohen MS, et al (eds): *Echocardiography in Pediatric and Congenital Heart Disease: From Fetus to Adult*, 2nd edition. Chichester, UK, Wiley-Blackwell, 2016, pp 37–39.
- Lopez L, Colan SD, Frommelt PC, et al: Recommendations for quantification methods during the performance of a pediatric echocardiogram: a report from the Pediatric Measurements Writing Group of the American Society of Echocardiography Pediatric and Congenital Heart Disease Council. J Am Soc Echocardiogr 23:465–495, 2010.

581. C. The image is not well centered in the right ventricle.

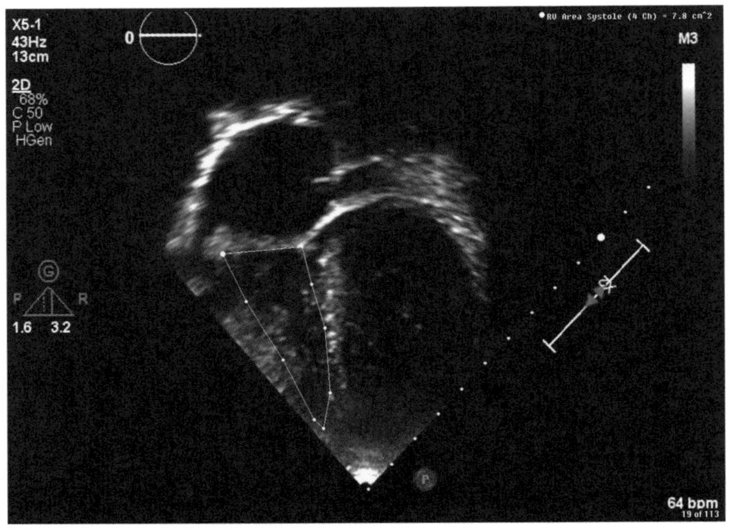

The apical four-chamber view seen here is tilted too far posterior. The outline has been set to measure the area of the right ventricle. The evidence of that is the presence in this image of the coronary sinus, a posterior structure in the heart, as well as the fact that the tricuspid valve is not visualized. Visualizing the coronary sinus or outflow tracts is a clue that the image is not centered in the right ventricle. When you calculate fractional area change (FAC), the image needs to be well centered in the right ventricle, and there should be adequate endocardial border definition.

- Lai WW, Mertens LL, Cohen MS, et al (eds): *Echocardiography in Pediatric and Congenital Heart Disease: From Fetus to Adult*, 2nd edition. Chichester, UK, Wiley-Blackwell, 2016, pp 118–120.
- Lopez L, Colan SD, Frommelt PC, et al: Recommendations for quantification methods during the performance of a pediatric echocardiogram: a report from the Pediatric Measurements Writing Group of the American Society of Echocardiography Pediatric and Congenital Heart Disease Council. J Am Soc Echocardiogr 23:465–495, 2010.

582. D. >35%.

Normal right ventricular fractional area change (RVFAC) is greater than 35%, but it is important to remember that it is a load-dependent measurement. In order to calculate RVFAC, you must image a well-centered right ventricle and well-defined endocardial borders. A normal FAC of greater than 40% has been proposed by Lai et al.

- Lai WW, Mertens LL, Cohen MS, et al (eds): *Echocardiography in Pediatric and Congenital Heart Disease: From Fetus to Adult*, 2nd edition. Chichester, UK, Wiley-Blackwell, 2016, p 120.

▶ Lopez L, Colan SD, Frommelt PC, et al: Recommendations for quantification methods during the performance of a pediatric echocardiogram: a report from the Pediatric Measurements Writing Group of the American Society of Echocardiography Pediatric and Congenital Heart Disease Council. J Am Soc Echocardiogr 23:465–495, 2010.

▶ Rudski LG, Lai WW, Afilalo J, et al: Guidelines for the echocardiographic assessment of the right heart in adults: a report from the American Society of Echocardiography endorsed by the European Association of Echocardiography, a registered branch of the European Society of Cardiology, and the Canadian Society of Echocardiography. J Am Soc Echocardiogr 23:685–713, 2010.

583. A. RVFAC (%) = [(RVEDA − RVESA)/RVEDA] × 100.

Subtracting the right ventricular end-systolic area (RVESA) from the right ventricular end-diastolic area (RVEDA), dividing the result by the RVEDA, and multiplying by 100 will yield the RVFAC expressed as a percentage (%).

▶ Lai WW, Mertens LL, Cohen MS, et al (eds): *Echocardiography in Pediatric and Congenital Heart Disease: From Fetus to Adult*, 2nd edition. Chichester, UK, Wiley-Blackwell, 2016, p 120.

▶ Lopez L, Colan SD, Frommelt PC, et al: Recommendations for quantification methods during the performance of a pediatric echocardiogram: a report from the Pediatric Measurements Writing Group of the American Society of Echocardiography Pediatric and Congenital Heart Disease Council. J Am Soc Echocardiogr 23:465–495, 2010.

Refer to video PER-Q584.

584. C. Hypoplasia of the right ventricle.

In superoinferior ventricles, right ventricular hypoplasia is commonly seen (video PER-Q584). Another feature of superoinferior ventricles is that the atrial and ventricular septa do not align as they do in normal hearts, and generally are perpendicular to each other, which results in the superoinferior orientation of the ventricles. Long cineloop times while performing the subcostal long-axis sweeps are very useful when evaluating superoinferior ventricles.

▶ Ezon DS, Goldberg JF, Kyle WB: *Atlas of Congenital Heart Disease Nomenclature: An Illustrated Guide to the Van Praagh and Anderson Approaches to Describing Congenital Cardiac Pathology*. Houston, Ezon Educational Services/CreateSpace, 2015, p 98.

585. C. Ejection fraction derived by biplane Simpson's method.

Of the available choices, ejection fraction derived by biplane Simpson's method is the best. The current scenario describes a regional wall motion abnormality that will not be evaluated when using the other three techniques. When assessing left ventricular function, it is essential to have good border detection at the endocardial border–to–blood pool interface. When performing biplane Simpson's method, do not trace around papillary muscles. Instead, the trace should follow the endocardial border through the papillary muscle heads.

- Lai WW, Mertens LL, Cohen MS, et al (eds): *Echocardiography in Pediatric and Congenital Heart Disease: From Fetus to Adult*, 2nd edition. Chichester, UK, Wiley-Blackwell, 2016, pp 101–103.
- Lopez L, Colan SD, Frommelt PC, et al: Recommendations for quantification methods during the performance of a pediatric echocardiogram: a report from the Pediatric Measurements Writing Group of the American Society of Echocardiography Pediatric and Congenital Heart Disease Council. J Am Soc Echocardiogr 23:465–495, 2010.

586. B. Ejection fraction by biplane Simpson's method.

The formula [(LVEDV − LVESV)/LVEDV] × 100 is used to determine ejection fraction by M-mode or biplane Simpson's method, where LVEDV is left ventricular end-diastolic volume and LVESV is left ventricular end-systolic volume. Assumptions about left ventricular geometry in M-mode inherently make the use of this technique a flawed method to calculate left ventricular ejection fraction, particularly when regional wall motion abnormalities are present. The fact that the biplane Simpson's method takes regional wall motion abnormalities into account makes it the best of the listed choices.

- Lai WW, Mertens LL, Cohen MS, et al (eds): *Echocardiography in Pediatric and Congenital Heart Disease: From Fetus to Adult*, 2nd edition. Chichester, UK, Wiley-Blackwell, 2016, pp 101–102.
- Lopez L, Colan SD, Frommelt PC, et al: Recommendations for quantification methods during the performance of a pediatric echocardiogram: a report from the Pediatric Measurements Writing Group of the American Society of Echocardiography Pediatric and Congenital Heart Disease Council. J Am Soc Echocardiogr 23:465–495, 2010.

587. C. Subcostal short-axis.

For the area-length method, the subcostal short-axis or parasternal short-axis view at the basal level of the left ventricle can be used to calculate left ventricular area.

- Lai WW, Mertens LL, Cohen MS, et al (eds): *Echocardiography in Pediatric and Congenital Heart Disease: From Fetus to Adult*, 2nd edition. Chichester, UK, Wiley-Blackwell, 2016, pp 102–103.
- Lopez L, Colan SD, Frommelt PC, et al: Recommendations for quantification methods during the performance of a pediatric echocardiogram: a report from the Pediatric Measurements Writing Group of the American Society of Echocardiography Pediatric and Congenital Heart Disease Council. J Am Soc Echocardiogr 23:465–495, 2010.

588. B. Subcostal long-axis.

The subcostal long-axis or apical four-chamber view is used to obtain left ventricular length. Care should be taken not to foreshorten the left ventricle, as that would skew measurements.

▶ Lai WW, Mertens LL, Cohen MS, et al (eds): *Echocardiography in Pediatric and Congenital Heart Disease: From Fetus to Adult*, 2nd edition. Chichester, UK, Wiley-Blackwell, 2016, pp 102–103.

589. A. 5/6 × short-axis basal area × LV length.

The equation used to calculate left ventricular volume using the area-length method is 5/6 × short-axis basal area (obtained in the subcostal or parasternal short-axis view) × LV length (subcostal long-axis or apical four-chamber view). This equation should first be used to calculate the left ventricular end-diastolic volume (LVEDV) and the left ventricular end-systolic volume (LVESV). With these two calculated volumes, an ejection fraction can be calculated using this equation:

$$\text{LV ejection fraction (as a percentage)} = [(LVEDV - LVESV)/LVEDV] \times 100$$

Good border detection of the left ventricular endocardial surface is essential, and care should be taken not to foreshorten the left ventricle (which would skew measurements).

▶ Lai WW, Mertens LL, Cohen MS, et al (eds): *Echocardiography in Pediatric and Congenital Heart Disease: From Fetus to Adult*, 2nd edition. Chichester, UK, Wiley-Blackwell, 2016, pp 102–103.

590. C. Mildly dilated ascending aorta.

A Z-score of +3.2 is in excess of two standard deviations above normal. The normal range of measurements is generally considered to be between a Z-score of –2 and +2; measurements beyond this range are considered abnormal. Therefore, in this patient an ascending aortic Z-score of +3.2 indicates that the ascending aorta is mildly dilated. The greater the Z-score, the more significant the dilatation of the ascending aorta. Aortic root and ascending aortic dilatation in Marfan syndrome can begin early in life. It is reported that by 19 years of age, close to 68% of patients diagnosed with Marfan syndrome will have developed some degree of aortic root dilatation.

▶ Allen HD, Shaddy RE, Penny DJ, et al: *Moss and Adams' Heart Disease in Infants, Children, and Adolescents, Including the Fetus and Young Adult*, 9th edition. Philadelphia, Wolters Kluwer, 2016, pp 800–801.

▶ Lai WW, Mertens LL, Cohen MS, et al (eds): *Echocardiography in Pediatric and Congenital Heart Disease: From Fetus to Adult*, 2nd edition. Chichester, UK, Wiley-Blackwell, 2016, pp 627–629.

591. B. B.

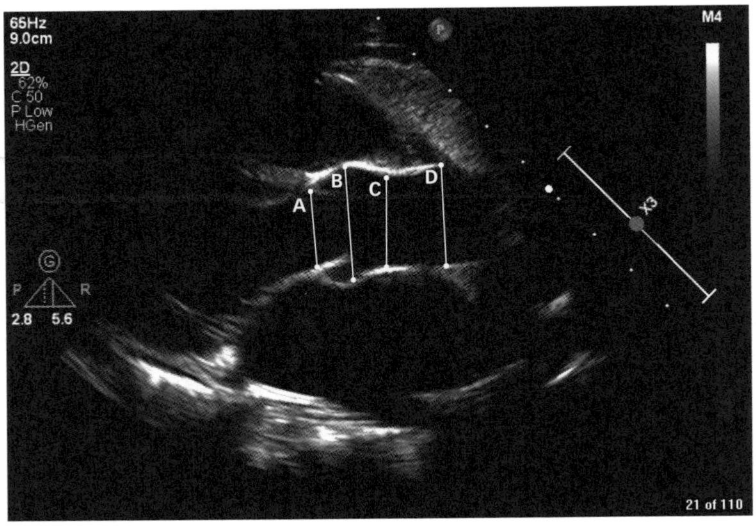

Choice B is at the level of the aortic sinuses of Valsalva, which is the most common site of dilatation by age 5 in Marfan syndrome. According to the standard guidelines for pediatric echocardiographic quantification published by the American Society of Echocardiography (ASE), the inner edge–to–inner edge technique at end systole is used to measure these values, which match measurements obtained with magnetic resonance imaging and computed tomography. This technique differs from the ASE's guidelines for adult echocardiography, which recommend a leading edge–to–leading edge technique.

- Allen HD, Shaddy RE, Penny DJ, et al: *Moss and Adams' Heart Disease in Infants, Children, and Adolescents, Including the Fetus and Young Adult*, 9th edition. Philadelphia, Wolters Kluwer, 2016, pp 800–801.
- Lai WW, Mertens LL, Cohen MS, et al (eds): *Echocardiography in Pediatric and Congenital Heart Disease: From Fetus to Adult*, 2nd edition. Chichester, UK, Wiley-Blackwell, 2016, pp 627–629.
- Lang RM, Badano LP, Mor-Avi V, et al: Recommendations for cardiac chamber quantification by echocardiography in adults: an update from the American Society of Echocardiography and the European Association of Cardiovascular Imaging. J Amer Soc Echocardiogr 28:1–39.e14, 2015.
- Lopez L, Colan SD, Frommelt PC, et al: Recommendations for quantification methods during the performance of a pediatric echocardiogram: a report from the Pediatric Measurements Writing Group of the American Society of Echocardiography Pediatric and Congenital Heart Disease Council. J Am Soc Echocardiogr 23:465–495, 2010.

Refer to video PER-Q592.

592. B. It is measured between the innominate artery and the left common carotid artery.

Video PER-Q592 shows an aortic arch. The proximal transverse arch is the aortic arch segment between the innominate (brachiocephalic) artery and the left common carotid artery. When evaluating the aortic arch by 2D echocardiography, the highest-frequency transducer available should be used; this will provide the best imaging for anatomic assessment and measurements. As with other measurements performed in pediatric echocardiography, the inner edge–to–inner edge technique should be applied.

- Lai WW, Mertens LL, Cohen MS, et al (eds): *Echocardiography in Pediatric and Congenital Heart Disease: From Fetus to Adult*, 2nd edition. Chichester, UK, Wiley-Blackwell, 2016, p 383.
- Lopez L, Colan SD, Frommelt PC, et al: Recommendations for quantification methods during the performance of a pediatric echocardiogram: a report from the Pediatric Measurements Writing Group of the American Society of Echocardiography Pediatric and Congenital Heart Disease Council. J Am Soc Echocardiogr 23:465–495, 2010.

593. A. Aortic isthmus.

Under normal circumstances the aortic isthmus is closest to the ductus arteriosus. In the case of coarctation of the aorta, it is believed that encirclement of the aortic isthmus by ductal tissue might induce development of the coarctation by ductal tissue constriction.

- Lai WW, Mertens LL, Cohen MS, et al (eds): *Echocardiography in Pediatric and Congenital Heart Disease: From Fetus to Adult*, 2nd edition. Chichester, UK, Wiley-Blackwell, 2016, pp 382–383.
- Lopez L, Colan SD, Frommelt PC, et al: Recommendations for quantification methods during the performance of a pediatric echocardiogram: a report from the Pediatric Measurements Writing Group of the American Society of Echocardiography Pediatric and Congenital Heart Disease Council. J Am Soc Echocardiogr 23:465–495, 2010.

594. C. C.

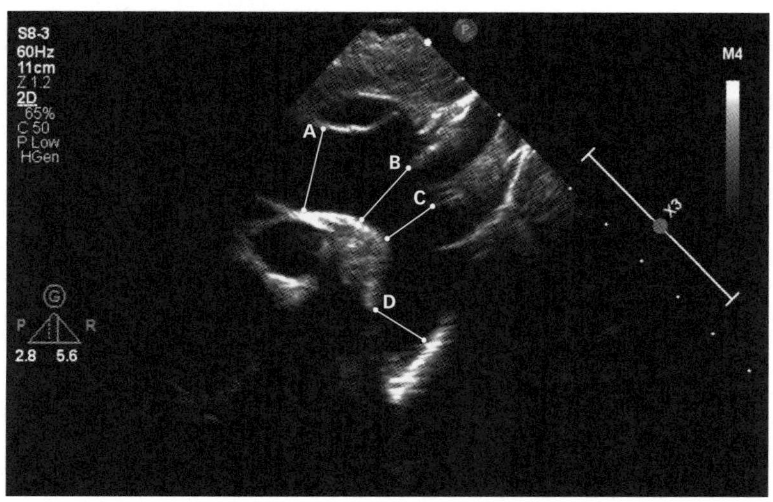

Choice C represents the distal transverse aortic arch, which is the segment between the left common carotid artery and left subclavian artery. When imaging the aortic arch, you should

use the highest-frequency transducer available to provide the best imaging possible. As with other measurements performed in pediatric echocardiography, the inner edge–to–inner edge technique should be applied.

▶ Lai WW, Mertens LL, Cohen MS, et al (eds): *Echocardiography in Pediatric and Congenital Heart Disease: From Fetus to Adult*, 2nd edition. Chichester, UK, Wiley-Blackwell, 2016, p 383.

▶ Lopez L, Colan SD, Frommelt PC, et al: Recommendations for quantification methods during the performance of a pediatric echocardiogram: a report from the Pediatric Measurements Writing Group of the American Society of Echocardiography Pediatric and Congenital Heart Disease Council. J Am Soc Echocardiogr 23:465–495, 2010.

ANSWERS

595. B. Hypoplastic distal transverse arch, elongation of the area between the left common carotid artery and left subclavian artery, and a narrowed aortic isthmus.

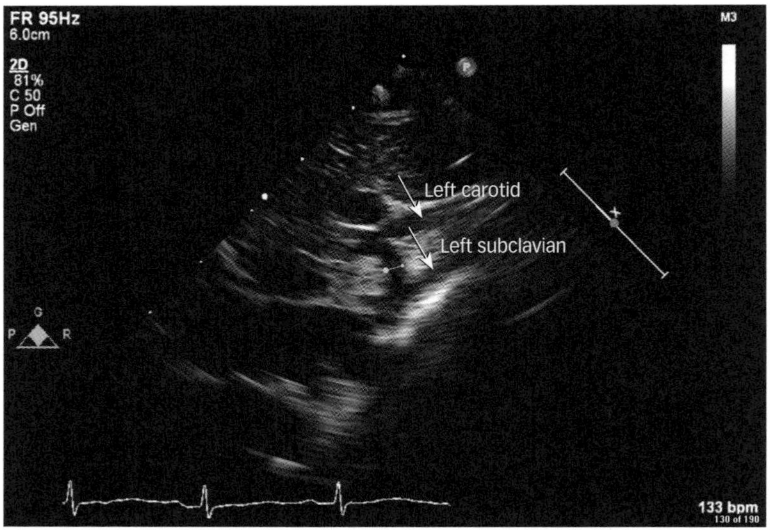

The term "tubular hypoplasia of the aortic arch" is used when the distal transverse arch is hypoplastic, the arch is elongated between the left common carotid and the left subclavian artery, and the aortic isthmus tapers down to become hypoplastic (similar to the isthmus hypoplasia seen with a more typical coarctation of the aorta).

▶ Lai WW, Mertens LL, Cohen MS, et al (eds): *Echocardiography in Pediatric and Congenital Heart Disease: From Fetus to Adult*, 2nd edition. Chichester, UK, Wiley-Blackwell, 2016, pp 382–383.

▶ Lopez L, Colan SD, Frommelt PC, et al: Recommendations for quantification methods during the performance of a pediatric echocardiogram: a report from the Pediatric Measurements Writing Group of the American Society of Echocardiography Pediatric and Congenital Heart Disease Council. J Am Soc Echocardiogr 23:465–495, 2010.

ANSWERS

596. A. Interventricular septal hypertrophy.

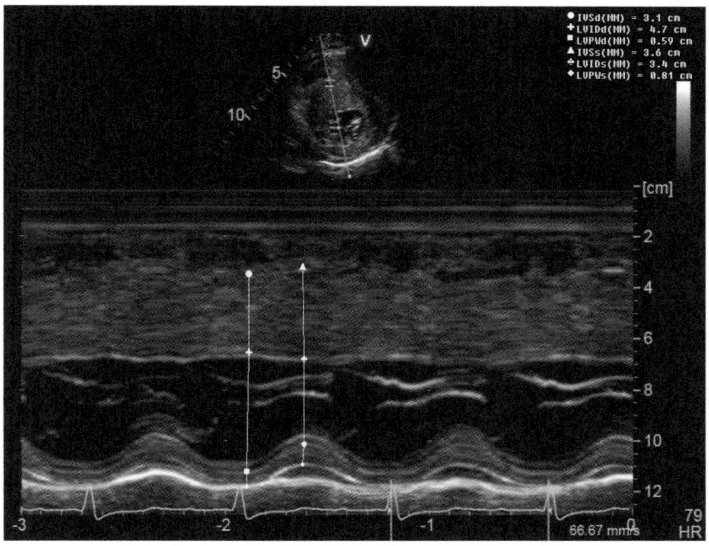

A Z-score that is less than or greater than 2 standard deviations is considered abnormal. The interventricular septum in this scenario has a Z-score of +6.0 and is considered hypertrophied. However, interventricular septal hypertrophy does not necessarily predict systolic anterior motion of the mitral valve.

▶ Lai WW, Mertens LL, Cohen MS, et al (eds): *Echocardiography in Pediatric and Congenital Heart Disease: From Fetus to Adult*, 2nd edition. Chichester, UK, Wiley-Blackwell, 2016, pp 68, 677–685.

▶ Lopez L, Colan SD, Frommelt PC, et al: Recommendations for quantification methods during the performance of a pediatric echocardiogram: a report from the Pediatric Measurements Writing Group of the American Society of Echocardiography Pediatric and Congenital Heart Disease Council. J Am Soc Echocardiogr 23:465–495, 2010.

597. B. Speed of left ventricular shortening, known as velocity of circumferential fiber shortening.

Velocity of circumferential fiber shortening (VCFc) is an estimate of the average rate of change of the left ventricular diameter per unit of time. It is relatively insensitive to preload changes but can be influenced by afterload. To correct for afterload, VCFc is evaluated in relation to afterload, which is measured by end-systolic wall stress (ESWS). The stress-velocity (ESWS-VCFc) relationship serves as a useful assessment of left ventricular myocardial contractility and is theoretically independent of loading conditions. VCFc and ESWS are used mostly as research tools, although in certain institutions they are routinely employed clinically to assess and follow left ventricular contractility in selected patient populations.

▶ Lai WW, Mertens LL, Cohen MS, et al (eds): *Echocardiography in Pediatric and Congenital Heart Disease: From Fetus to Adult*, 2nd edition. Chichester, UK, Wiley-Blackwell, 2016, p 105.

598. C. Is negative when normal.

Normal global left ventricular longitudinal strain (GLS) is –20%. Here is an example that helps with understanding the principles of GLS: If a myocardium that measures 10 mm in diastole deforms to 8 mm in systole in the apical four-chamber view, it has undergone a 20% deformation, and the GLS would be reported as –20%. A positive deformation value is considered abnormal, as myocardium should shorten toward the apex and not elongate when you are measuring GLS in the apical views.

- Levy PT, Machefsky A, Sanchez AA, et al: Reference ranges of left ventricular strain measures by two-dimensional speckle-tracking echocardiography in children: a systematic review and meta-analysis. J Am Soc Echocardiogr 29:209–225, 2016.

Refer to video PER-Q599.

599. D. Muscular VSD with shunting seen in systole.

The ventricular septal defect (VSD) seen in video PER-Q599 is a muscular VSD that is shunting left to right in systole. The typical inlet VSD has a scooped-out appearance and is usually visualized with both atrioventricular valves in view; no such defect is seen in this video clip. A perimembranous VSD is located adjacent to the septal leaflet of the tricuspid valve and just below the aortic valve, and it is generally well demonstrated from the parasternal short-axis view with the aortic valve seen en face. In this view, when the aortic valve is considered as the face of a clock, the perimembranous VSD can be visualized between the 9 and 11 o'clock positions. A subpulmonary VSD (also known as supracristal, doubly committed, or subarterial VSD) represents significant deficiency or absence of the infundibular (conal) septum, which is the portion of ventricular septum located between the aortic and pulmonary valves. Using the analogy of the clock face described above, this type of VSD can be visualized between the 12 and 2 o'clock positions in the parasternal short-axis view. In this video clip, neither a perimembranous nor a subpulmonary VSD can be seen.

- Ezon DS, Goldberg JF, Kyle WB: *Atlas of Congenital Heart Disease Nomenclature: An Illustrated Guide to the Van Praagh and Anderson Approaches to Describing Congenital Cardiac Pathology*. Houston, Ezon Educational Services/CreateSpace, 2015, pp 54–55.
- Lai WW, Mertens LL, Cohen MS, et al (eds): *Echocardiography in Pediatric and Congenital Heart Disease: From Fetus to Adult*, 2nd edition. Chichester, UK, Wiley-Blackwell, 2016, pp 215–230.

600. D. –20%.

Normal global left ventricular longitudinal strain (GLS) is –20%. A positive deformation value (such as choice A) is considered abnormal, as myocardium should shorten toward the apex and not elongate when you are measuring GLS in the apical views. Although choices B and C are negative values, they are considered abnormal values for GLS.

▸ Levy PT, Machefsky A, Sanchez AA, et al: Reference ranges of left ventricular strain measures by two-dimensional speckle-tracking echocardiography in children: a systematic review and meta-analysis. J Am Soc Echocardiogr 29:209–225, 2016.

Refer to video PER-Q601.

601. B. At ventricular systole, closest to the QRS complex.

In almost all instances (see video PER-Q601) mitral valve regurgitation occurs during ventricular systole. All of the other possible answers describe events occurring during ventricular diastole. It is important to note that having an electrocardiogram tracing is not only a laboratory standard but also crucial when defining the timing of events within the heart as demonstrated by echocardiography.

▸ Lai WW, Mertens LL, Cohen MS, et al (eds): *Echocardiography in Pediatric and Congenital Heart Disease: From Fetus to Adult*, 2nd edition. Chichester, UK, Wiley-Blackwell, 2016, p 107.

602. C. C.

See Color Plate 33 on page xxxv.

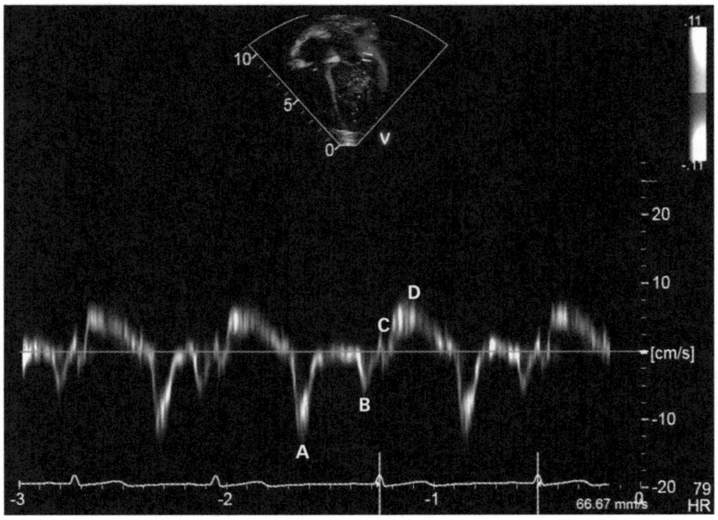

This image is a tissue Doppler image (TDI) at the level of the lateral mitral valve annulus. The letter C corresponds with isovolumic contraction time (ICT), which is the time interval between termination of the a′ wave (atrial contraction) and the initiation of the s′ wave (systolic mitral annular motion

toward the apex). During this time, there is a rapid increase in left ventricular pressure (due to myocardial contraction), but there is no change in ventricular volume until the aortic valve opens and left ventricular ejection begins. Hence, the term "isovolumic" refers to the fact that there is no change in ventricular volume during this period.

▶ Lai WW, Mertens LL, Cohen MS, et al (eds): *Echocardiography in Pediatric and Congenital Heart Disease: From Fetus to Adult*, 2nd edition. Chichester, UK, Wiley-Blackwell, 2016, pp 132–139.

603. A. R wave to R wave interval.

The myocardial performance index (MPI) is a measure of global left ventricular function. The formula for calculating the MPI (also known as the Tei index) is:

$$(ICT + IRT)/ET$$

Notice that in the formula both systolic and diastolic intervals are used to evaluate left ventricular function. It is helpful to remember the time interval definitions when calculating MPI: Isovolumic contraction time (ICT) for the left ventricle is the period in systole when the left ventricle contracts but no forward flow crosses the aortic valve. Isovolumic relaxation time (IRT) is the period after aortic valve closure and before early mitral valve opening, prior to left ventricular filling. The normal value for left ventricular MPI is 0.35 ± 0.03.

▶ Lai WW, Mertens LL, Cohen MS, et al (eds): *Echocardiography in Pediatric and Congenital Heart Disease: From Fetus to Adult*, 2nd edition. Chichester, UK, Wiley-Blackwell, 2016, pp 106–107.

PART 8

Application for CME Credit

Pediatric Echocardiography Review

Objectives of This Activity

How to Obtain CME Credit

Applicant Information

Evaluation—You Grade Us!

Answer Sheet

CME Quiz

This continuing medical educational (CME) activity is approved for 12 hours of credit by the Society of Diagnostic Medical Sonography. This credit may be applied as follows:

- Echocardiographers and sonographers may apply these Category A hours toward the CME requirements of the ARDMS, APCA, and/or CCI as well as to the CME requirements of most other organizations that may accredit your facility.
- SDMS-approved credit is not applicable toward the AMA Physician's Recognition Award but may be applicable to the CME requirements for physicians associated with accredited ultrasound facilities. Be sure to confirm requirements with the pertinent organizations.
- If you have any questions whatsoever about CME requirements that affect you, please contact the organization that governs your credential directly for current information. CME requirements can and sometimes do change.

Objectives of This Activity

Upon completion of this educational activity, you will be able to:

1. Describe and identify the echocardiographic appearances of normal and abnormal pediatric cardiac anatomy and physiology.
2. Describe how, why, and when pediatric echocardiography is used.
3. Differentiate normal from abnormal findings and explain the correlations between these findings and pertinent laboratory and imaging studies.
4. Describe how, when, why, and what types of measurements are made using pediatric echocardiography.
5. Explain the applications of pediatric echocardiography to the diagnosis and management of congenital cardiac conditions.
6. Describe the echocardiographic findings in the presence of specific pediatric diseases, conditions, complications, associated disorders, and postoperative anatomy.
7. Explain how to prepare for, perform, and explain the techniques of pediatric echocardiography.

How to Obtain CME Credit

To apply for credit, please do all of the following:

1. Read and study the mock exam questions.
2. Be sure to make photocopies of the blank forms below. Then use those photocopies to fill in your information and circle the answers. Keep the original forms in this book blank, and do not share your answers with others. That way you will always have the original set of blank forms in case you wish to make this CME activity available to others for their use.
3. Return the completed "Applicant Information" form, "Evaluation—You Grade Us!" questionnaire, and CME Answer Sheet, together with payment of the administrative processing fee of $39.50 (if you are the book's original purchaser) or $49.50 (for borrowers or purchasers of used books), by one of these methods:

Mail with enclosed paper check or credit card information to:

Davies Publishing, Inc.
CME Coordinator
32 South Raymond Avenue, Suite 4
Pasadena, California 91105-1961

Fax the appropriate pages to 626-792-5308 and pay by credit card. Include credit card information on the applicant information form OR call in your credit card after faxing.

Email to cme@daviespublishing.com and pay by credit card. Include credit card information on the applicant information form OR call in your credit card after emailing.

We grade quizzes within 24 business hours of receipt and will email your certificate to the email address you provide in your application form. Questions? Please call us at 626-792-3046 or toll-free (within the continental United States) at 877-792-0005.

Applicant Information

Pediatric Echocardiography Review

Name ______________________________ Date of birth ____________

Your degrees and credentials ______________________________

Address ______________________________

City/State/ZIP ______________________________

Telephone ______________ Email (required) ______________

ARDMS # ____________ ARRT # ____________ CCI # ____________

SDMS # ____________ Sonography Canada # ____________

Payment Information

❑ I am the original purchaser of an unused (new) copy of this book (fee is $39.50).

❑ I borrowed the book or purchased it used (fee is $49.50).

Credit card # ______________ Exp date ______ 3- or 4-digit code ____

Name and address on credit card (if different from above):

Name ______________________________

Address ______________________________

City/State/ZIP ______________________________

Signature and date certifying your completion of the activity:

____

NOTE: The original purchaser of this CME activity is entitled to submit this CME application for an administrative fee of $39.50. Please enclose a check payable to Davies Publishing, Inc., or include credit card information with your application. Others may also submit applications for CME credits by completing the activity for an administrative fee of $49.50. The CME administrative fee helps to defray the cost of processing, evaluating, and maintaining a record of your application and the credit you earn. Fees may change without notice. For the current fee, call us at 626-792-3046, email us at **cme@daviespublishing.com**, or write to us at the aforementioned address. We will be happy to help!

Evaluation—You Grade Us!

Please let us know what you think of *Pediatric Echocardiography Review*. Participating in this quality survey is a requirement for CME applicants, and it benefits future readers by ensuring that current readers are satisfied or, if not, that their comments and opinions are heard and taken into account.

1. Why did you purchase *Pediatric Echocardiography Review*? (Check your primary reason.)

   ❑ Registry review ❑ Course text

   ❑ Clinical reference ❑ CME activity

2. Have you used *Pediatric Echocardiography Review* for other reasons, too? (Check all that apply.)

   ❑ Registry review ❑ Course text

   ❑ Clinical reference ❑ CME activity

3. To what extent did *Pediatric Echocardiography Review* meet its stated objectives and your needs? (Check one.)

   ❑ Greatly ❑ Moderately

   ❑ Minimally ❑ Insignificantly

4. The content of *Pediatric Echocardiography Review* was (check one):

   ❑ Just right ❑ Too basic

   ❑ Too advanced

5. The quality of the questions, explanations, illustrations, and case examples was mainly (check one):

   ❑ Excellent ❑ Good

   ❑ Fair ❑ Poor

6. The manner in which *Pediatric Echocardiography Review* presents the material is mainly (check one):

   ❑ Excellent ❑ Good

   ❑ Fair ❑ Poor

7. If you used *Pediatric Echocardiography Review* to prepare for the registry exam, did you also use other materials or take any exam-preparation courses?

   ❑ No ❑ Yes

   If yes, please specify what materials and courses:

   ____

   ____

   ____

8. If you used *Pediatric Echocardiography Review* for a course, please list the course name, the instructor's name, the name of the school or program, and any other textbooks you may have used:

   Course/instructor/school or program:

   ____

   ____

9. What did you like best about *Pediatric Echocardiography Review*?

   ____

   ____

   ____

   ____

10. What did you like least about *Pediatric Echocardiography Review*?

   ____

   ____

   ____

   ____

11. If you used *Pediatric Echocardiography Review* to prepare for your registry exam please answer these questions:

    Which exam did you take?

    ❑ ARDMS's PE exam

    ❑ Other: ______________________________

    Did you pass?

    ❑ Yes ❑ No ❑ Haven't yet taken it

12. May we quote any of your comments in our catalogs or promotional material?

    ❑ Yes ❑ No

    ❑ Further comment:

    ____

    ____

    ____

    ____

    ____

    ____

    ____

    ____

    ____

    ____

    ____

    ____

Answer Sheet

Pediatric Echocardiography Review

Circle the correct answer below and return this sheet to Davies Publishing, Inc. Passing criterion is 70% for attempt 1 and (for those who do not pass on the first attempt) 75% for attempts 2 and 3. The applicant may not have more than 3 attempts to pass.

1. A B C D
2. A B C D
3. A B C D
4. A B C D
5. A B C D
6. A B C D
7. A B C D
8. A B C D
9. A B C D
10. A B C D
11. A B C D
12. A B C D
13. A B C D
14. A B C D
15. A B C D
16. A B C D
17. A B C D
18. A B C D
19. A B C D
20. A B C D
21. A B C D
22. A B C D
23. A B C D
24. A B C D
25. A B C D
26. A B C D
27. A B C D
28. A B C D
29. A B C D
30. A B C D
31. A B C D
32. A B C D
33. A B C D
34. A B C D
35. A B C D
36. A B C D
37. A B C D
38. A B C D
39. A B C D
40. A B C D
41. A B C D
42. A B C D
43. A B C D
44. A B C D
45. A B C D
46. A B C D
47. A B C D
48. A B C D
49. A B C D
50. A B C D
51. A B C D
52. A B C D
53. A B C D
54. A B C D
55. A B C D
56. A B C D
57. A B C D
58. A B C D
59. A B C D
60. A B C D
61. A B C D
62. A B C D
63. A B C D
64. A B C D
65. A B C D
66. A B C D
67. A B C D
68. A B C D
69. A B C D
70. A B C D
71. A B C D
72. A B C D
73. A B C D
74. A B C D
75. A B C D
76. A B C D
77. A B C D
78. A B C D
79. A B C D
80. A B C D
81. A B C D
82. A B C D
83. A B C D
84. A B C D
85. A B C D
86. A B C D
87. A B C D
88. A B C D
89. A B C D
90. A B C D
91. A B C D
92. A B C D
93. A B C D
94. A B C D
95. A B C D
96. A B C D
97. A B C D
98. A B C D
99. A B C D
100. A B C D
101. A B C D
102. A B C D
103. A B C D
104. A B C D
105. A B C D
106. A B C D
107. A B C D
108. A B C D
109. A B C D
110. A B C D
111. A B C D
112. A B C D
113. A B C D
114. A B C D
115. A B C D
116. A B C D
117. A B C D
118. A B C D
119. A B C D
120. A B C D

CME Quiz

Pediatric Echocardiography Review

Please answer the following questions after you have completed the CME activity. There is one best answer for each question. Circle it on the answer sheet. The passing criterion is 70% for attempt 1 and (for those who do not pass on the first attempt) 75% for attempts 2 and 3. The applicant may not have more than 3 attempts to pass.

1. Measuring the mean gradient across the atrial septum is important in acute clinical management of:

   A. Atrial septal defect
   B. Congenitally corrected transposition of the great arteries (ccTGA)
   C. Transposition of the great arteries (d-TGA) with intact ventricular septum
   D. Double-inlet left ventricle

2. In which of the following scan planes would the view of the left atrium be most obscured?

   A. Parasternal long-axis view in the presence of mechanical aortic and mitral valves, using transthoracic echocardiography
   B. Mid-esophageal four-chamber view with a prosthetic mitral valve closed, using transesophageal echocardiography
   C. Mid-esophageal two-chamber view with a prosthetic mitral valve open, using transesophageal echocardiography
   D. Parasternal long-axis view with a closed bioprosthetic mitral valve in the presence of a normal aortic valve, using transthoracic echocardiography

3. Sinus venosus atrial septal defect is best visualized in which view?

   A. Apical four-chamber view
   B. Parasternal short-axis view
   C. Subxiphoid sagittal (short-axis) view
   D. Subxiphoid coronal (long-axis) view

4. You should measure the right ventricular free wall thickness:

   A. Just below the pulmonary valve
   B. With heavy trabeculations included
   C. Just past the QRS complex on the electrocardiogram tracing
   D. At end diastole

5. Echocardiographic findings in a newborn baby include dextrocardia, double-outlet right ventricle (DORV), unbalanced complete atrioventricular canal (right dominant, with a small left ventricular chamber), common atrium, unroofed coronary sinus, infradiaphragmatic total anomalous pulmonary venous connection (TAPVC), and pulmonary atresia. The liver is noted in midline. What is the most likely diagnosis?

   A. Asplenia syndrome (right atrial isomerism)
   B. Loeys-Dietz syndrome
   C. Complete atrioventricular block
   D. Polysplenia syndrome (left atrial isomerism)

6. Your patient has Marfan syndrome with an ascending aortic Z-score of +3.2. What does this finding most likely signify?

   A. Normal value
   B. Severely dilated ascending aorta
   C. Nothing of significance; Z-scores are not considered useful in echocardiography.
   D. Mildly dilated ascending aorta

7. Your patient is a newborn who has undergone a transannular patch repair of tetralogy of Fallot without complication. What course is expected for this patient?

   A. No anticipated future cardiac interventions
   B. Anticipated pulmonary valve replacement before 18 years of age
   C. Possible secondary aortic regurgitation due to a size discrepancy when the aorta and pulmonary artery were moved during surgery
   D. Potential development of a vascular ring during this patient's adolescence

8. Last year, your patient with tetralogy of Fallot (TOF) had a pulmonary artery stent placed to correct stenosis in the left pulmonary artery (LPA). On today's follow-up exam the LPA stent is not well seen on echocardiography, and no flow can be demonstrated in the LPA. Also, the right pulmonary artery (RPA) appears larger, with increased flow noted at a peak velocity of 2 m/sec. What are you looking for on the echocardiogram?

   A. Cardiac dysfunction
   B. Residual ventricular septal defect
   C. LPA stent obstruction
   D. RPA stenosis

9. What forms the left aortic arch in the developing embryo?

   A. The right fourth aortic arch and left dorsal aorta
   B. Persistence of the fifth aortic arch and seventh intersegmental artery
   C. Involution of the left dorsal aorta
   D. The left fourth aortic arch and left dorsal aorta

10. In calculating left ventricular mass using M-mode measurements, which of the following parameters would NOT be applied?

    A. Heart rate
    B. Left ventricular end-diastolic dimension
    C. Posterior left ventricular wall thickness in end diastole
    D. Interventricular septum wall thickness in end diastole

11. Secondary hypertrophic cardiomyopathy is LEAST likely to be associated with:

    A. Mitochondrial disease
    B. Noonan syndrome
    C. Duchenne muscular dystrophy
    D. LEOPARD syndrome

12. Transposition of the great arteries (d-TGA) most commonly coexists with:

    A. Ventricular septal defect
    B. Coarctation of the aorta
    C. Vascular ring
    D. Total anomalous pulmonary venous connection

13. To calculate left ventricular ejection fraction using the area-length method, which view should you use to obtain the left ventricular area?

    A. Parasternal long-axis
    B. Subcostal short-axis
    C. Apical two-chamber
    D. Subcostal long-axis

14. A rocking prosthetic mitral valve (PMV):

    A. Is indicative of valve dehiscence
    B. Is normal in the setting of size mismatch between the patient and the PMV
    C. Is seen with washing regurgitation jets in normally operating PMVs
    D. Is often seen in pediatric prosthetic valve placement

15. Myocardial ischemia in anomalous left coronary artery from the pulmonary artery is caused by:

    A. Deoxygenated blood from the pulmonary artery
    B. High pulmonary vascular resistance
    C. Coronary artery steal
    D. Severe mitral regurgitation

16. Which of the following parameters is most useful for evaluating early rejection of a transplanted heart?

    A. Pulsed-wave tissue Doppler evaluation of the lateral mitral annulus
    B. Measurement of the left ventricular ejection fraction
    C. Measurement of the left ventricular shortening fraction
    D. Measurement of the tricuspid valve regurgitant velocity

17. An infant was diagnosed with physiologically "corrected" transposition of the great arteries without pulmonary outflow tract obstruction. Echocardiography reveals mild tricuspid valve regurgitation with a velocity of 4.0 m/sec and mild mitral valve regurgitation with a velocity of 3.0 m/sec. What is the pulmonary artery systolic pressure?

    A. 16 mmHg + right atrial pressure
    B. 18 mmHg + right atrial pressure
    C. 36 mmHg + right atrial pressure
    D. 64 mmHg + right atrial pressure

18. With echocardiography, left atrial volume is best determined by which of the following methods?

    A. Simpson's method
    B. M-mode
    C. Inclusion of the left atrial appendage
    D. Inclusion of the proximal pulmonary veins

19. What maneuver from the apical four-chamber view was performed to obtain the following image?

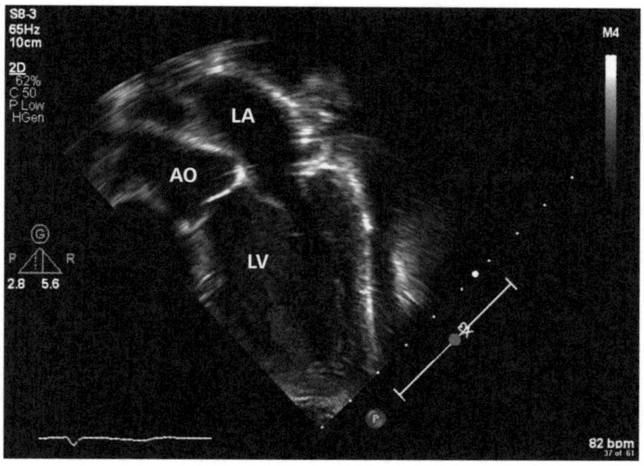

    A. Posterior angulation of the transducer
    B. Rotation of the transducer clockwise with the notch/dot at 4 o'clock
    C. Anterior angulation of the transducer
    D. Rotation of the transducer counterclockwise with the notch/dot at 12–1 o'clock

20. With the subcostal long-axis sweep, more superior angulation of the transducer is most useful to evaluate which of the following?

    A. Individual pulmonary veins
    B. Anatomy of the ductus arteriosus
    C. Right and left ventricular outflow tracts
    D. Semilunar valve morphology

21. Which duct-dependent lesion listed below is most likely to be an echocardiographic finding in a female neonatal patient with Turner syndrome?

    A. Tetralogy of Fallot
    B. Interrupted aortic arch with a posterior malalignment ventricular septal defect
    C. Pulmonary atresia with intact ventricular septum
    D. Hypoplastic left heart syndrome

22. Agitated saline during echocardiography is helpful for diagnosing all EXCEPT:

    A. An unroofed coronary sinus
    B. Aortopulmonary collaterals
    C. Atrial septal defects
    D. Pulmonary arteriovenous fistulae

23. The most common location for the terminal end of a coronary-cameral fistula is the:

    A. Right ventricle
    B. Left ventricle
    C. Left atrium
    D. Coronary sinus

24. Underestimation of the severity of mitral valve stenosis is most likely in the presence of which coexisting cardiac defect?

    A. Mitral valve regurgitation
    B. Ventricular septal defect
    C. Patent ductus arteriosus
    D. Atrial septal defect

25. What type of artifact is associated with the atrial septum seen in this image?

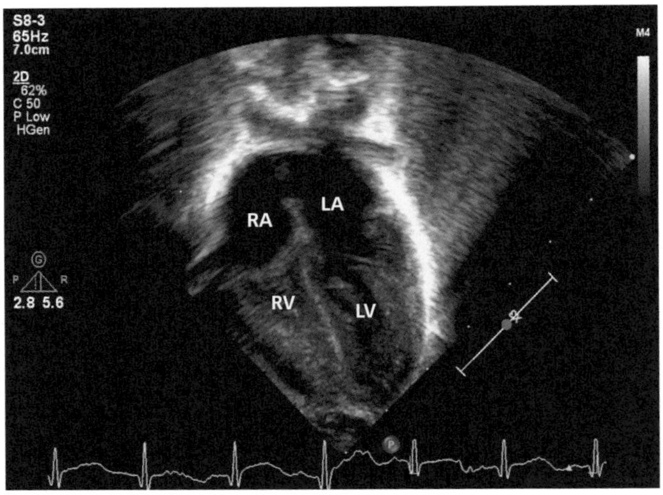

    A. Side lobe artifact
    B. Slice-thickness artifact
    C. Image dropout artifact
    D. There is no artifact; there is a secundum atrial septal defect.

26. Identify the valve of the coronary sinus:
    A. Thebesian valve
    B. Eustachian valve
    C. Crista terminalis
    D. Chiari network

27. Your patient has a patent ductus arteriosus (PDA) device closure. The patient has differential blood pressures between the upper and lower extremities, based on noninvasive assessment. What do you think this patient might have?
    A. Residual PDA
    B. Poor left ventricular function
    C. It is a normal finding.
    D. Coarctation

28. Which of the following surgically correctable lesions is the most likely to result in a clinical picture of dilated cardiomyopathy?
    A. Bacterial myocarditis
    B. Juvenile rheumatoid arthritis
    C. Right coronary artery to pulmonary artery fistula
    D. Anomalous left coronary artery from the pulmonary artery

29. What is the most common complication after the atrial switch operation (Mustard or Senning) for transposition of the great arteries (d-TGA)?
    A. Superior vena cava pathway obstruction
    B. Supravalvular neopulmonary stenosis
    C. Inferior vena cava pathway obstruction
    D. Subaortic obstruction

30. Your patient is a newborn with coarctation of the aorta. Which transducer would you use to obtain the best 2D image of the aortic arch?
    A. 3D matrix
    B. 5 MHz
    C. 8 MHz
    D. 12 MHz

31. Which of the following syndromes is associated with the findings in this image?

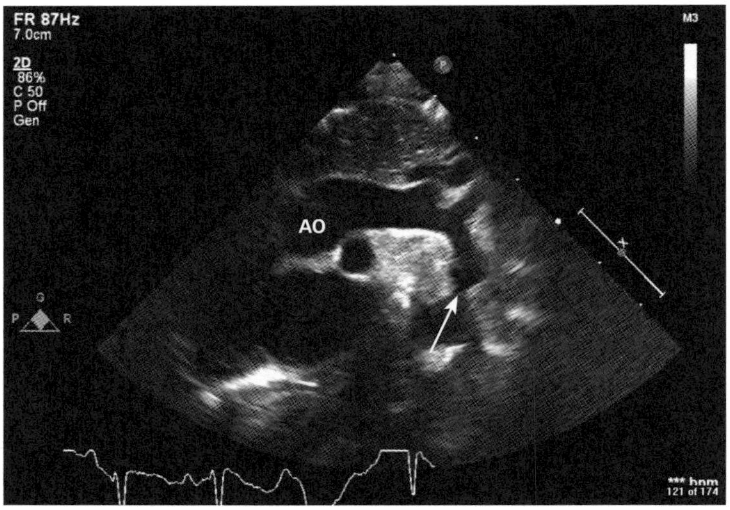

A. Down syndrome
B. Turner syndrome
C. Patau syndrome
D. Holt-Oram syndrome

32. Which type of cardiac defect is most likely to be found with DiGeorge syndrome?

A. Supramitral valve ring
B. Pulmonary venous abnormality
C. Levoatrial cardinal vein
D. Tetralogy of Fallot

33. Which of the following echocardiographic parameters can be used to evaluate acute, moderate to severe aortic valve regurgitation?

A. Reversal of flow in the descending aorta
B. Left ventricle tissue Doppler
C. Left ventricle dimension
D. Left ventricular ejection fraction

34. Spectral Doppler reference values for diastolic dysfunction differ in the pediatric population as compared with the adult population. What defines the difference?

A. They are the same for both pediatric and adult patients.
B. They vary by age.
C. They differ only for the neonatal population.
D. They do not exist for the neonatal population.

35. Which anatomic component of the heart is most likely to require surgical reintervention to correct post-procedure complications following the Ross procedure?

A. Aortic arch
B. Coronary arteries
C. Neoaortic valve (autograft)
D. Right ventricle-to-pulmonary artery conduit

36. A 6-month-old infant who has had pulmonary artery (PA) banding to address multiple large muscular ventricular septal defects (VSDs) now presents with worsening cyanosis. The echocardiogram reveals the PA band in good position between the pulmonary valve and branch pulmonary arteries, with an increased peak systolic Doppler gradient across the PA band of 100 mmHg compared to 60 mmHg at the prior visit. What do you suspect is the primary problem?

A. Pulmonary hypertension
B. Pulmonary valve insufficiency
C. Slipped PA band causing branch pulmonary artery stenosis
D. PA band that is too tight

37. Which atrioventricular (AV) valve is the arrow in this image pointing to?

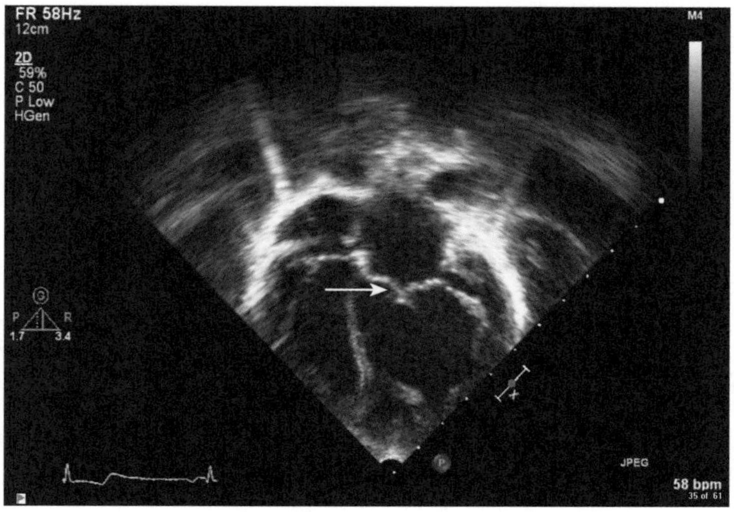

A. Tricuspid valve
B. Pulmonary valve
C. Aortic valve
D. Mitral valve

38. Which of the following correctly describes a type A interrupted left aortic arch?

    A. Interruption between the right and left common carotid arteries
    B. Interruption between the left common carotid and left subclavian arteries
    C. Often associated with aberrant origin of the right subclavian artery
    D. Interruption after the left subclavian artery

39. Which condition has the potential for biventricular circulation without the need for Fontan palliation?

    A. Hypoplastic left heart syndrome with mitral atresia
    B. Pulmonary atresia with intact ventricular septum and mild tricuspid valve/right ventricular hypoplasia
    C. Tricuspid atresia, nonrestrictive ventricular septal defect, and normally related great arteries
    D. Double-outlet right ventricle (DORV) with mitral atresia

40. Which of the following will help you identify the pulmonary artery in a neonate?

    A. Presence of a carina
    B. Trileaflet semilunar valve
    C. Patent ductus arteriosus (PDA)
    D. Bifurcation of the great artery

41. The patent ductus arteriosus (PDA) closes after birth due to an increase in:

    A. Pulmonary venous return to the left atrium
    B. Arterial oxygen
    C. Prostaglandin E1 (PGE1)
    D. Pulmonary vascular resistance

42. Sudden cardiac death (SCD) in children and young adults is most commonly caused by:

    A. Ventricular septal defect
    B. Hypertrophic cardiomyopathy
    C. Bicuspid aortic valve
    D. Pericardial effusion

43. While performing presurgical echocardiography on a patient who was diagnosed with moderate pulmonary stenosis, you find that the peak pulmonary valve gradient is 15 mmHg. The pulmonary valve appears dysplastic with a pulmonary annulus Z-score of −3.3. Which factor below best explains the low peak pulmonary gradient?

    A. Depressed right ventricular systolic function
    B. Right ventricular hypertrophy
    C. Right ventricular dilatation
    D. Mitral valve regurgitation

44. In the equations below, RVEDA = right ventricular end-diastolic area and RVESA = right ventricular end-systolic area. Which equation is used to calculate right ventricular fractional area change (RVFAC)?

    A. RVFAC (%) = [(RVEDA/RVESA) + RVEDA] × 100
    B. RVFAC (%) = [(RVEDA + RVESA)/RVEDA] × 100
    C. RVFAC (%) = [(RVEDA − RVESA)/RVEDA] × 100
    D. RVFAC (%) = [(RVEDA + RVESA) × RVEDA] × 100

45. When would you see an E/A ratio of less than 1?

    A. With restrictive cardiomyopathy
    B. In an athlete
    C. With abnormal relaxation and normal left atrial pressure
    D. In a young adult

46. This image displays the spectral recording of a pulmonary vein Doppler tracing. What is the arrow pointing to?

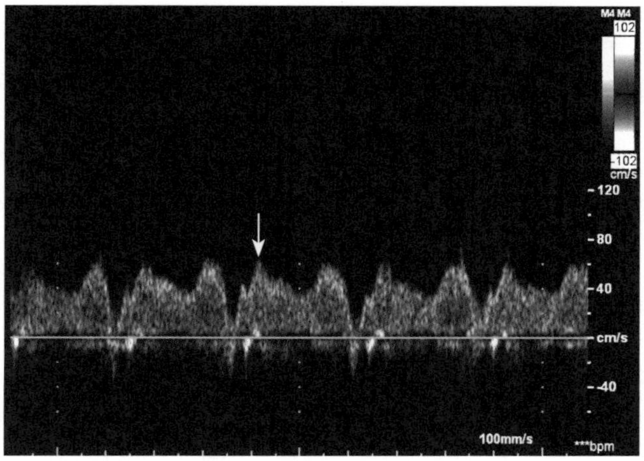

A. A wave
B. D wave
C. E wave
D. S wave

47. Which dimension of the tricuspid valve is being measured in this image?

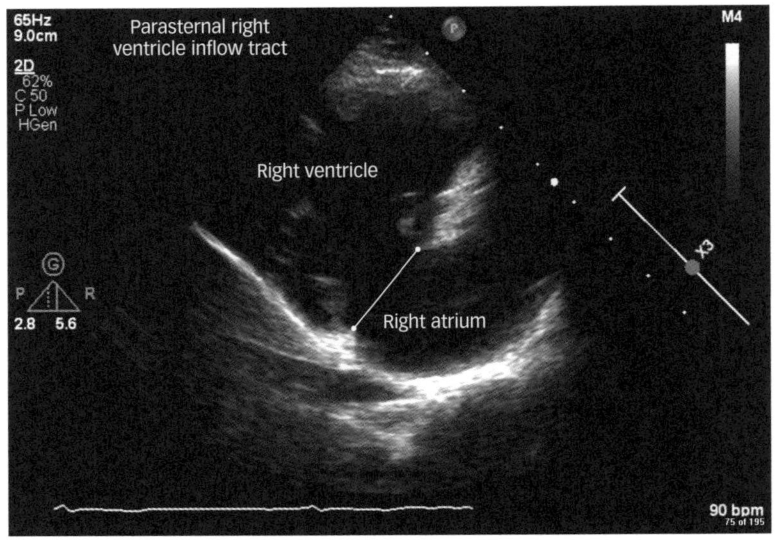

A. Septal-lateral diameter
B. Anterior-septal diameter
C. Anterior-posterior diameter
D. Posterior-septal diameter

48. Your 5-year-old patient has thickened, rolled leaflets and short chordae tendineae. Which measurement will you perform to evaluate for mitral valve stenosis?

A. Mean mitral valve gradient with continuous-wave Doppler
B. Mean mitral valve gradient with pulsed-wave Doppler
C. Pressure half-time (PHT) to determine mitral valve area
D. Mitral valve area using 2D planimetry in the parasternal short-axis plane

49. A left-sided superior vena cava (SVC) usually drains to the:

A. Left atrium
B. Coronary sinus
C. Coronary artery
D. Left pulmonary vein

50. In a patient who has an atrial septal defect with left-to-right shunting, which Qp/Qs ratio is most likely?

A. 1:1
B. 1:1.3
C. 0.7:1
D. 1.5:1

51. What statement is most likely to be true of a vertical vein coursing between the left pulmonary artery and left mainstem bronchus in total anomalous pulmonary venous connection?

A. The vein is obstructed.
B. The vein is not obstructed.
C. The vertical vein is not clinically significant.
D. Vertical veins do not course between the left pulmonary artery and left mainstem bronchus.

52. What is indicated by an increase in duration of the pulmonary vein Ar wave (atrial reversal with atrial contraction) as compared to the duration of the mitral valve inflow A wave (late left ventricular filling)?

A. Decreased left ventricular filling pressure
B. Normal left ventricular filling pressure
C. Normal left atrial pressure
D. Increased left ventricular filling pressure

53. An infant with hypoplastic left heart syndrome was palliated with a Norwood procedure with a modified Blalock-Taussig (BT) shunt. Initial postoperative oxygen saturation was 75%, and echocardiography was performed while the patient was on inotropic support and mechanical ventilation was demonstrating a peak velocity across the BT shunt of 2.3 m/sec. Two weeks later, following clinical improvement of the patient that included extubation and cessation of inotropic support, pulse oximetry demonstrates an oxygen saturation of 85% and a routine echocardiogram demonstrates a modified BT shunt velocity of 3.5 m/sec. What is the most likely cause of this difference?

A. Aortopulmonary collateral flow
B. Coarctation of the distal Norwood anastomosis
C. Reduction in pulmonary vascular resistance
D. BT shunt obstruction

54. With rupture of a sinus of Valsalva aneurysm, which heart chamber most commonly receives the left-to-right shunt through the aneurysm?

A. Right ventricle
B. Left ventricle
C. Right atrium
D. Left atrium

55. You have calculated the aortic valve area in your young adult patient to be 0.9 cm^2. The condition of this patient's aortic valve is best described as:

A. Mildly stenotic
B. Severely stenotic
C. Moderately stenotic
D. Normal

56. To detect and evaluate an anterior muscular ventricular septal defect by color Doppler, which echocardiographic view is best?

A. Suprasternal coronal view
B. Apical four-chamber view
C. Subcostal coronal view
D. Parasternal short-axis view

57. Which of the following characteristics best establishes left atrial morphology?

A. Finger-like appendage
B. Site of pulmonary venous connection
C. Crista terminalis
D. Septum secundum

58. Which statement about mirror-image artifacts is true?

A. Incorrect time gain compensation produces mirror-image artifacts.
B. The artifact appears deeper than the real structure.
C. A mechanical mitral valve can cause a mirror-image artifact.
D. The real structure appears deeper than the artifact.

59. All of the following conditions will affect accurate assessment of aortic valve stenosis EXCEPT:

    A. Mild pulmonary valve stenosis
    B. A large patent ductus arteriosus
    C. A dilated left ventricle with a shortening fraction of 20% and an ejection fraction of 40%
    D. Anemia

60. A cleft in the anterior leaflet of the mitral valve is best demonstrated by which of the following echocardiographic views of the left ventricle?

    A. Subcostal long-axis view
    B. Parasternal short-axis view
    C. Apical four-chamber view
    D. Parasternal long-axis view

61. In tetralogy of Fallot with an absent pulmonary valve, which of the following echocardiographic features will NOT be present?

    A. Aneurysmal pulmonary arteries
    B. Overriding aorta
    C. Mild right ventricular outflow tract obstruction
    D. Large patent ductus arteriosus

62. The azygos vein draining into the superior vena cava is best demonstrated by the:

    A. Suprasternal coronal view
    B. Subcostal sagittal view
    C. Subcostal coronal view
    D. Suprasternal sagittal view

63. A vascular ring is produced by which anatomic arrangement of the aortic arch?

    A. Right aortic arch with mirror-image branching
    B. Left aortic arch with an aberrant right subclavian artery
    C. Right aortic arch with a retroesophageal left subclavian artery and a left ductal ligament
    D. Left aortic arch with normal branching and a left ductal ligament

64. A right-sided morphologic right atrium and left-sided morphologic left atrium are known as:

    A. Situs solitus
    B. Asplenia
    C. Polysplenia
    D. Situs inversus

65. A 3-year-old boy presents with a history of aortic stenosis and coarctation of the aorta status post coarctation repair during infancy. The velocity across the isthmus of the aorta is 4 m/sec. What is the best estimation of the re-coarctation peak gradient?

    A. 16 mmHg
    B. 64 mmHg
    C. 64 mmHg plus aortic valve velocity
    D. More information is needed to make this calculation.

66. *Preload* is best defined as:

    A. The load at the end of diastole and before contraction
    B. The pressure at the beginning of systole
    C. The time elapsed during ventricular contraction
    D. The load at the end of systole

67. On echocardiography, a larger than usual amount of blood flow returning from the superior vena cava to the right atrium characterizes which of the following conditions?

    A. Large atrial septal defect
    B. Tetralogy of Fallot
    C. Truncus arteriosus
    D. Supracardiac total anomalous pulmonary venous connection

68. Which is the higher-pressure chamber in double-chambered right ventricle?

    A. Infundibulum
    B. Right ventricular sinus
    C. Conus arteriosus
    D. Main pulmonary artery

69. What echocardiographic finding would you look for in a young patient diagnosed with rheumatic fever?

    A. Clot
    B. Mitral valve regurgitation
    C. Pulmonary valve stenosis
    D. Vegetation

70. You should obtain all of the following measurements in patients with a history of surgically repaired tetralogy of Fallot EXCEPT:

    A. Velocity across the pulmonary valve using pulsed-wave Doppler
    B. Velocity across the pulmonary valve using continuous-wave Doppler
    C. Left upper pulmonary vein diameter
    D. Left pulmonary artery diameter

71. The most common coronary artery abnormality associated with supravalvular aortic stenosis is:

    A. Anomalous left coronary artery from the pulmonary artery
    B. Anomalous right coronary artery from the pulmonary artery
    C. Coronary ostial stenosis
    D. Coronary-cameral fistula

72. Straddling mitral valve (SMV):

    A. Exists in the absence of a ventricular septal defect
    B. Consists of abnormal mitral valve chordae attaching to both the right and left ventricles
    C. Is defined as straddling chordae attaching to the aortic valve
    D. Is the same as an overriding mitral valve

73. After Rastelli repair, percutaneous intervention with or without stent placement or repeat heart surgery may be required in the presence of certain complications. Which of the following complications most commonly requires such postoperative intervention?

    A. Right ventricle–to–pulmonary artery conduit stenosis
    B. Right ventricle–to–pulmonary artery conduit insufficiency

C. Atrioventricular valve regurgitation
D. Decreased left ventricular systolic function

74. A 5 MHz curvilinear array transducer is best suited for which of these tasks?

A. Vascular imaging
B. Neonatal imaging
C. Obstetric/fetal imaging
D. Imaging of an adult with a limited transthoracic window

75. Which of these findings suggests pulmonary hypertension?

A. Mitral valve vibration in diastole
B. Pulmonary valve motion with an absent A-dip on M-mode
C. Aortic valve reopening in late systole
D. Mitral valve systolic anterior motion

76. You are performing a stat bedside echocardiogram in the intensive care unit on a 10-year-old patient who has undergone aortic valve repair secondary to aortic stenosis. The pulsed-wave Doppler velocity across the aortic valve is 1.3 m/sec. There is trivial aortic insufficiency. The fractional shortening is 10%. The cardiologist asks you for your assessment of the echocardiogram. What do you tell her?

A. There may be significant residual aortic stenosis in the setting of poor cardiac output.
B. There is subaortic stenosis.
C. There is poor left ventricular systolic function with no aortic stenosis.
D. There is depressed left ventricular systolic function and mild aortic stenosis based on the velocity obtained.

77. In cor triatriatum, which structure has failed to be fully incorporated into the left atrium?

A. Left cardinal vein
B. Azygos vein
C. Common pulmonary vein
D. Crista terminalis

78. In this image the arrow is pointing to which anatomic structure?

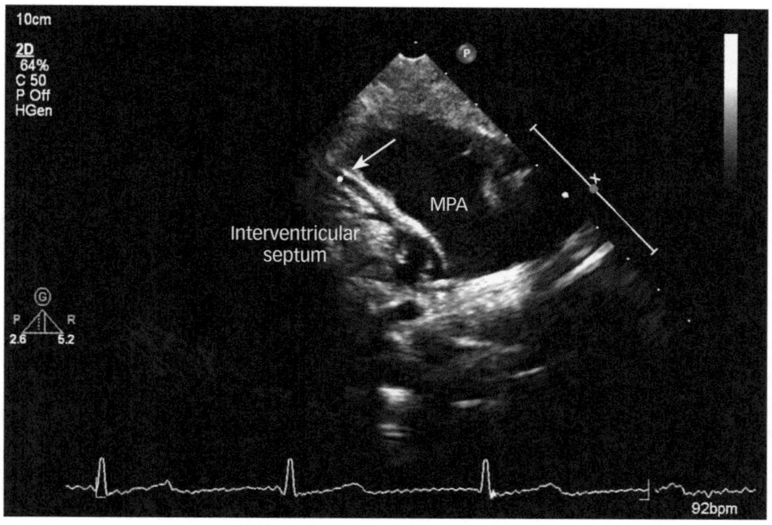

A. Left main coronary artery (LMCA)
B. Circumflex coronary artery (Cx)
C. Left main coronary artery fistula
D. Left anterior descending coronary artery (LAD)

79. What is the appropriate point in the cardiac cycle to measure left atrial volume?

A. At end systole before mitral valve opening
B. At the onset of the P wave on the electrocardiogram (ECG)
C. At end diastole during late ventricular filling with the mitral valve open
D. At the onset of the QRS complex on the ECG

80. The ductus arteriosus usually closes:

A. 36–48 hours after birth
B. 24 hours after birth
C. 48–72 hours after birth
D. 72–96 hours after birth

81. A patient with a single ventricle has undergone a Norwood procedure with a modified Blalock-Taussig shunt. Spectral Doppler is not reliable for postoperative assessment of the descending aorta because:

A. There is diastolic runoff through the shunt
B. There is diastolic runoff in the Norwood anastomosis
C. Cyanotic children develop aortopulmonary collaterals
D. Patch material is used for the aortic arch repair

82. An arterial switch operation is needed to correct:

    A. Tricuspid atresia
    B. Transposition of the great arteries (d-TGA)
    C. Ebstein anomaly
    D. Double aortic arch

83. Maternal diabetes is most strongly associated with which of the following congenital cardiac malformations?

    A. Sinus venosus atrial septal defects
    B. Total anomalous pulmonary venous connection
    C. Tetralogy of Fallot
    D. Aortopulmonary window

84. Why is it important to obtain an echocardiogram of a prosthetic valve immediately after implantation?

    A. Gradients recorded soon after implantation are the highest that will be recorded during the lifetime of the valve and can be used as a baseline.
    B. Early post-implantation echocardiography can exclude perivalvular leaks; a perivalvular leak that manifests later in the postoperative period would then be considered a normal finding.
    C. The first echocardiographic exam will document bioprosthetic valve clicks with spectral Doppler.
    D. Early post-implantation echocardiography provides baselines for many aspects of valve function, including (and not limited to) gradients, regurgitation, and leaflet motion.

85. What proximal aortic arch diameter is considered hypoplastic if the ascending aortic diameter is 12 mm?

    A. 7 mm
    B. 8 mm
    C. 9 mm
    D. 10 mm

86. The third stage of hypoplastic left heart palliation is:

    A. Redirection of inferior vena cava blood directly to the pulmonary arteries
    B. Complete bilateral superior vena cava connection to the pulmonary arteries

C. Reconstruction of the aortic arch
D. Reconstruction of the atrial septum

87. Echocardiography demonstrates a complete atrioventricular canal defect (AVCD) with the anterior-superior bridging leaflet partially divided and inserting into a papillary muscle in the right ventricle. This type of AVCD is known as:

A. Rastelli A
B. Rastelli B
C. Rastelli C
D. Rastelli D

88. What value, expressed as a percentage, is calculated by this formula:

$$(LVEDV - LVESV)/LVEDV \times 100$$

where LVEDV = left ventricular end-diastolic volume and LVESV = left ventricular end-systolic volume?

A. Left ventricular mass
B. Fractional shortening using M-mode
C. Fractional shortening using 2D technique
D. Ejection fraction by biplane Simpson's method

89. You are performing echocardiography on a boy who sustained blunt trauma to the chest during a football game. Which part of the heart are you especially concerned with?

A. Left ventricle
B. Left atrium
C. Right ventricle
D. Right atrium

90. Assuming that left ventricular contractility is normal, what will happen to the shortening fraction when left ventricular volume acutely increases?

A. SF will increase.
B. SF will stay the same.
C. SF will decrease.
D. More information is needed.

91. How does the Starnes procedure address Ebstein anomaly?

    A. Replaces the tricuspid valve using a specific type of suturing technique.
    B. Closes the tricuspid valve with a fenestrated patch, thereby excluding the right ventricle.
    C. Moves the tricuspid valve annulus to the normal position.
    D. Sutures the septal and posterior leaflets together to create a competent valve.

92. Spectral Doppler shows a peak velocity of 4 m/sec across a perimembranous ventricular septal defect (VSD). What is the peak gradient through the defect?

    A. 8 mmHg
    B. 16 mmHg
    C. 32 mmHg
    D. 64 mmHg

93. In a patient with an interrupted inferior vena cava the most likely finding is:

    A. Dilated coronary sinus
    B. Dilated superior vena cava
    C. Dilated hepatic veins
    D. Dilated innominate vein

94. Which type of ventricular septal defect (VSD) is associated with a mitral valve cleft?

    A. Perimembranous VSD
    B. Outlet VSD
    C. Supracristal VSD
    D. Atrioventricular canal type VSD

95. What is the most important factor in determining whether a pericardial effusion will cause tamponade physiology?

    A. The location of the effusion
    B. The volume of the effusion
    C. The rapidity of the effusion's development
    D. The duration of the effusion

96. Your patient is a 2-year-old boy with a 10-day history of high fever and symptoms including cracked lips and a red, swollen tongue. Based on the findings in this image and the boy's history and symptoms, you suspect:

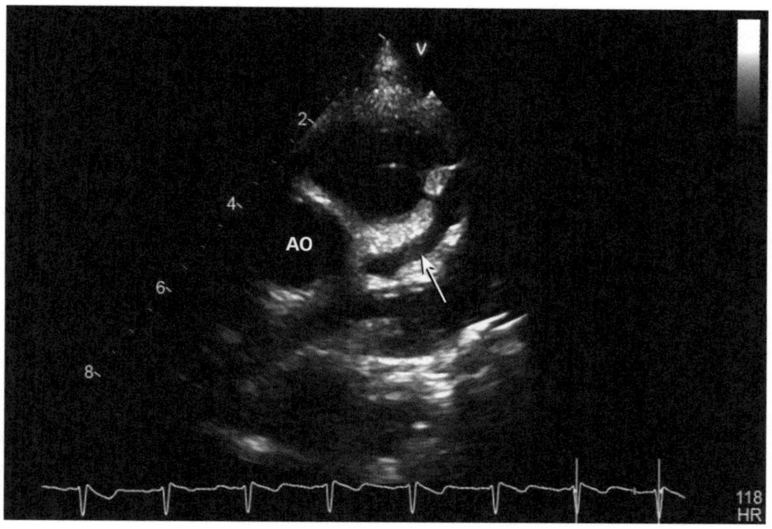

A. Viral syndrome with fever
B. Kawasaki disease
C. Endocarditis
D. Rheumatic fever

97. What is LEAST likely to be associated with tricuspid valve stenosis?

A. Hepatomegaly
B. Obligatory left-to-right atrial shunting
C. Right atrial hypertrophy
D. Right ventricular outflow tract obstruction

98. What atrial-level shunting pattern would you most likely see in a neonate with tricuspid atresia with transposition of the great arteries?

A. No atrial-level shunting by color flow Doppler
B. A morphologic right atrial to morphologic left atrial shunt
C. A morphologic left atrial to morphologic right atrial shunt
D. Bidirectional atrial-level shunting

99. A diagnosis of restrictive cardiomyopathy would be supported by which echo finding?

    A. Dilated right and left atria
    B. Pericardial effusion
    C. Dilated left ventricle
    D. Respiratory variations in atrioventricular valve inflow

100. To assess future morbidity in a child who has undergone the arterial switch operation to correct d-TGA, which of the following coronary artery patterns would suggest the highest risk of complications and mortality?

    A. Inverted pattern
    B. Single right coronary artery
    C. Intramural left coronary artery
    D. Circumflex from the right coronary artery

101. Azygos continuation of the inferior vena cava (IVC) occurs when there is:

    A. Interruption of the hepatic portion of the IVC
    B. Interruption of the levoatrial cardinal vein
    C. Interruption of the right anterior cardinal vein
    D. Interruption of the left vitelline vein

102. For which of the following congenital heart defects would you be most likely to choose a subcostal view?

    A. Supracardiac total anomalous pulmonary venous connection (TAPVC)
    B. Coarctation of the aorta
    C. Infradiaphragmatic TAPVC
    D. Double aortic arch

103. The segmental approach to congenital heart disease describes the following three segments:

    A. Ventricles, atrioventricular junction, and great arteries
    B. Ventricles, ventriculoarterial connection, and great arteries
    C. Atria, ventricles, and great arteries
    D. Atria, atrioventricular canal, and ventricles

104. You are examining a postoperative coarctation patient with a re-coarctation. Using Doppler to interrogate the descending aorta, which waveform do you expect to see?

A. Early-peaking Doppler or reverse dagger
B. Double envelope Doppler waveform
C. Late-peaking dagger-shaped Doppler waveform
D. Rounded Doppler envelope

105. Your 5-year-old patient has mitral stenosis due to a parachute mitral valve and no other form of congenital heart disease is noted. On the echocardiogram the mitral valve mean pressure gradient was recorded as 8 mmHg. What do these findings suggest?

A. Normal
B. Mild
C. Moderate
D. Severe

106. Following a Mustard atrial switch procedure, the best view for assessing the superior vena cava would be the:

A. Parasternal short-axis view
B. Apical five-chamber view
C. Apical four-chamber view
D. Suprasternal notch view

107. Which condition is commonly associated with rhabdomyoma?

A. Tuberous sclerosis
B. Down syndrome
C. DiGeorge syndrome
D. Turner syndrome

108. Your patient has total anomalous pulmonary venous connection. To use color flow Doppler to visualize flow in the individual veins returning to the pulmonary venous confluence, what maneuver is most helpful?

A. Reducing the color flow Doppler scale
B. Increasing color flow Doppler gain
C. Decreasing 2D imaging gains
D. Changing from brightness to variance mode

109. What is the best transducer position and maneuver to optimize visualization of the innominate (brachiocephalic) vein?

 A. Suprasternal sagittal view with the transducer notch/dot at 1–2 o'clock; axis from the left should point to the patient's right hip.
 B. Suprasternal coronal view with the transducer notch/dot at 3 o'clock; transducer should be angled anteriorly.
 C. High right parasternal parasagittal view with the transducer notch/dot at 12 o'clock; transducer should be angled to the patient's right side.
 D. High left parasternal view with the transducer notch/dot at 3 o'clock; transducer should be angled superiorly.

110. Your patient has a history of aortic valve regurgitation. A recent echocardiogram shows the left ventricle more dilated compared to the previous study. When you measure the aortic valve regurgitation by spectral Doppler, what pressure half-time (PHT) finding do you expect?

 A. Longer PHT
 B. Same PHT
 C. Shorter PHT
 D. PHT is not used to evaluate aortic valve regurgitation.

111. Vascular Ehlers-Danlos syndrome, Loeys-Dietz syndrome, and arterial tortuosity syndrome are all forms of:

 A. Connective tissue disorders
 B. Nervous system disorders
 C. Takayasu's syndrome
 D. Immune system disorders

112. Which structure is characterized by a smooth septal surface and fine ventricular trabeculations?

 A. Univentricular sinus
 B. Right ventricle
 C. Left ventricle
 D. Right ventricular infundibular chamber

113. In this image the aortic arch is marked by the letter:

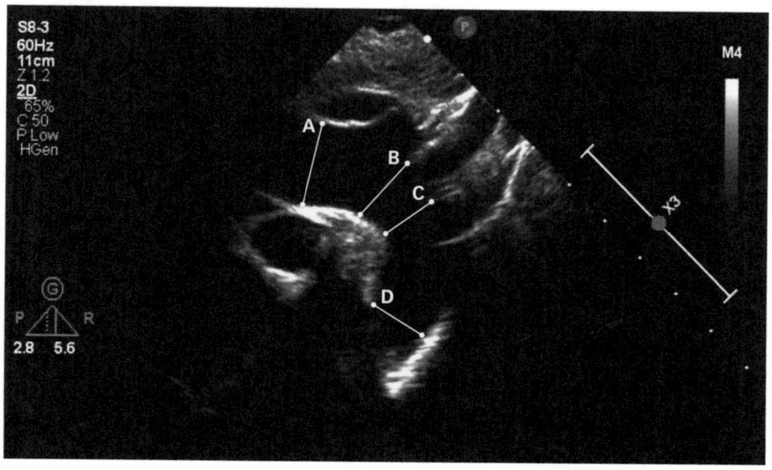

A. A
B. B
C. C
D. D

114. Up to 25% of patients with tetralogy of Fallot will also have:

A. Double aortic arch
B. Right aortic arch
C. Persistence of the fifth aortic arch
D. Left aortic arch with aberrant right subclavian artery

115. The most important technique for accurately estimating left atrial volume is:

A. Including the pulmonary vein ostia and excluding the left atrial appendage
B. Including both the pulmonary vein ostia and the left atrial appendage
C. Measuring atrial lengths in both the apical four-chamber and two-chamber views
D. Using the longest atrial length obtained from either the apical two-chamber or apical four-chamber view

116. If ascending aorta velocity is 2 m/sec and aortic isthmus velocity is 4 m/sec, what is the true peak gradient across the aortic isthmus?

A. 16 mmHg
B. 36 mmHg
C. 48 mmHg
D. 64 mmHg

117. For which condition is pulmonary artery (PA) banding surgery NOT appropriate?

A. Single ventricle with unguarded pulmonary blood flow
B. Double-outlet right ventricle
C. Tetralogy of Fallot
D. Multiple ventricular septal defects

118. The most commonly encountered variant of the aortic arch is a:

A. Double aortic arch
B. Right aortic arch with anomalous left subclavian artery
C. Left aortic arch with anomalous right subclavian artery
D. Persistent fifth aortic arch

119. An extracardiac Fontan conduit is sewn to which vessel?

A. Celiac artery
B. Abdominal aorta
C. Superior vena cava
D. Inferior vena cava

120. In the presence of Ebstein anomaly, what is indicated by a Celermajer index greater than 1?

A. Normal cardiac function in the setting of tricuspid valve regurgitation
B. Poor prognosis in the setting of Ebstein anomaly of the tricuspid valve
C. Poor prognosis in the setting of Ebstein anomaly of the mitral valve
D. Good prognosis in the setting of borderline pulmonary pressures

PART 9

Suggested Readings

Publications

Allen HD, Shaddy RE, Penny DJ, et al: *Moss and Adams' Heart Disease in Infants, Children, and Adolescents, Including the Fetus and Young Adult*, 9th edition. Philadelphia, Wolters Kluwer, 2016.

Anderson RH, Baker EJ, Penny D, et al: *Paediatric Cardiology*, 3rd edition. Philadelphia, Churchill Livingstone/Elsevier, 2010.

Armstrong WF, Ryan T: *Feigenbaum's Echocardiography*, 8th edition. Philadelphia, Lippincott Williams & Wilkins, 2019.

Drose JA: *Fetal Echocardiography*, 2nd edition. St. Louis, Saunders Elsevier, 2010.

Ezon DS, Goldberg JF, Kyle WB: *Atlas of Congenital Heart Disease Nomenclature: An Illustrated Guide to the Van Praagh and Anderson Approaches to Describing Congenital Cardiac Pathology*. Houston, Ezon Educational Services/ CreateSpace, 2015.

Kremkau FW: *Sonography: Principles and Instruments*, 9th edition. St. Louis, Elsevier, 2016.

Lai WW, Geva T, Shirali GS, et al: *Guidelines and Standards for Performance of a Pediatric Echocardiogram: A Report from the Task Force of the Pediatric Council of the American Society of Echocardiography*. JASE 19:1413–1430, 2006.

Lai WW, Mertens LL, Cohen MS, et al (eds): *Echocardiography in Pediatric and Congenital Heart Disease: From Fetus to Adult*, 2nd edition. Chichester, UK, Wiley-Blackwell, 2016.

Lewin MB, Stout K (eds): *Echocardiography in Congenital Heart Disease*. Philadelphia, Elsevier Saunders, 2012.

Moore KL, Persaud TVN, Torchia MG: *The Developing Human: Clinically Oriented Embryology*, 9th edition. Philadelphia, Elsevier Saunders, 2013.

Nagueh SF, Appleton CP, Gillebert TC, et al: Recommendations for the evaluation of left ventricular diastolic function by echocardiography. J Am Soc Echocardiogr 22:107–133, 2009.

Nagueh SF, Smiseth OA, Appleton CP, et al: Recommendations for the evaluation of left ventricular diastolic function by echocardiography: an update from the American Society of Echocardiography and the European Association of Cardiovascular Imaging. J Am Soc Echocardiogr 29:277–314, 2016.

Nichols DG, Ungerleider RM, Spevak PJ, et al: *Critical Heart Disease in Infants and Children*, 2nd edition. Philadelphia, Mosby Elsevier, 2006.

Park MK: *Park's Pediatric Cardiology for Practitioners*, 6th edition. Philadelphia, Saunders, 2014.

Rudolph AM: *Congenital Diseases of the Heart: Clinical-Physiological Considerations*, 3rd edition. Chichester, UK, Wiley Blackwell, 2009.

Wong PC, Miller-Hance WC (eds): *Transesophageal Echocardiography for Congenital Heart Disease*. London, Springer-Verlag, 2014.

Yagel S, Silverman NH, Gembruch U (eds): *Fetal Cardiology: Embryology, Genetics, Physiology, Echocardiographic Evaluation, Diagnosis and Perinatal Management of Cardiac Diseases*, 2nd edition. New York, Taylor & Francis, 2009.

Websites

American Registry for Diagnostic Medical Sonography (ARDMS). Pediatric Echocardiography page. https://www.ardms.org/get-certified/rdcs/pediatric-echocardiography-pe/.

American Society of Echocardiography (ASE). www.asecho.org.

Echocardiographer.org. www.echocardiographer.org.

University of Minnesota: Atlas of human cardiac anatomy. www.vhlab.umn.edu/atlas/echocardiography-tutorial/what-is-echocardiography.shtml.

PART 10

ARDMS Exam Content Outline: Tasks Cross-Referenced to Mock Exam Questions

Publisher's note: *For your convenience, question numbers in this mock exam are arranged below under the task-related topics and subtopics of the latest ARDMS exam content outline for the Pediatric Echocardiography (PE) specialty exam. The questions and/or the explanations of the answers refer to the tasks for which they are listed. And if a question is relevant to more than one task, it is listed for every task to which it pertains. Why? To provide you with a framework for targeting study on specific clinical tasks.*

Remember that the ARDMS exam content outlines may be updated every few years. Always be sure to visit the ARDMS "Get Certified" page at www.ardms.org to view the latest exam content outlines.

Anatomy and Physiology—10%

Identify great artery anatomy and flow patterns (i.e., aorta; aortic arch sidedness and branching; main and branch pulmonary arteries): *See questions* 1, 2, 3, 4, 5, 6, 7, 13, 98, 452, 466, 482, 483, 486, 487, 536, 593.

Identify normal valve structure, motion, and flow patterns: *See questions* 20, 29, 59.

Identify normal ventricular morphology and motion: *See questions* 1, 8, 9, 11, 46, 47, 49.

Identify normal transitional circulation (e.g., patent foramen ovale [PFO], patent ductus arteriosus [PDA], decreasing pulmonary vascular resistance): *See questions* 4, 16, 17, 18, 21, 23, 24, 41, 58, 265.

Identify coronary artery origins, proximal branches, and color flow pattern: *See questions* 25, 26, 27, 28, 30, 31, 32, 80, 445, 481.

Identify normal systemic and pulmonary venous anatomy and flow patterns (i.e., superior vena cava, inferior vena cava, innominate vein, coronary sinus, azygos vein, pulmonary veins): *See questions* 33, 34, 35, 36, 37, 40, 54, 56, 286, 292, 459, 476, 478, 479, 480, 484.

Identify normal abdominal situs and segmental cardiac anatomy: *See questions* 1, 19, 44, 45, 47, 48, 50, 51, 52, 55, 460, 462, 464, 472.

Identify normal right and left atrial morphology (i.e., Eustachian valve, Chiari network, appendages): *See questions* 1, 14, 15, 19, 38, 39, 43, 53, 57, 159, 257, 279, 287, 460, 485.

Pathology and Pathophysiology—12%

Assess cardiomyopathies (e.g., dilated, hypertrophic, restrictive): *See questions* 60, 61, 62, 63, 64, 65, 66, 67, 68, 69, 70, 71, 87, 112, 400, 557, 579.

Assess findings associated with pulmonary hypertension: *See questions* 10, 72, 73, 74, 75, 76, 77, 78, 134, 224, 317, 384, 386, 389, 393.

Assess pericardial effusion: *See questions* 81, 82, 83, 84, 85, 86, 294.

Assess coronary artery abnormalities associated with Kawasaki disease: *See questions* 79, 80.

Identify findings associated with infective endocarditis (e.g., valvular regurgitation, vegetation, abscess): *See questions* 88, 89, 90, 423.

Identify intracardiac and vascular thrombus: *See questions* 120, 122, 123, 362, 400, 401, 404, 434.

Assess functional abnormalities associated with drug toxicity (e.g., Adriamycin chemotherapy): *See questions* 91, 92, 113, 546.

Assess findings associated with rheumatic fever: *See question* 90.

Assess features associated with cardiac transplantation and rejection: *See questions* 93, 94, 540.

Assess lesions associated with gestational or maternal diabetes: *See questions* 112, 115.

Assess pleural effusions: *See question* 82.

Identify possible echocardiographic abnormalities associated with systemic hypertension in children: *See questions* 117, 118, 119, 558.

Identify lesions associated with connective tissue disorders (e.g., Marfan syndrome, Ehlers-Danlos syndrome, Loeys-Dietz syndrome): *See questions* 109, 110, 111, 590, 591.

Identify lesions associated with syndromes (e.g., Turner, Williams, DiGeorge, Noonan): *See questions* 69, 99, 100, 101, 102, 103, 104, 105, 106, 108, 114, 124, 125, 126, 127, 222, 243, 246, 266, 274, 282, 296, 297, 307, 336.

Identify lesions associated with Down syndrome: *See questions* 95, 96, 97, 142, 150, 151.

Congenital Anomalies—22%

Assess aortic arch anomalies (e.g., coarctation, interruption, anomalous branching patterns): *See questions* 42, 98, 99, 104, 105, 117, 118, 128, 129, 131, 132, 133, 134, 136, 139, 140, 142, 143, 161, 173, 324, 325, 407, 438, 441, 442, 495, 595.

Assess conotruncal defects (e.g., tetralogy of Fallot [TOF], double-outlet right ventricle [DORV], truncus arteriosus, and aortopulmonary [AP] window): *See questions* 77, 78, 100, 101, 107, 115, 144, 145, 146, 147, 148, 149, 150, 151, 152, 153, 154, 155, 156, 157, 158, 159, 161, 162, 164, 231, 233, 237, 238, 245, 252, 261, 272, 321, 354, 374, 394, 402.

Assess abnormalities of the aortic valve: *See questions* 12, 143, 145, 165, 166, 167, 169, 202, 309, 313, 328, 334, 335, 338, 341, 437, 439, 579.

Assess abnormal atrioventricular and ventriculoarterial connections (e.g., dextro-transposition of the great arteries [d-TGA], levo-transposition of the great arteries [l-TGA], or physiologically corrected TGA): *See questions* 22, 28, 124, 175, 176, 177, 178, 179, 180, 181, 182, 183, 184, 185, 186, 188, 256, 361, 374, 375, 390, 395, 398, 412, 501.

Assess atrioventricular septal defects (e.g., endocardial cushion defect, atrioventricular canal defect): *See questions* 95, 96, 206, 207, 208, 209, 210.

Assess ventricular outflow tract abnormalities (e.g., subvalvular obstructive lesions): *See questions* 174, 182, 210, 239, 240, 241, 395, 465, 468, 470.

Assess atrial and ventricular septal defects: *See questions* 75, 144, 148, 157, 160, 163, 167, 168, 173, 179, 181, 185, 189, 190, 191, 192, 193, 194, 195, 196, 197, 198, 199, 200, 201, 202, 203, 204, 205, 231, 233, 238, 242, 260, 311, 312, 328, 403, 404, 408, 409, 496, 497, 499, 501, 502, 535, 539, 574, 599.

Assess pulmonary venous anomalies (i.e., partially and totally anomalous connection/drainage; pulmonary vein stenosis): *See questions* 106, 108, 124, 125, 192, 195, 205, 211, 212, 213, 214, 215, 216, 217, 218, 219, 220, 221, 222, 223, 224, 284, 298, 300, 301, 384, 385, 386, 387, 388, 405, 448, 463.

Assess pulmonary artery (PA) abnormalities (i.e., supravalvar and peripheral PA stenosis; dilated PAs; discontinuous PAs): *See questions* 149, 154, 155, 156, 238, 243, 244, 245, 262, 263, 410.

Assess abnormalities of the mitral valve: *See questions* 88, 163, 169, 193, 200, 201, 225, 226, 227, 228, 229, 231, 287, 310, 336, 337, 533, 579.

Assess patent ductus arteriosus and aortopulmonary collaterals: *See questions* 232, 255, 264, 265, 271, 272, 273, 309, 406, 510, 521, 593.

Assess abnormalities of the pulmonic valve: *See questions* 74, 116, 149, 232, 234, 235, 236, 237, 238, 246, 252, 254, 255, 315, 316, 317, 318, 339, 342.

Assess supravalvular aortic stenosis: *See questions* 274, 275, 276, 277.

Assess coronary artery abnormalities (i.e., sinusoids, fistulae, anomalous origins): *See questions* 61, 146, 147, 170, 171, 177, 247, 248, 249, 250, 251, 267, 268, 269, 270, 370, 376.

Assess abnormalities of the tricuspid valve: *See questions* 72, 113, 256, 257, 259, 260, 314, 340, 572, 573, 575, 576, 577.

Assess abnormalities of abdominal and cardiac situs/position: *See questions* 124, 125, 126, 127, 180, 183, 222, 258, 266, 295, 296, 297, 304, 305.

Assess vascular rings and slings (i.e., double aortic arch, right arch with aberrant subclavian artery, pulmonary sling): *See questions* 42, 130, 135, 136, 137, 138, 139, 141.

Assess systemic venous anomalies (i.e., interrupted inferior vena cava, bilateral superior vena cava): *See questions* 278, 280, 286, 290, 291, 293, 303, 305, 306, 436.

Assess cardiac tumors: *See questions* 281, 282, 283, 288, 294.

Assess cor triatriatum: *See questions* 230, 285, 287, 289, 302.

Postoperative Anatomy—20%

Assess tetralogy of Fallot repair: *See questions* 315, 316, 317, 319, 320, 322, 323.

Assess valve repair/replacement: *See questions* 88, 89, 335, 337, 338, 340, 372, 422, 423, 424, 425, 426, 427, 428, 429, 430, 431, 432, 433, 434, 435.

Assess surgical repair for coarctation of the aorta: *See questions* 324, 325, 327, 328, 330, 331, 333, 336.

Assess atrial and ventricular septal defect surgical repairs: *See questions* 189, 195, 408, 409.

Assess shunt closure devices (i.e., atrial septal defect, patent ductus arteriosus, and ventricular septal defect devices/coils): *See questions* 195, 403, 404, 405, 406, 407.

Assess Fontan palliation procedure with and without fenestration: *See questions* 349, 351, 362, 369, 373, 417, 418, 419, 421, 522.

Assess bidirectional Glenn anastomosis: *See questions* 299, 350, 353, 356, 357, 362, 365, 366, 367, 416.

Assess arterial/atrial switch operation: *See questions* 187, 188, 358, 359, 360, 361, 370, 371, 374, 376, 377, 390, 410, 411, 412, 420, 585.

Assess patients after balloon dilation of valves and great vessels: *See questions* 326, 329, 332, 339, 341.

Assess modified Blalock-Taussig shunt or central shunt: *See questions* 346, 348, 354, 355, 368, 413, 414, 415, 523.

Assess Norwood stage 1 procedure and modifications: *See questions* 344, 345, 347, 348, 352, 355, 368, 413, 414.

Assess Ross procedure: *See questions* 343, 378, 379, 380, 381, 382, 383.

Assess repair of total/partial anomalous pulmonary venous connection: *See questions* 384, 385, 386, 387, 388.

Assess pulmonary artery banding: *See questions* 363, 364, 389, 390, 391, 392, 393, 394.

Assess Rastelli repair: *See questions* 375, 395, 396, 397, 398.

Assess implantable devices and lines (e.g., catheters, pacemaker/defibrillator leads, cannulae, stents): *See questions* 122, 363, 364, 399, 400, 401, 402, 403, 404, 405, 406, 407, 435.

Clinical Standards and Guidelines—8%

Obtain a parasternal view (i.e., short axis, long axis, right, high left): *See questions* 178, 197, 198, 264, 432, 471, 472, 475, 476, 477, 479, 481, 482, 536.

Obtain a suprasternal view (i.e., short axis, long axis): *See questions* 358, 439, 459, 478, 480, 483, 484, 485, 486, 487.

Obtain an apical view (i.e., two-chamber, three-chamber/long axis, four-chamber with apex down, five-chamber): *See questions* 187, 469, 470, 471, 473, 474.

Obtain a subcostal/subxiphoid view (i.e., sagittal/long axis, coronal/long axis): *See questions* 189, 191, 239, 329, 460, 461, 462, 463, 464, 465, 466, 467, 468.

Select appropriate settings to optimize image quality and Doppler information: *See questions* 440, 445, 448, 449, 450, 451, 543.

Select appropriate transducer(s) for patient size, window, and modality: *See questions* 437, 438, 439, 441, 442, 443, 444, 446, 447.

Identify imaging artifacts: *See questions* 435, 452, 453, 454, 455, 456, 457, 458, 543.

Measurement Techniques and Quantification—28%

Interrogate the aortic arch using color and spectral Doppler: *See questions* 133, 273, 330, 331, 363, 488, 489, 490, 491, 495, 510, 591, 592, 593, 594, 595.

Interrogate the atrial and ventricular septum using color Doppler: *See questions* 189, 190, 194, 197, 254, 311, 312, 387, 388, 499.

Assess aortic stenosis and grade severity: *See questions* 334, 493, 494, 503, 504, 505, 512.

Interrogate the pulmonary venous return using color and spectral Doppler: *See questions* 223, 387, 388, 520, 521, 524, 525, 526, 527, 528, 537, 538.

Interrogate the pulmonary artery and branches using color and spectral Doppler: *See questions* 265, 273, 352, 415, 511.

Assess right ventricular pressure using tricuspid and pulmonary regurgitant jet velocities: *See questions* 72, 76, 185, 253, 317, 321, 498.

Assess pulmonary stenosis and grade severity: *See questions* 116, 232, 234, 342, 393, 492.

Interrogate systemic venous return using color and spectral Doppler: *See questions* 76, 122, 187, 219, 293, 298, 387, 436, 479.

Assess tricuspid regurgitation and grade severity: *See questions* 72, 184, 318, 518, 519, 535.

Assess aortic regurgitation and grade severity: *See questions* 60, 168, 172, 203, 341, 380, 381, 382, 383, 411, 506, 507, 508, 509, 512.

Analyze ventricular regional wall motion qualitatively using two-dimensional imaging and/or M-mode: *See questions* 60, 121, 185, 465, 474, 598.

Assess mitral regurgitation and grade severity: *See questions* 184, 533, 534, 601.

Assess mitral stenosis and grade severity: *See questions* 169, 337, 500, 529, 530, 531, 532, 568, 569, 570, 571, 574, 579.

Assess ventricular septal defect gradients: *See questions* 168, 185, 496, 497, 499, 535, 599.

Calculate maximal pressure gradients using the modified Bernoulli equation: *See questions* 72, 325, 327, 490, 492.

Assess pulmonary regurgitation and grade severity: *See questions* 236, 321, 343, 511.

Demonstrate echocardiographic findings at specific times during the electrocardiogram (cardiac) cycle: *See questions* 186, 371, 562, 601.

Assess atrial septal shunting gradients: *See questions* 308, 501, 502, 539.

Assess tricuspid stenosis and grade severity: *See questions* 253, 572, 573, 577.

Measure chamber sizes and wall thickness using M-mode: *See questions* 60, 68, 516, 517, 578, 596.

Calculate fractional shortening using M-mode: *See questions* 513, 514, 515, 568, 597.

Perform linear measurements using two-dimensional imaging methods: *See questions* 434, 566, 568, 575, 581, 585, 586, 590, 591.

Calculate ejection fraction using two-dimensional imaging methods: *See questions* 471, 585, 586, 587, 588, 589, 600.

Calculate indices of diastolic function (e.g., E/A ratio, E/E′ ratio, mitral valve inflow pattern, pulmonary venous flow pattern): *See questions* 67, 85, 87, 94, 498, 541, 542, 544, 545, 546, 547, 548, 549, 552, 553, 555, 556, 557, 560, 561, 563, 564, 565, 569, 602, 603.

Measure chamber sizes and wall thickness using two-dimensional imaging methods: *See questions* 68, 471, 550, 551, 558, 559, 566, 567, 579, 580, 581, 582, 583, 584.